Fix Pain

Hi Nicole,
If I had my life to do over I think it would be great — provided I had the attitudes — to be just where you are!
Thanks for your help — Fred 3/18

Fix Pain

Bodywork Protocols for Myofascial Pain Syndromes

John Harris
Fred Kenyon

Illustrations by Patricia Zavagno West

First Printing 2002

Photography – Fred Kenyon
Illustrations – Patty Zavagno-West
Book and jacket design – Frank Goad
Editors – Fred Harwood, Byron (Pete) Evans and Kathleen Dickenson Sullivan
Printed in Korea by asianprinting.com

ISBN Number 0-9665843-1-7

Library of Congress Catalog Card Number 2002100324

1. Massage and bodywork
2. Health and fitness
3. Sports injuries
4. Trigger point pain

DISCLAIMER

This manual presents a general guide to therapeutic protocols. We have attempted to be as accurate as possible in our descriptions. Although the manual is based on over fifty years of experience, we do anticipate that we will learn more as the years go by, and invite the reader to send us their comments to improve our protocols in the future. The authors refuse to accept either responsibility for or liability to anyone regarding any loss or damage alleged to be either directly or indirectly caused by his/her utilization of the information contained in this manual. If you can't agree with this disclaimer, please return the manual for a full refund.

Press4Health LLC
133 E. De La Guerra, Ste. 23
Santa Barbara, CA 93101

To Nikki Allyn Grosso, who kept me alive,
literally, during this long process

John Harris

To Avery Kenyon-Wilmanns for achievement,
Len Lamensdorf for insight and
my wife Carol for support

Fred Kenyon

Table of Contents

PART 4 – REGIONAL PROTOCOLS

PART 5 – APPENDICES AND OVERVIEWS

Foreword

NANCY DELUCREZIA

I HAVE HAD THE BLESSING of receiving, practicing and teaching massage and various advanced forms of bodywork since the early 1980s. One thing that has become increasingly clear to me over these years is that each session that occurs is a sacred exchange, a dialog, a communion of energy, and a release of that which blocks its flow. The practitioner doesn't "work on" the client; rather each person works with his/her own body during the session regardless of which role each plays. With this in mind, it seems clear to me that the practitioner should share in the benefits of the session and actually feel better afterwards.

When practitioners complain that they feel tired or drained after working, or that their fingers, wrists or lower backs bother them, I ask to watch them work. Invariably, they display some form of poor body mechanics, especially misuse or overuse of their own body parts. It's imperative to understand the importance of using the right tool for any given job – you would no more use a sledgehammer to place a push pin into a cork board than you would try to drive a stake into the ground with your finger. Yet bodyworkers continuously misuse their thumbs, wrists and even elbows (driving pressure into the shoulder girdle, upper ribs and thoracic outlet) to create more pressure than these body parts are designed to handle. I advise them to lower their table, get into a position over the client, and work with body weight rather than just muscle power from upper limbs. Putting someone on the floor and using your feet is the obvious and ultimate extension of this advice. DeeperWork protocols will show you how.

Remember to be patient and receptive as you begin to explore this new way of working. You may have no idea of the level of palpation skills possible with your feet, but that will quickly change. After you get a sense of what your feet can accomplish, you'll wonder how you ever worked without them, and your fingers, wrists and elbows will thrive on work more appropriate to their capabilities. This manual also instructs you in the proper use of hands when only they will do.

The concepts and techniques presented in this book are revolutionary in that they will expand your capacity as a bodyworker the way the industrial revolution expanded mechanical technology. The inclusion of your feet as a tool will nearly double your repertoire of techniques and allow you more ease, efficiency and success in your work with less effort. They will, more than any other technique I've seen, support you in letting go of the "I'm the giver, they're the receiver" mode which so depletes the practitioner. You will experience each session as a miraculous dance that energizes and restores both people involved.

—NANCY DELUCREZIA, Director
Kali Institute for Massage & Somatic Therapies
Ventura, California

Preface

THIS IS A HOW-TO-DO-IT MANUAL designed for people who practice massage and bodywork. It contains effective protocols that address myofascial pain and dysfunction – an all too common source of misery for people from all walks of life. In this manual, we share with you what we've learned from our extensive work with both chronic and acute pain sufferers.

By adding a perfect weight-bearing pressure tool, the foot, to your therapeutic armatorium, you can remedy your clients' problems and eliminate injury to yourself. We call this marriage of Eastern bodywork (using the foot) with Western scientific manual medicine DeeperWork™. DeeperWork uses deep compressions to circumvent the problems you've had with your hands and shoulders. You can still give sports or restorative massage, trigger point therapy, fascial stretching and deep tissue work, but now without hurting yourself. By showing you how to use your feet, we offer you a revolution in massage therapy

Chronic pain is complex. Thousands of intelligent, dedicated scientists study the perplexing problem of pain, but they've yet to completely resolve the question of "what to do to make everyone better".

How the physiologic mechanisms work is less important than that we empirically know that our work serves our clients well; many no longer hurt. We offer you these "fix-it" protocols with the assurance that they will work.

To better prepare you, this manual balances logical, sequential protocols and art. To round out the presentation, we've followed notable success stories with unusual anomalies or goofs.

This manual is for massage therapists, bodyworkers, physical therapists, athletic trainers, chiropractors, osteopaths and others with sufficient training and experience to work safely, sensibly and effectively with the public. We recommend that you receive training in DeeperWork. Do not use this manual unless you have requisite understanding of anatomy, physiology, pathology and contraindications to work safely.

We have borrowed heavily from the experience, innovation and hard work of the following mavens of palpatory and applied anatomy and pain alleviation:

JANET G. TRAVELL, M.D.
DAVID G. SIMONS, M.D.
JAMES CYRIAX, M.D., M.R.C.P.
RAYMOND L. NIMMO, D.C.
BLANDINE CALAIS-GERMAIN
STANLEY HOPPENFELD, M.D.
LEON CHAITOW, N.D., D.O., M.B.N.O.A.
PHILIP E. GREENMAN, D.O., F.A.A.O.

What follows is our bodywork adaptations of their work. Any mistakes, errors, or faults in this manual are probably ours and not theirs.

–JOHN HARRIS

–FRED KENYON

PART 1

Introduction

CHAPTER 1

Indications

When To Use DeeperWork

Most generally healthy, normally muscled clients will benefit from DeeperWork. It is an ideal protocol for those large, well-muscled, dense, "difficult to get deep enough" types – exactly the kind of clients who can take a toll on our hands. If they are suffering from stress, tension, or chronic myofascial pain syndromes and appreciate strong, deep pressure, so much the better, because DeeperWork was designed with their needs in mind.

Tense, tight, lean clients, while not so heavily muscled, are also good candidates. Just remember to use moderate, broad pressure and a soft foot. DeeperWork is powerful and you will need to use it judiciously. But aside from a few conditions and standard contraindications, most clients will love this work.

Read the prerequisites (Chapter 2 through Chapter 5) before beginning the WALKAROUND.

CHAPTER 2

Model Client Intake and Session Guide

I. Pre-visit:

A. Advise your client to wear loose-fitting, comfortable clothing without belts, jewelry etc.

B. Review cautions and contraindications. Ask your client about varicose veins as they may be hidden from view.

II. Records:

A. Take a Client Health History – a client's history guides us in ascertaining local, regional and absolute bars to our work. Referral for evaluation and medical clearance is always an option. When in doubt, refer.

Health History

Name______________________________

Address______________________________

Phone______________ Occupation______________

Emergency Contact______________________________

Physician(s) + phone(s)______________________________

Surgeries______________________________

Injuries______________________________

Illness - acute______________________________

Illness - chronic______________________________

Medications______________________________

Supplements______________________________

Current state of health – statement from client:

Physical______________________________

____

Emotional______________________________

Hobbies/Sports______________________________

Client comments______________________________

B. I have been informed that:

1. This is not a medical treatment.
2. I may be required to receive my doctor's clearance for some bodywork treatments.
3. There should be positive changes in my problem within 3 to 5 sessions, or, following consultation, I will be referred for evaluation.
4. I have been briefed to assume responsibility for feedback, and I will give full disclosure of relevant information that effects the treatment.
5. It is my responsibility to stop any treatment that feels invasive or painful.

____
Client Signature / Date

C. Body Illustrations - have client mark chart with the location of their pain.

D. Listen carefully to and record your client's description of their problem(s) and follow with a discussion of treatment goals and probable outcomes.

III. Three items to be discussed with clients regarding therapy protocol:

A. Time involved:
1. We recommend 20 to 30 minutes as the maximum time used for trigger point or friction treatments per session.
2. Compression Massage can be used to warm up muscles and round out your treatment.

B. Possible side effects of therapy:
1. Bruising is possible – use care to properly warm the tissues before treatment to lessen chances of bruising.
2. Post treatment soreness – this soreness should not last longer than 2 days. Instruct client to do some gentle passive stretches if soreness is noted.
3. Possible (temporary) exacerbation of symptoms – note to client that this is probably a good sign. We've located the offending trigger points and successive sessions will eliminate their problems.

C. Schedule computation: Trigger points can continue to refer up to 24 hours, even after a successful treatment – schedule sessions on alternate days.

IV. Visual Evaluation:

A. Pay close attention the client's movements, posture and compensatory patterns.

B. Check for limitations in range-of-motion.

C. Note which movements amplify pain.

V. Position client on mat:

A. Watch your client carefully as they get into position on the mat for treatment – note weaknesses and apparent problems.

B. Bolster as needed to find a position of safety and comfort for the client and biomechanical ease for yourself.

C. Remember to warm muscles before trigger point or other therapeutic work.

VI. Following therapy:

A. Give your client a brief overview of self-care – identify and instruct proper stretching or strengthening procedures.

(or)

B. Refer your client to a trainer or therapist qualified to brief these stretching or strengthening procedures.

CHAPTER 3

Cautions and Contraindications

When To Be Careful or When Not To Use DeeperWork Protocols

In a nutshell, those who are generally frail, debilitated, weak, hypermobile, easily bruised, flaccid or emotionally labile should be treated cautiously, if at all, with deep compressions. Persons with chronic diseases can often be helped by this type of work, but only after consultation among you, your clients and their primary physicians.

On occasion you will have to make an informed judgment as to how deep and when and where to work. An informed judgment might include client consultation, medical consultation and/or consulting with more experienced massage therapists.

Remember our Three-Treatment Rule: If the work doesn't provide a cure or result in significant improvement within three sessions, look for another source of the pain, or refer. Our admonition to clients for years has been, "I don't diagnose, prescribe or treat. I just rub it, and if it gets better, great."

> **PAY ATTENTION TO YOUR CLIENTS**
>
> Even with the best of intentions, clients have been damaged by deep work. Medical journals from throughout the world document serious injuries to clients from deep work by therapists who ignored their clients' feedback. In many cases of injury, clients stated that they were being hurt. Listen to your clients.
>
> For a list of notorious cases in the 1990s, check out "Adverse Effects of Pressure" on pg. 73 of *Therapeutic Massage, A Scientific Approach* by Ross Turchaninov, M.D.

Cautions

Cautions indicate that you should be careful and think before acting. Use caution when working with:

1. Hypermobile clients – bolster them carefully as they over-stretch easily.
2. Post-surgical clients – work only after a physician consult.
3. Indications of peripheral vascular disease or varicose veins – never step on these areas.
4. Posttraumatic stress disorder or other psychological "nonorganic" problems – work only after conferring with their therapist or M.D.
5. Clients taking anticoagulants such as Aspirin, Coumadin, Lavanox or Heparin should check with their Doctor prior to treatment – deep bruising and clots are a possibility.
6. Osteoporosis (brittle bone disease), associated with nutritional osteomalacia in older women, requires special care.
7. When you intuitively feel the work is too strong for a client either before or during a session – abstain, trust and follow your "gut" instinct.

Contraindications – divided into two groups:.
(Remember, when in doubt, refer or withhold treatment)

Local Contraindications = do not work in affected area.

1. Fresh bruises
2. Skin lesions / wounds
3. Fractures
4. Varicosities
5. Phlebitis / cellulitis
6. Acute (recent) injuries
7. Any suspected compartment syndrome
8. Endangerment sites – those areas (often close to the suface) where veins and nerves are unprotected

General Contraindications = do not work with this particular client at this time.

1. Unconfirmed or undiagnosed injuries – e.g., blows to the head or neck, "whiplash," etc.
2. Rheumatoid arthritis – in the inflammatory stage
3. Inflammatory conditions of the bowel, joints, veins, etc. (should be first cleared by a physician)
4. Cancer – consult physician
5. Inebriation
6. Use of recreational or other drugs
7. Infectious diseases, especially if accompanied by abnormal body temperature

Visceral Pain

Visceral disease can refer pain to surface areas of the body and yet appear to be muscular in origin. Some bodyworkers will attempt to treat this referred pain with musculoskeletal approaches – usually ineffective and a mistake. These problems (coming from internal organs) can be serious – occasionally life theatening.

Muscular problems appearing with sudden onset and with no apparent physical cause (with or without intense pain) that don't resolve or shift in intensity or location with our soft-tissue intervention are all suspect. Remember the Three-Treatment Rule.

If there are any concomitant signs of illness such as excessive fatigue, a low-grade fever, or nausea accompanying the pain, refer for medical evaluation. Prolonged massage treatment can mask symptoms and prevent clients from receiving timely medical treatment. Some very specific forms of medical massage, e.g., segment reflex massage, can be useful adjuncts to standard medical treatments.

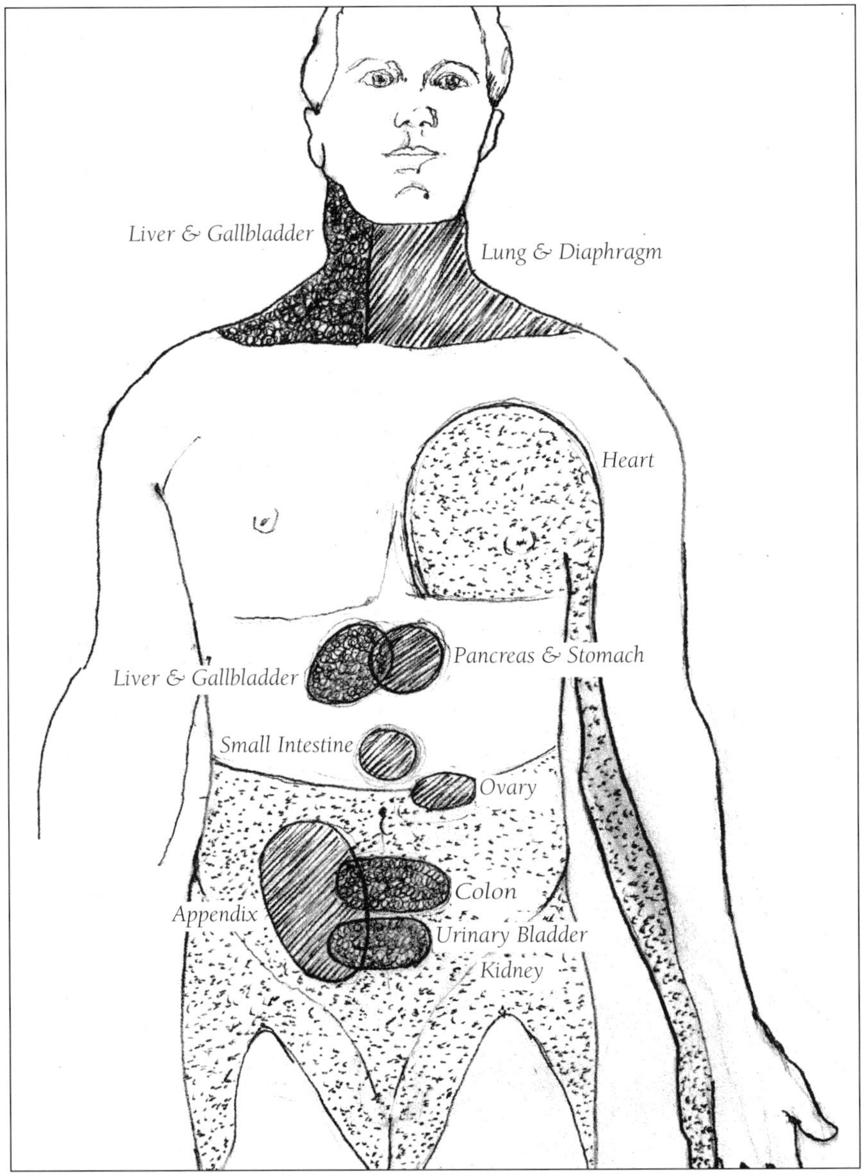

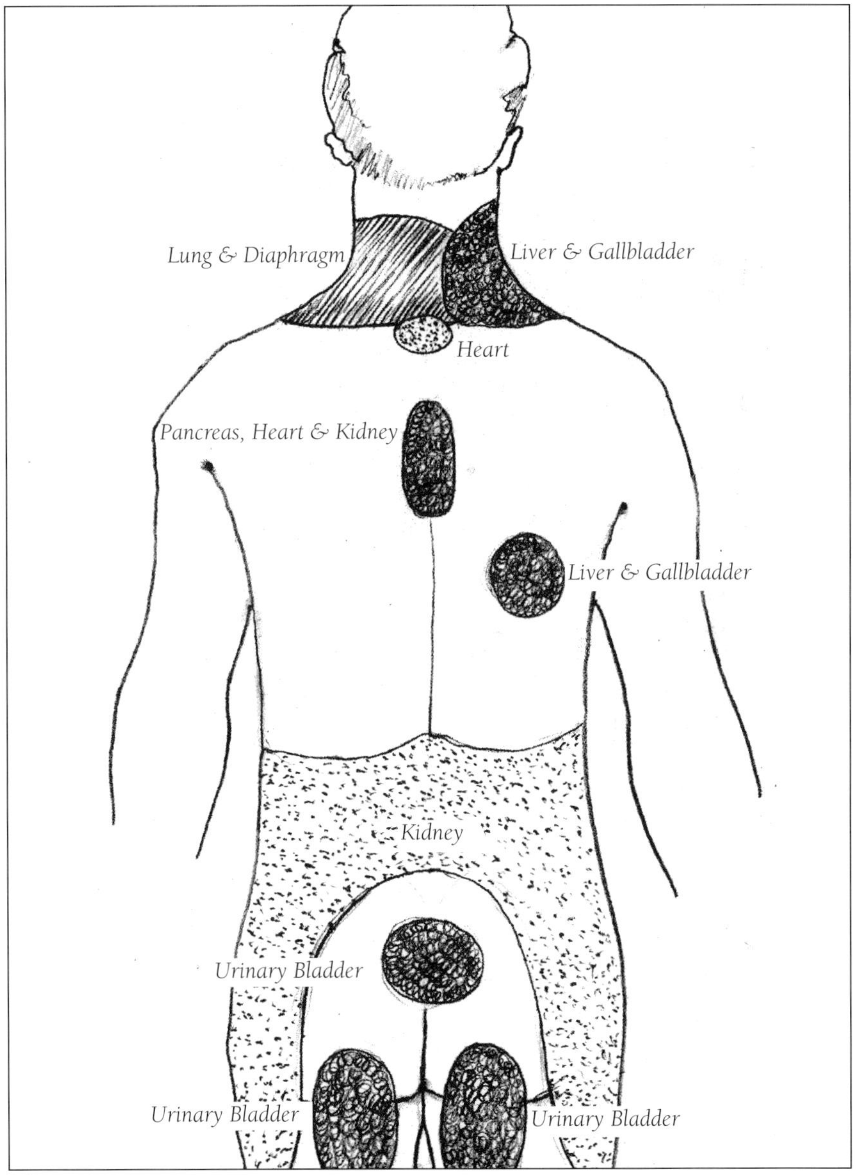

CHAPTER 4

Endangerment Sites, Joint Cavities and Bony Prominences

Areas To Avoid

1. Head/Neck
2. Axillary Area
3. Elbow Joint
4. Viscera, External Iliac Arteries
5. Wrist
6. Groin/Inguinal Triangle
7. Knee

7a. Knee Joint/Popliteal Fosia

8. Kidney/Floating Ribs
9. Sciatic Notch (between Ischial Tuberosity and Greater Trocanter of Femur)
10. Spinous Processes
11. Hunters Canal
12. Ankle
13. Deltopectoral Groove
14. Breast
15. Posterior Femor (Sciatic Nerve Lateral to Ischial Tuberosity)
16. Coccyx
17. Posterior Shoulder Joint

C = Use caution
X = Avoid deep, strong or heavy pressure

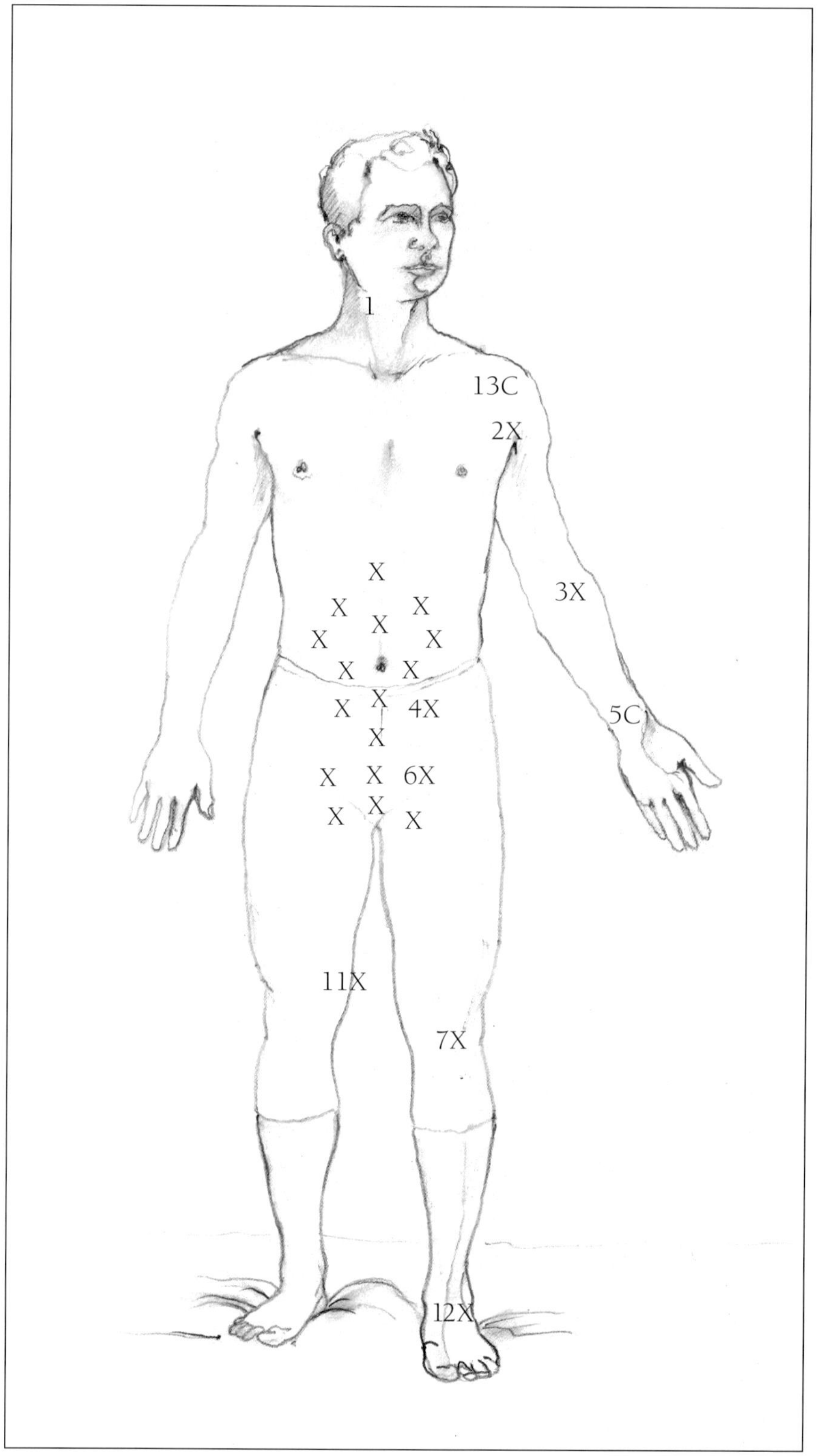

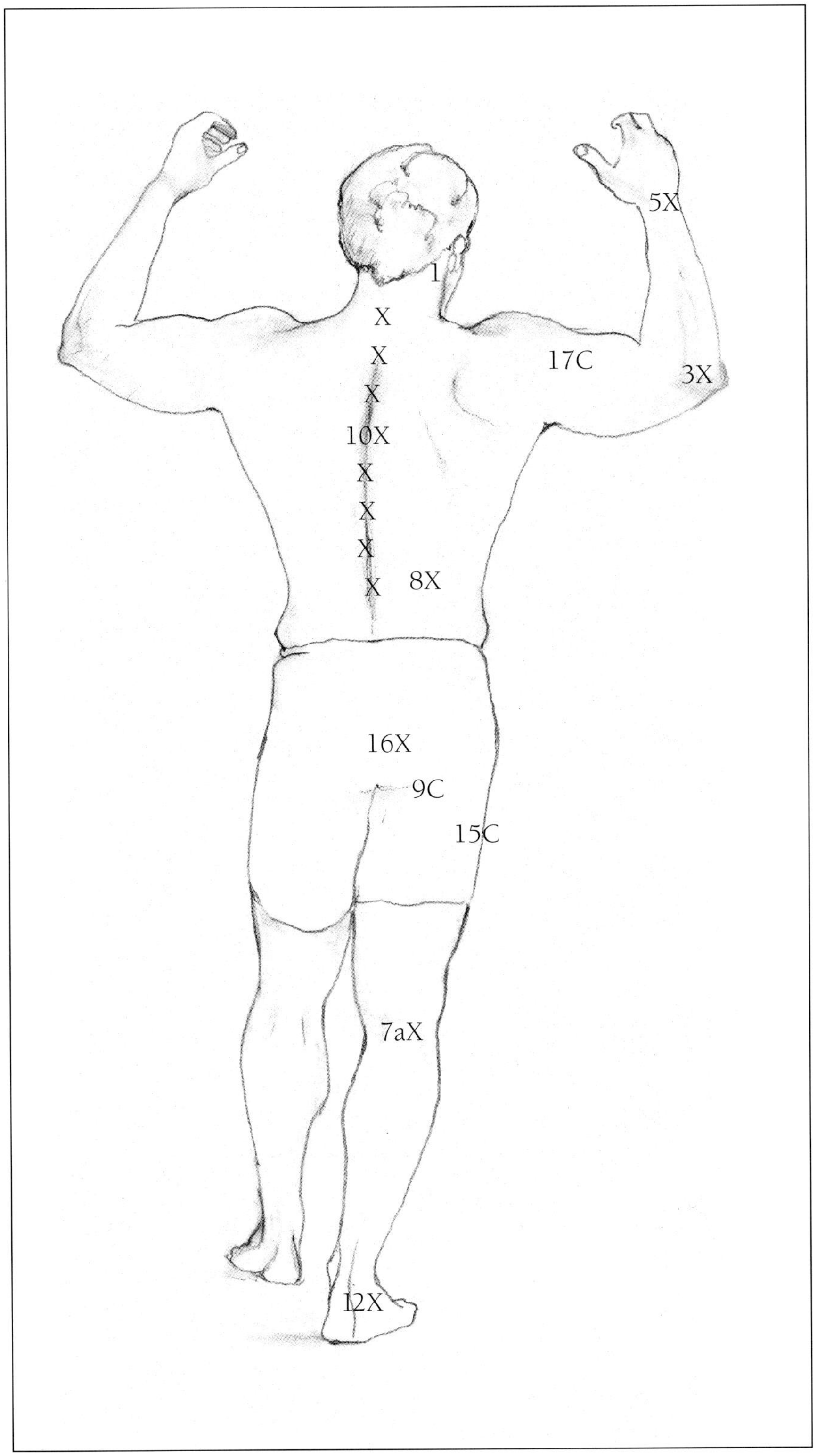
5X
1
X
X
17C
3X
X
10X
X
X
X
8X
X
16X
9C
15C
7aX
12X

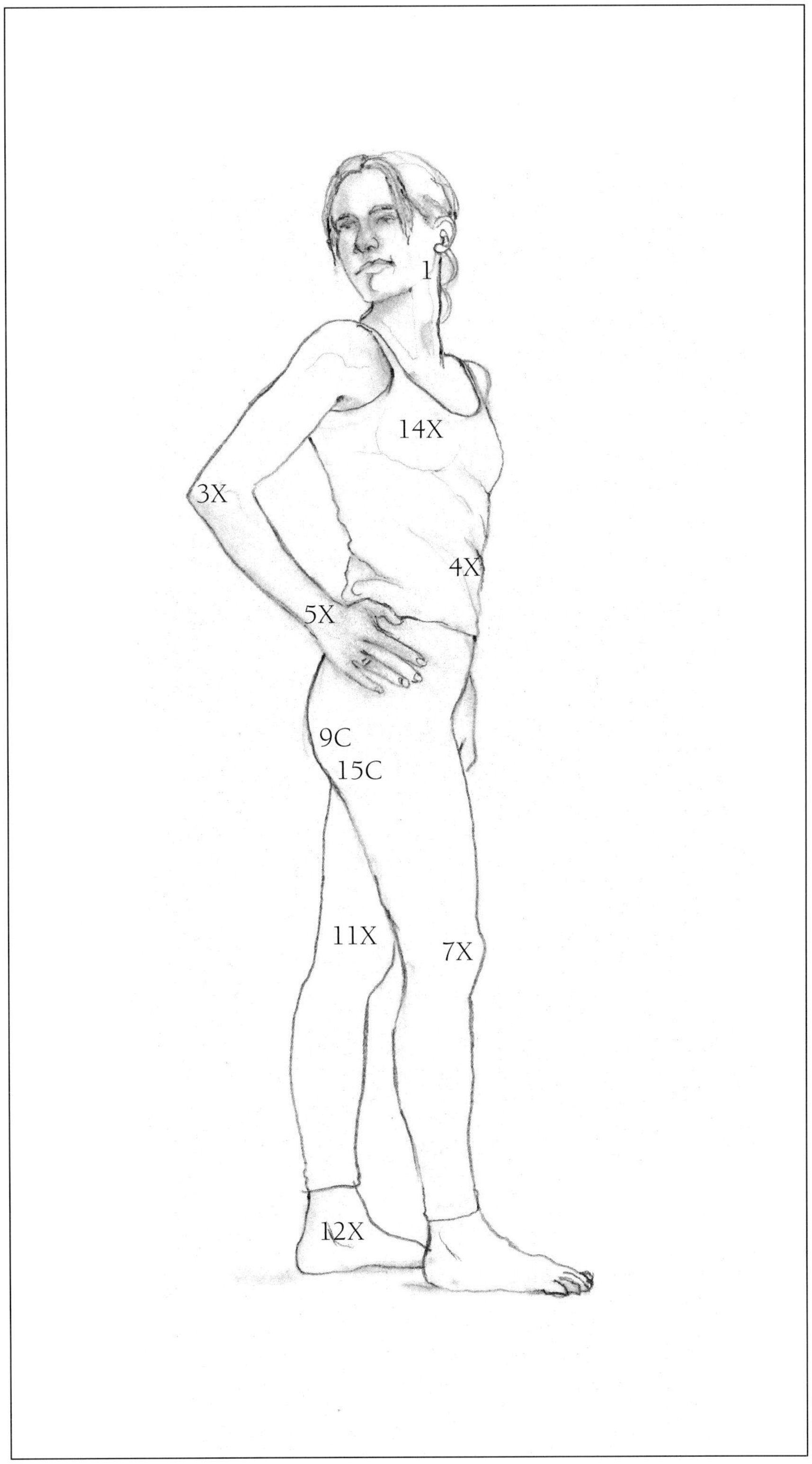
1
14X
3X
4X
5X
9C
15C
11X
7X
12X

CHAPTER 5

Psychological "Nonorganic" and Special Advisements

SHOCK

Shock (often associated with trauma) is an unexpected disturbance of mental or emotional balance that can result in physiologic responses including a dramatic lowering of blood pressure.

Clients in shock may require medical attention. Vital processes can be depressed. If you are not certified in First Aid and CPA, use emergency services (911).

While awaiting emergency help, lie client down, elevate their feet, and keep them warm.

Hypersensitive Clients

Some hypersensitive clients (particularly those with posttraumatic hyperirritability syndrome) can faint or go into shock when treated with even moderate direct pressure. Clues to this impending condition (it can happen almost instantaneously) are extremely strong jump-signs, a full-body glistening sweat, or an impulse to vomit or defecate.

We recommend you STOP treatment immediately. Firm direct pressure is not appropriate for these clients. Even though they may respond well to light direct pressure administered by hand, some clients will have strong emotional responses to direct pressure. These clients should not be treated with direct pressure. Delicate, fragile and some elder-probably not be treated with direct pressure. Delicate, fragile, and some elderly clients should be treated with even more caution.

Posttraumatic Stress Disorder

Clients with posttraumatic stress disorder are susceptible to dissociative states and flashbacks. Because this can be a delicate or frightening subject to broach for both the client and therapist, we recommend that you receive training to help you to recognize posttraumatic stress disorder and alert the client as necessary. See Posttraumatic Stress Disorder discussion in the Appendix under "What To Do."

Clients with Hypoglycemia

Clients with hypoglycemia should eat about 1 hour before treatment. Strong cathartic releases (sobbing, shaking, raging) following awareness of suppressed material may initiate hypoglycemic shock in this population.

Maintaining sugar levels will also often stop the washed-out, shaky, spaced-out feelings that can follow catharsis. A readily absorbable source of sugar (juice, barley sugar etc.) to use post-catharsis can often prevent this problem.

Tetany & Hyperventilation

Some clients are extremely anxious and tend to hyperventilate. This produces unpleasant symptoms. Highly anxious clients need to be addressed by trained, experienced therapists. Clients moving into tetany (spasm), shock or deep dissociative states can be unnerving to inexperienced therapists. For both your and their well-being, refer these clients if you are not experienced in working with these conditions.

PART 2

COMPRESSION MASSAGE

CHAPTER 6

Compression Massage The WALKAROUND

AKA DEEP COMPRESSIVE MASSAGE COMPRESSIVE DEEP TISSUE MASSAGE

Overview

COMPRESSION MASSAGE IS SIMPLE, powerful, effective and unfortunately, physically demanding on therapists. Whether administered with a flat palm, a loose fist, a forearm or a thumb pad, compressions take a severe toll on wrists and hands. Our contribution to client and therapist well-being is to couple the therapeutic benefits of compression with prolonged and effortless application.

The WALKAROUND uses nature's perfectly designed weight bearing structure (the foot) to effectively warm, stretch and hydrate fascia and muscle.

Use compressions to improve function, enhance health and release, relieve and remove many of the effects of common myofascial pain syndromes. While we use and respect the gentler bodywork approaches, our experience suggests that prolonged, deep compressions best address many chronic problems (trigger points, fascial restrictions and/or adhesions).

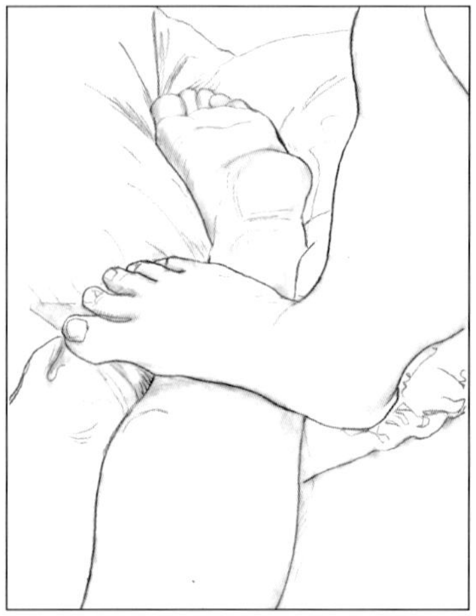

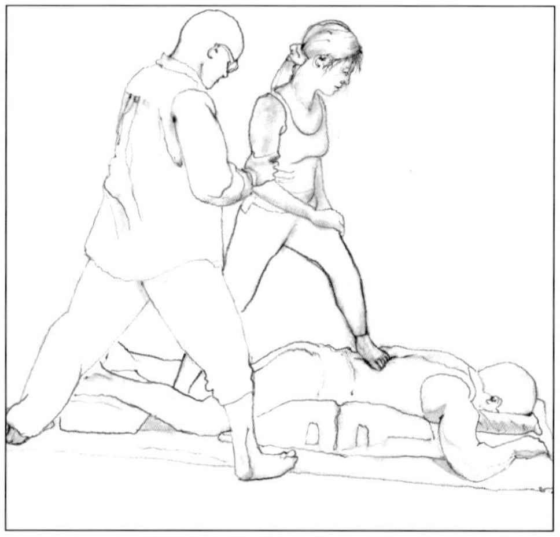

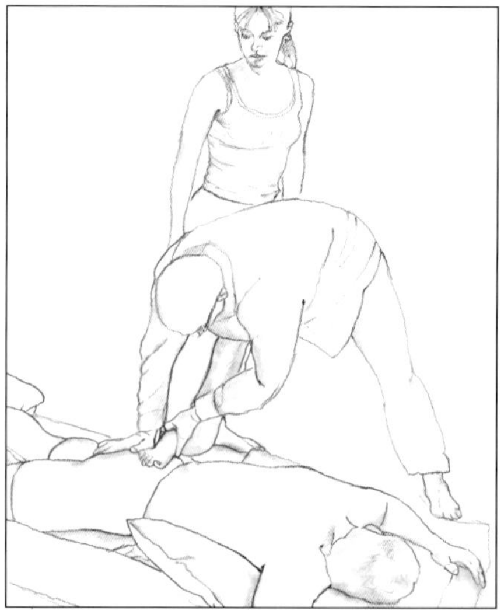

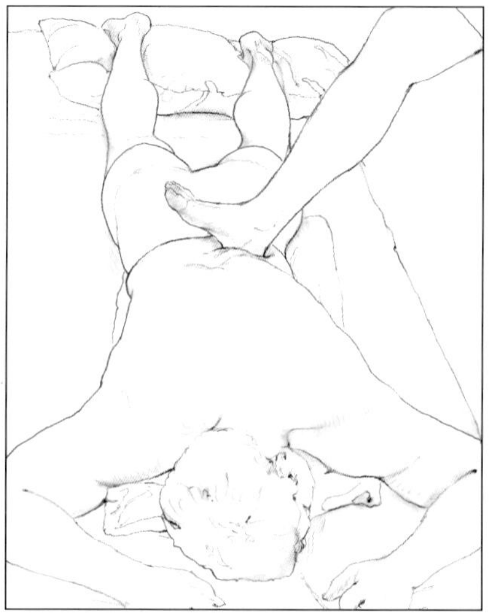

Hypermobility of the thumb is one of the most common and difficult problems associated with ischemic direct pressure. One expert on hand-care for massage therapists even suggests that therapists just stop doing deep work and switch to easier-to-administer Swedish strokes. Unfortunately, many clients (perhaps most now) want deeper work. Practitioners with small, hyperflexible and delicate hands and wrists are particularly prone to injury. Most of us don't have the hands to work many hours a day on large, bulky clients, even with gentle Swedish strokes.

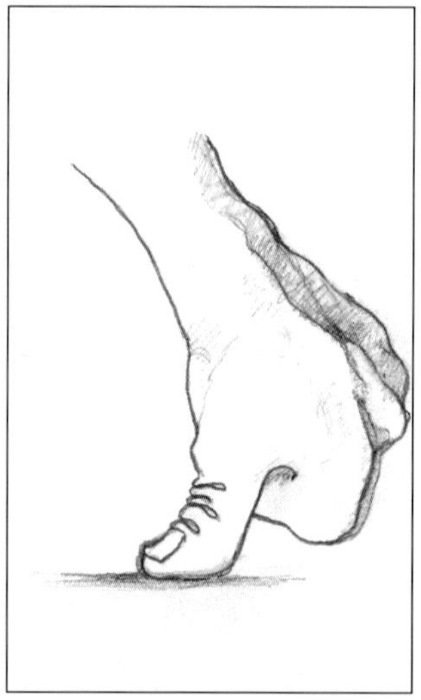

The bane of bodyworkers – a hypermobile thumb. Direct pressure compresses the joint and can lead to osteoarthritis.

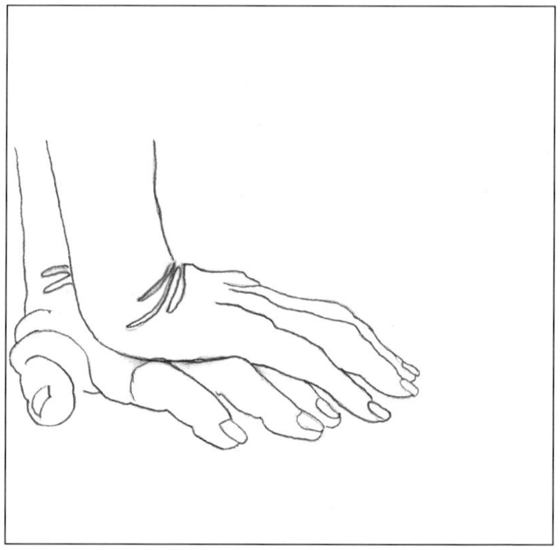

Extreme wrist extension combined with the strong downward pressure is hard on a therapist's wrists. Extensive use can lead to severe joint and ligament problems often taking more than a year to heal.

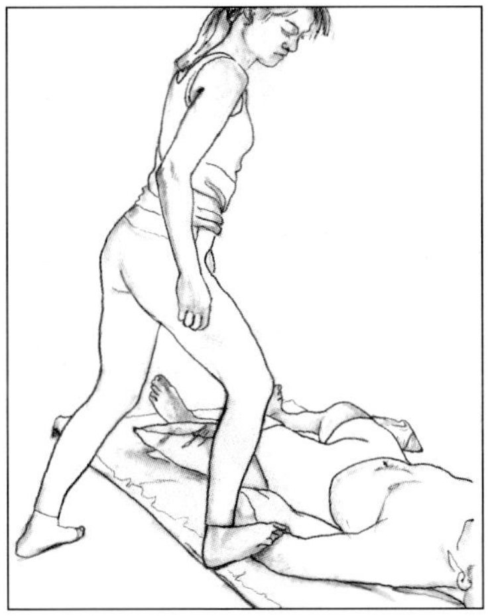

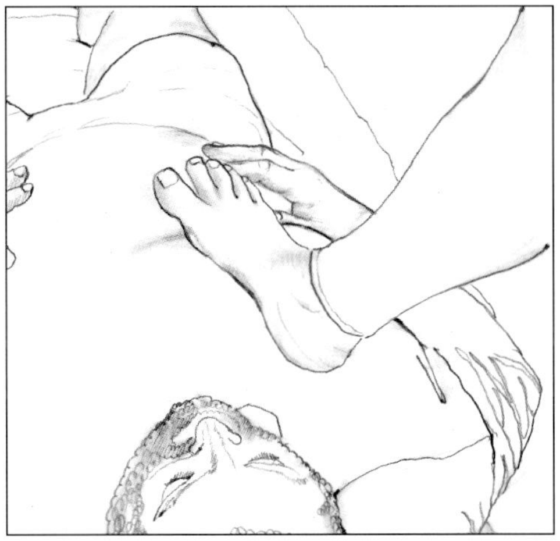

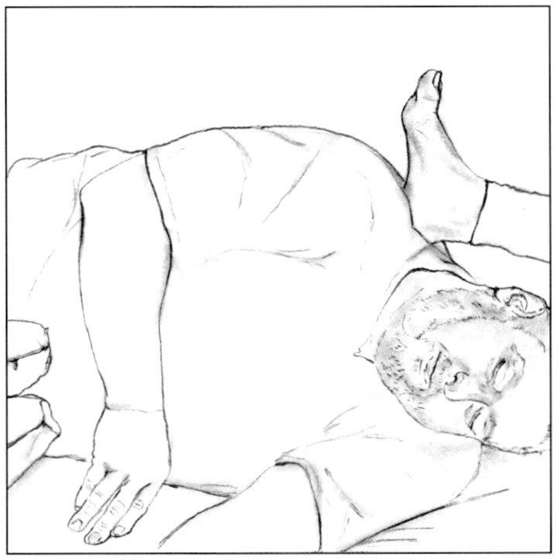

Employ good biomechanics, body weight and proper client positioning to effortlessly treat chronic myofascial pain syndromes of the major muscles of the torso and extremities.

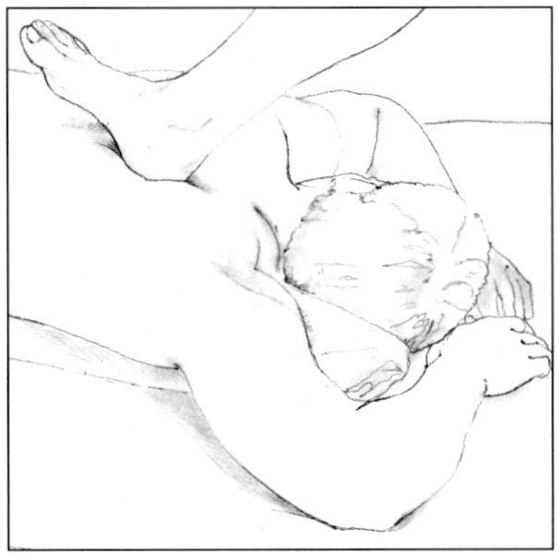

Heels are broad and mitigate the intensity of treatment. When applying pressure to a trigger point, your foot is much less invasive than an elbow or thumb. The heel also provides some of the stretch needed to complete a trigger point treatment.

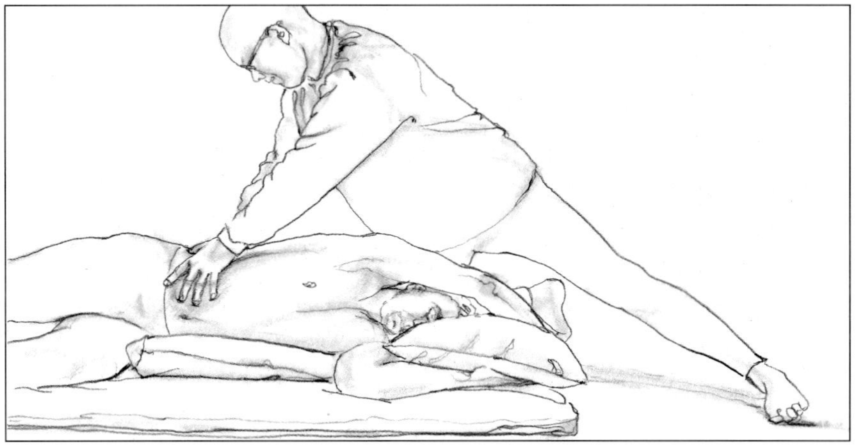

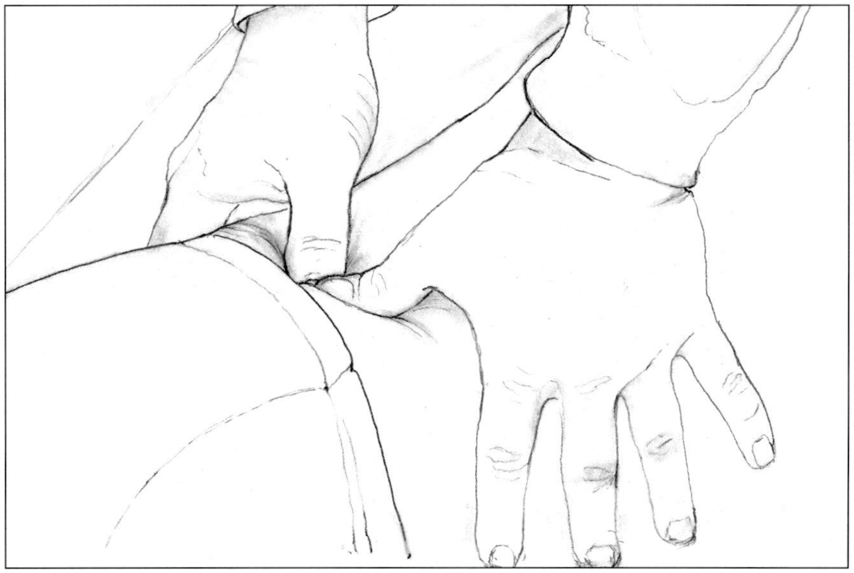

Hand approaches are used where feet won't do.

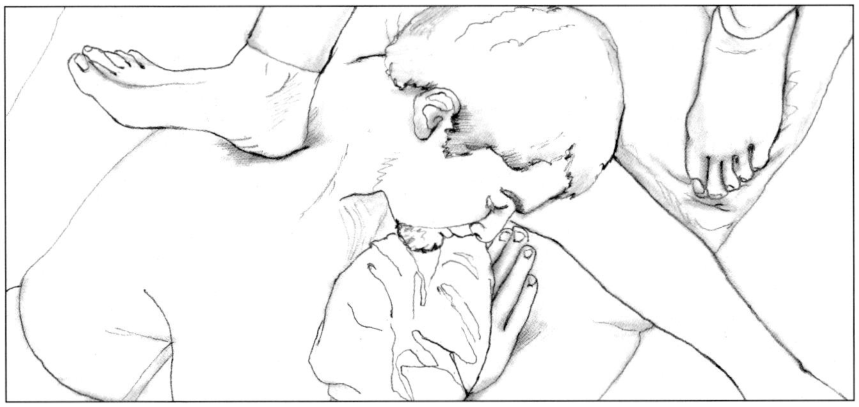

The WALKAROUND

THE WALKAROUND (the name derives from Fred's flying days and is analagous to the preflight inspection preformed prior to flight) is a fullbody compression massage that is useful as a pre-therapy evaluation tool. It fosters parasympathetic dominance, relaxes hypertonic muscles, reduces or relieves post-exercise soreness, effectively stretches soft tissues and, in general, promotes good health. While this compression massage is best learned in a workshop or from our video, studying the 101 photos included will suffice for many.

APPROACH

Rhythm and Depth

Start your session slowly and step moderately. The most common errors made with hands are also the ones made with feet. Working too deeply and too quickly are the two most frequent mistakes. Both lessen your ability to process feedback from the touch receptors in your foot. Excessive and rapid compressions also over-stimulate and irritate your clients.

Clients armor when you step too hard. This fear or pain-invoked tightening-up can ruin your session. Listen to the tissues. Older or debilitated people generally require a lighter touch. The pressure transmitted through your feet is significantly greater than you can achieve using your hands. Inattention to the strong forces generated by compressions leads to haphazard or sloppy work that can hurt your client.

When your client is ready to receive deeper work, shift your weight from the balance leg to the application leg by moving your center of gravity towards the point of compression. Apply/increase pressure gradually. Steady rhythm and your compression's depth maximize effectiveness and induce a deep relaxation. Sink slowly into the soft tissues. Allow adequate time to move capillary blood and lymph, flush metabolites and promote the infusion of health-enhancing arterial blood.

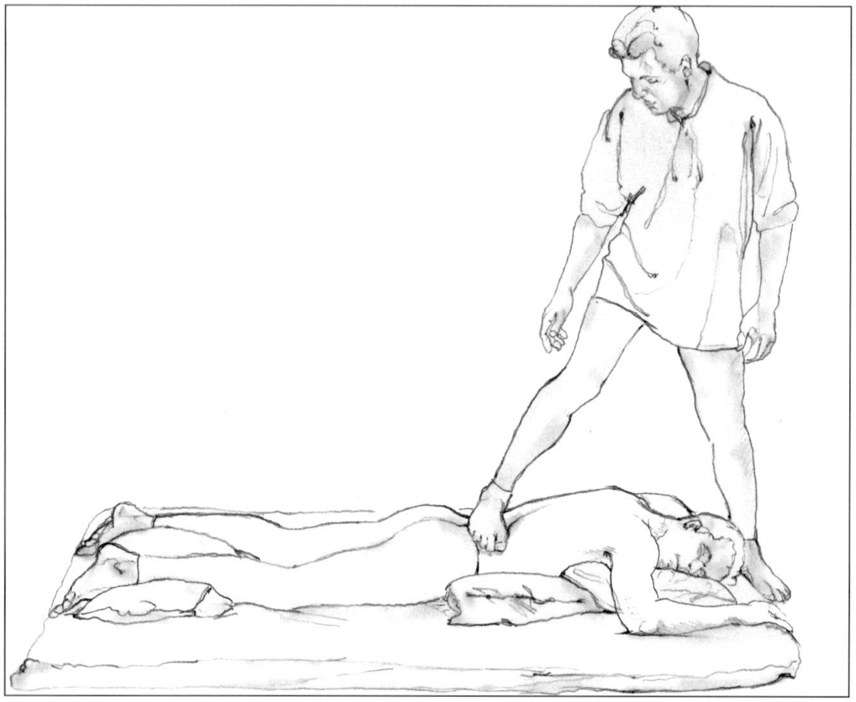

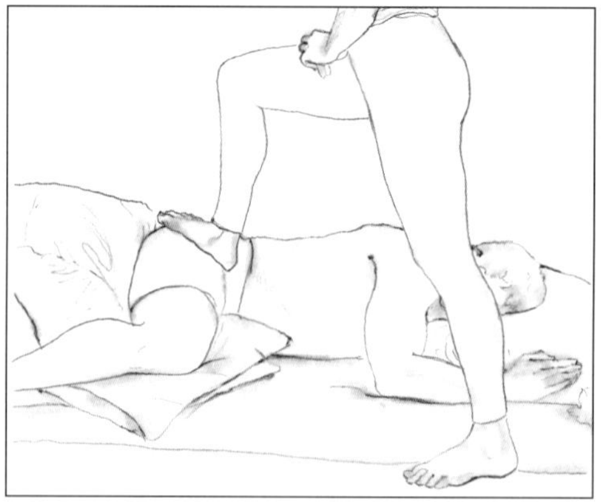

Focus on your client's response – especially while learning this new skill. Practice will quickly improve your balance and efficacy. After a short while, clients won't be able to distinguish between contact made by your hand or foot, except that footwork is firmer, deeper and often more satisfying.

Balance

You can quickly improve your balance by the daily practice of standing on one foot with your eyes closed. Physical therapists use it to rehab feet after nerve damage or surgery.

Wearing shoes diminishes stirrup muscle tone and intrinsic foot muscle strength. Over-support (wearing rigid footgear) reduces muscle tone. Going barefoot, particularly on uneven surfaces, will quickly help you develop better balance. We've found that going barefoot is also a good tip to offer older clients who are becoming uncertain of their balance.

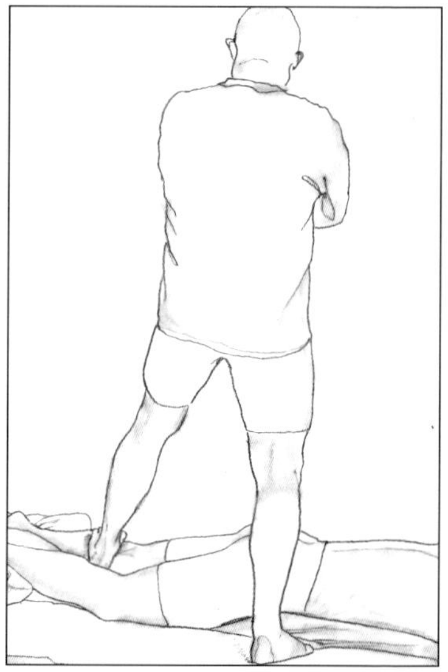

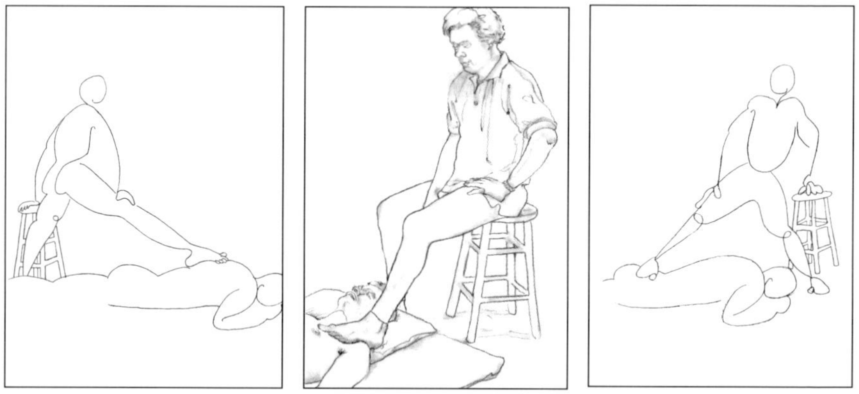

If your balance is uncertain – try using a stool or a walking stick.

Your feet should observe the same hygienic care as your hands.

Soft Foot

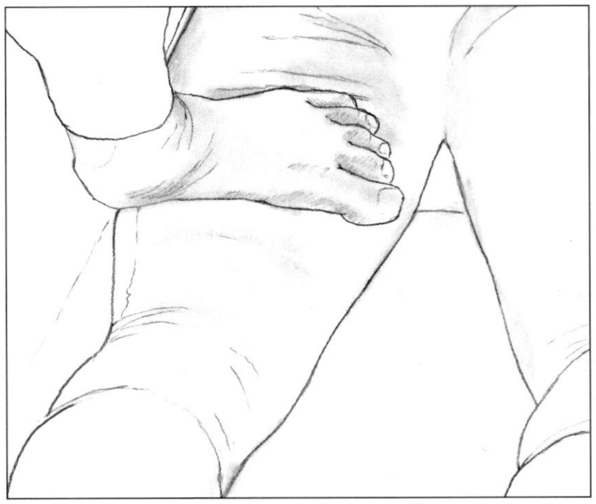

In many ways, feet are analogous to hands. For best results, use a relaxed, soft foot held in a neutral position, not pronated or supinated. Your toes should be relaxed, not extended or flexed. You'll know you're using a soft foot when your whole foot forms to the tissue beneath it.

Posture

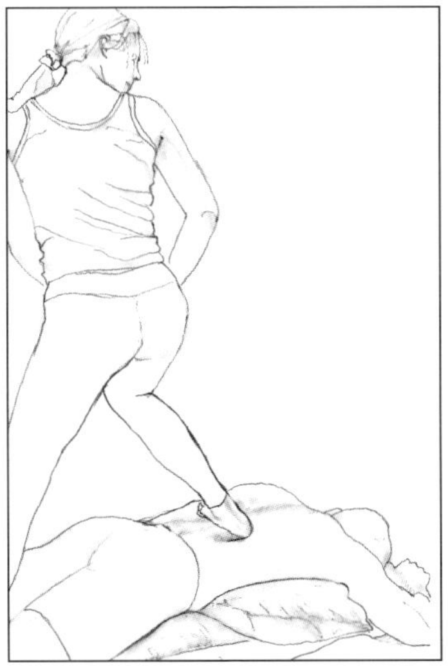

Protect yourself. By not rotating your thigh medially, you avoid a possible medial collateral ligament strain. Good biomechanics also demand you avoid "hiking" the supporting leg's hip joint.

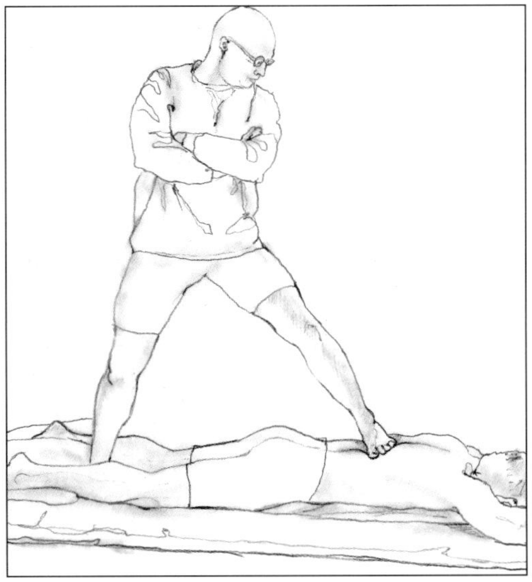

Balanced, elegant posture promotes effective work. Take every advantage of gravity. Visualize and assume "straight" postural attitudes. Position yourself so that undue strain is not transmitted through your bent joints.

The Session

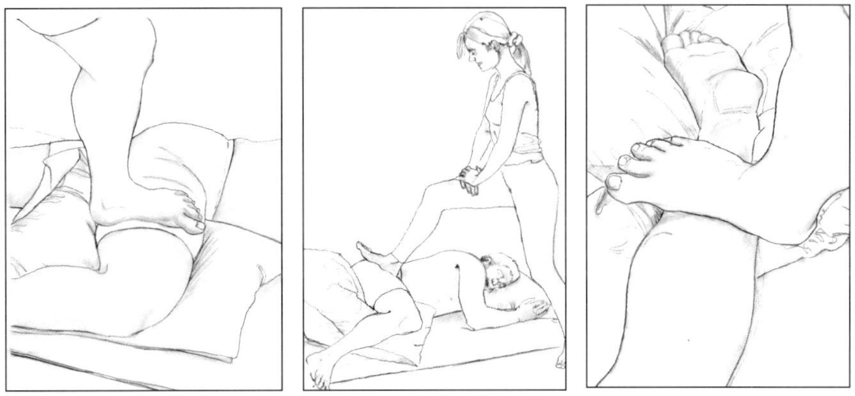

Each session is unique. Be creative and tailor your session to cater to the particular needs of your client. While a rote application of these principles works, over time you will develop a much more "organic" approach.

Feedback

You can use a numeric feedback mechanism to help determine optimal pressure. Promote feedback from your clients. Let them know that they should guide you to proper depth and pressure, and that they are responsible for their own well-being during the session. Therapists who use client feedback get better results and fewer complaints.

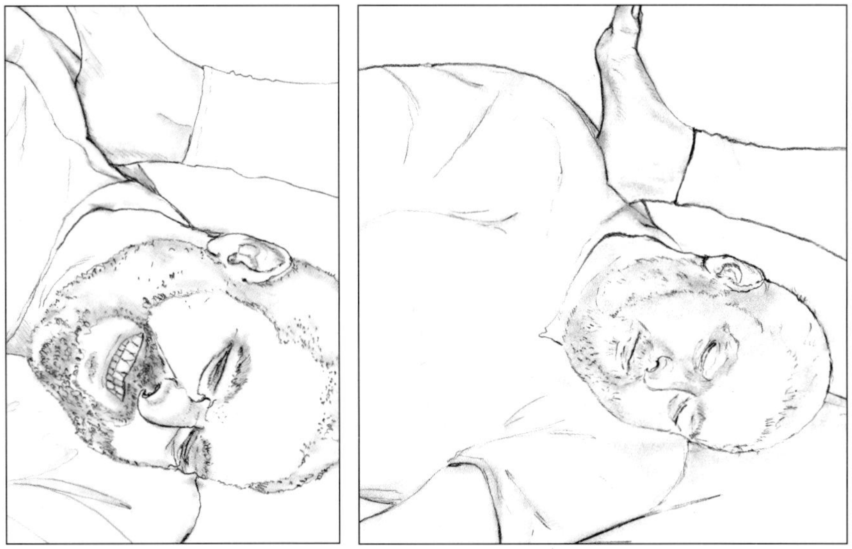

Clients are briefed to use a 1 to 10 scale for pressure or pain. One is defined as light touch. Ten really hurts (it's the level of pressure that causes your client to severely tighten up).

Seven is theraputic pressure. It feels good, even with some pain. Seven is more exactly defined as the pressure leading to diminishing sensitivity when held for 10 to 12 seconds. Diminishing means falling off – not necessarily eliminated. Extremely literal clients will be unable to work with this scale. These clients can rely on "it hurts good" or "it hurts bad" or "it feels therapeutic" or "it feels invasive."

If your client indicates an 8 (or more), decrease your pressure. More is not necessarily better. Too much pressure increases your workload and slows therapeutic progress.

Work within a therapeutic range. If, however, there are no problems in the area being compressed, there is no need for feedback.

> You will notice that the pressure required to reach a level of 7 increases with each session. In time (assuming stress levels and health-in-general remain constant), your client will have pain-free sessions. Healthy tissues do not hurt when compressed.

When Your Clients Hurt

Pain indicates problems. Reduce pressure and slow down if your client hurts. Sensitive areas often indicate old adhesions, trigger points or hypertonicity. Add some jostling (shaking and gentle joint manipulations) by rolling your foot back and forth over the affected site. Add some glides, slides, vibrations. You can apply gentle stretches to the painful tissues by simply twisting your foot to promote quicker, more thorough and deeper releases. It takes time for tissue to release. Gradually increase the depth with each succeeding round of compressions. Three passes are usually adequate.

One approach to combining deep compressive massage with therapy would be to conduct a 30 to 45 minute WALKAROUND to allow examination of the whole body while simultaneously relaxing your client. Then address the presenting complaint.

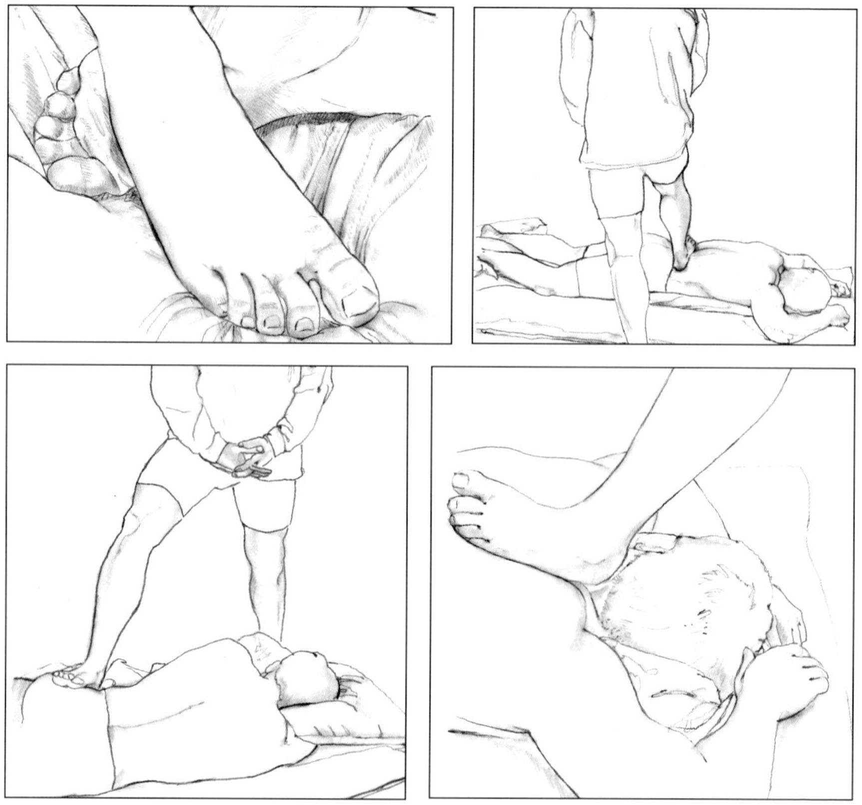

> Before putting your feet to work, take time to review the indications, contraindications and client intake procedures.

Therapist Quick Review

1. Bolster to insure client safety and comfort and proper treatment biomechanics for yourself.

2. Work with feedback. Do not exceed 7 on a therapeutic pressure scale.

3. Sink in – use 10 to 15 second compressions for warming tissue.

4. Increase compressions gradually. Listen to the tissues. Think hydraulically.

5. To maximize benefits, increase pressure to work at 7 on each round of compressions. Three compressions or three passes per muscle group are usually adequate.

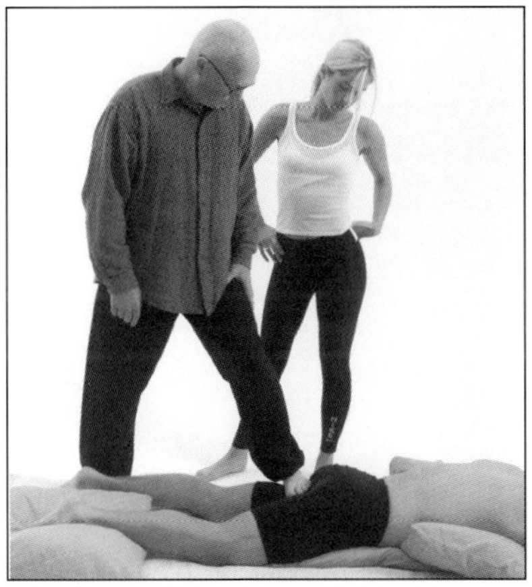

1. Start just below the gluteal fold.

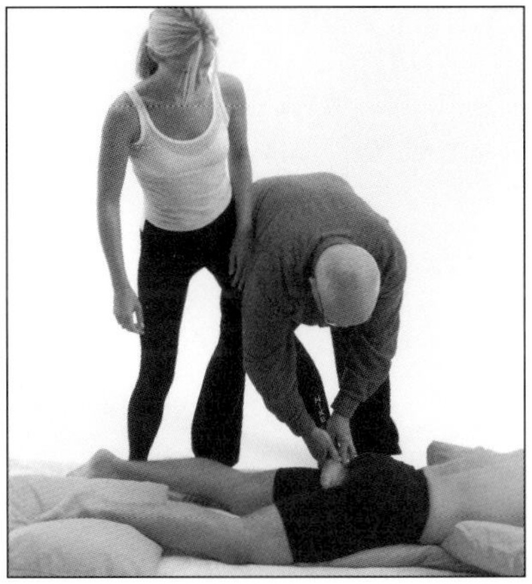

2. Start at the ischial tuberosity.

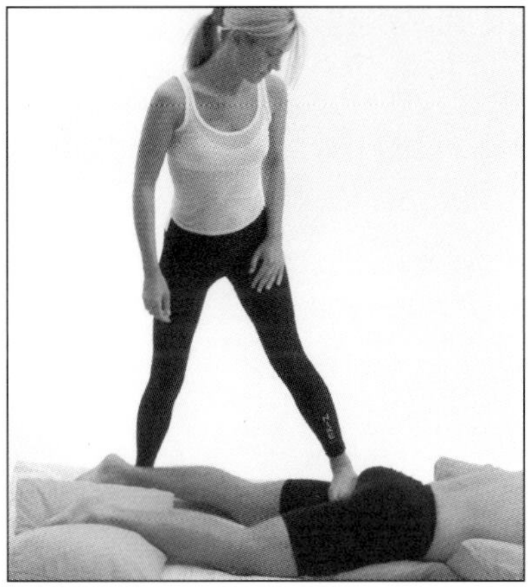

3. Enter slowly.

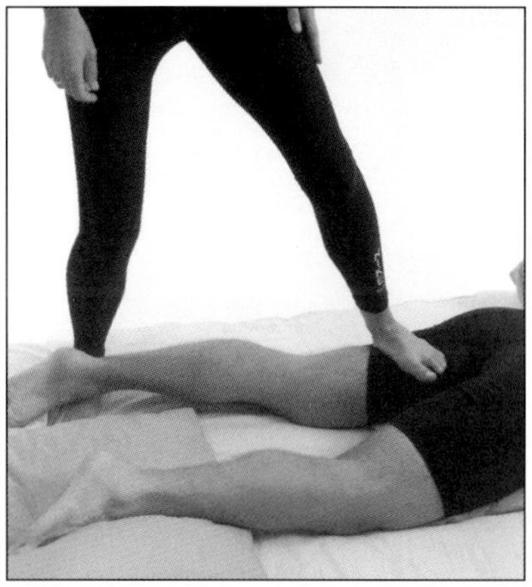

4. Lean forward to increase pressure.

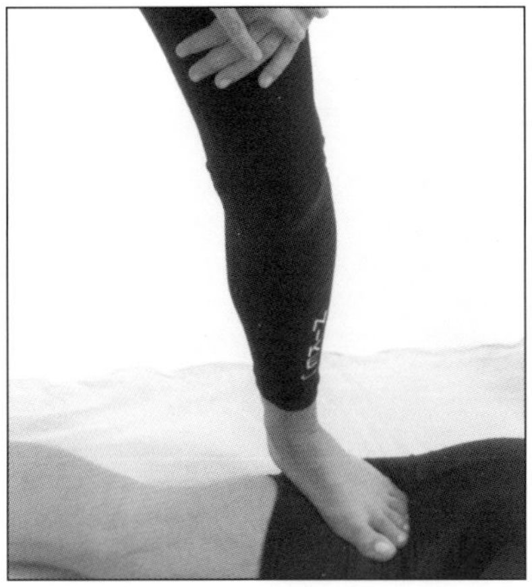

5. Bend further for more pressure.

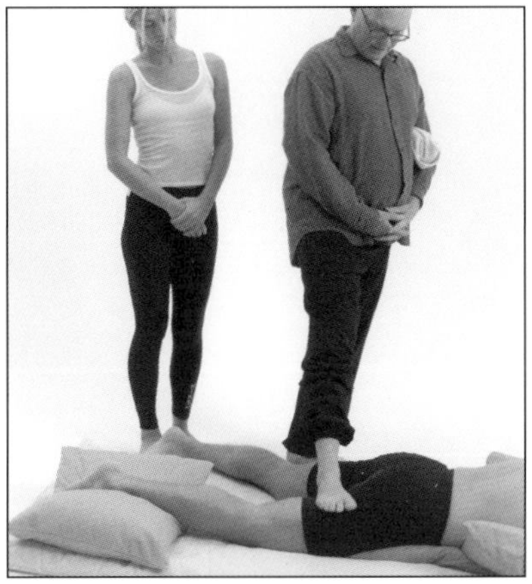

6. Step across to the medial hams.

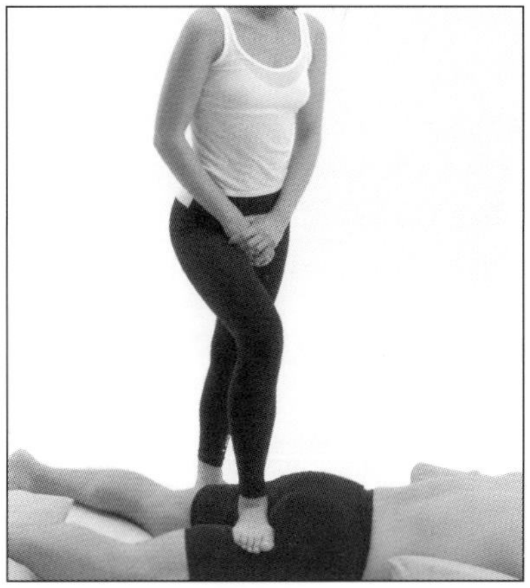

7. Smile?

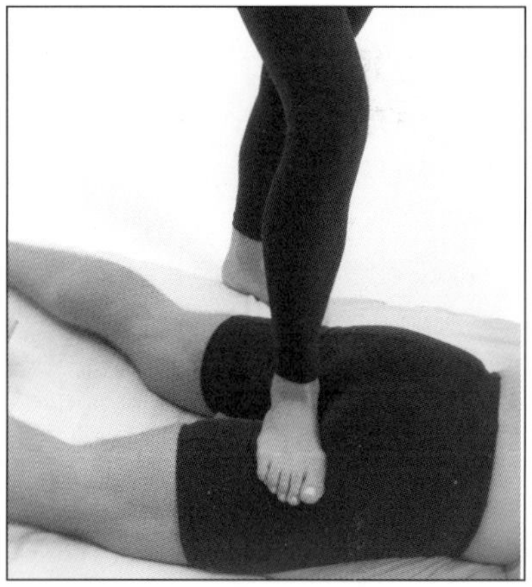

8. Deeper.

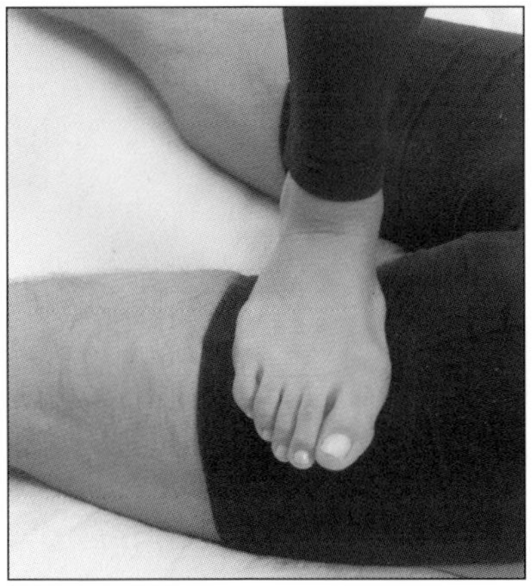

9. Lower.

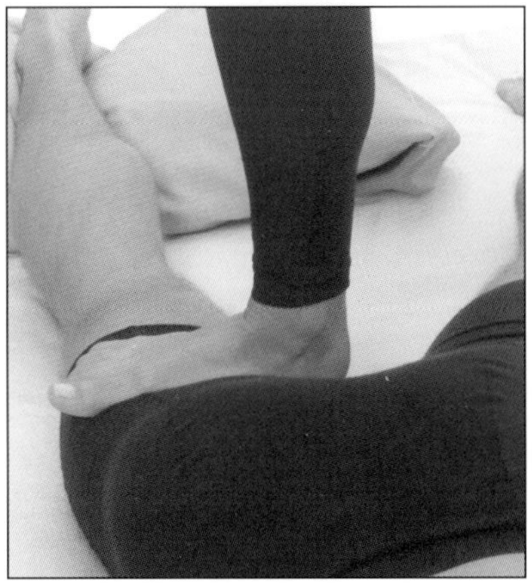

10. Deeper.

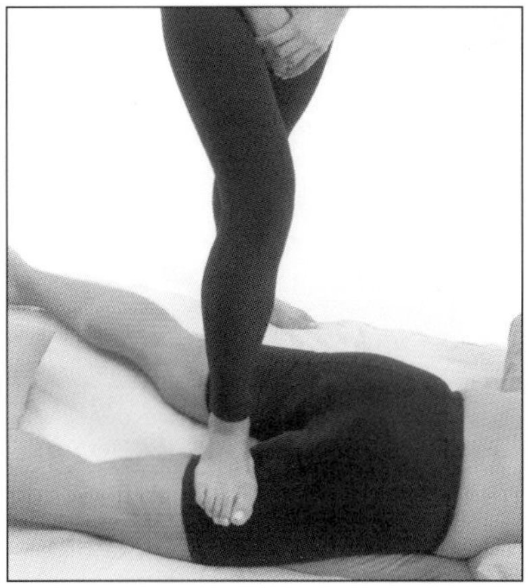

11. Lower.

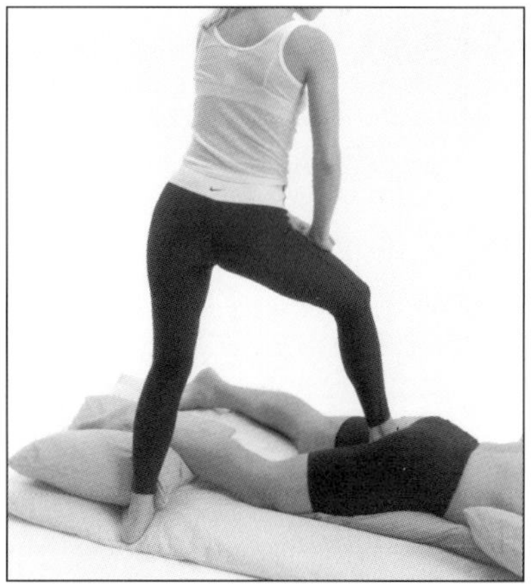

12. Wait.

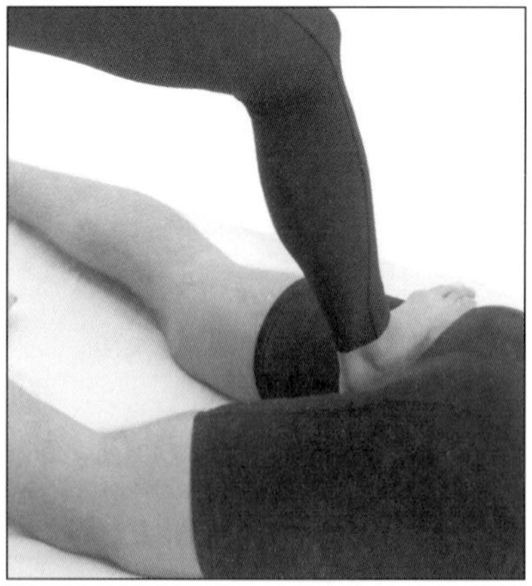

13. Sink.

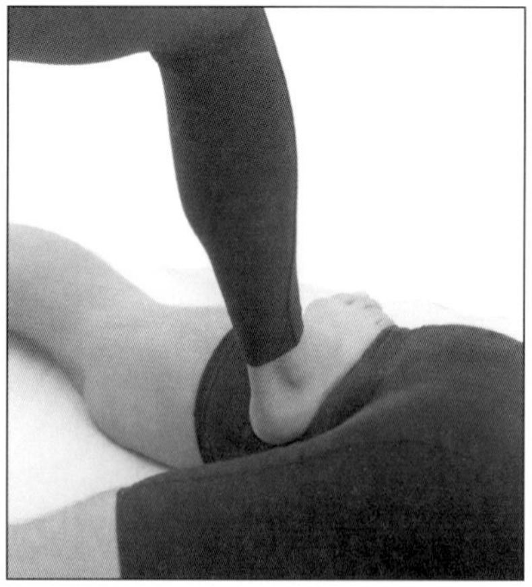

14. Conform.

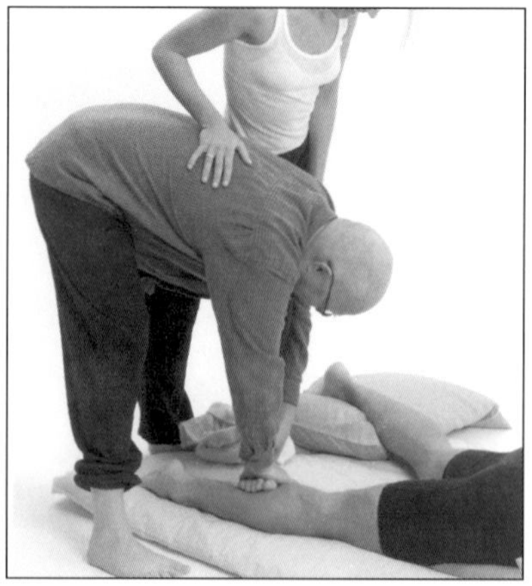

15. Medial.

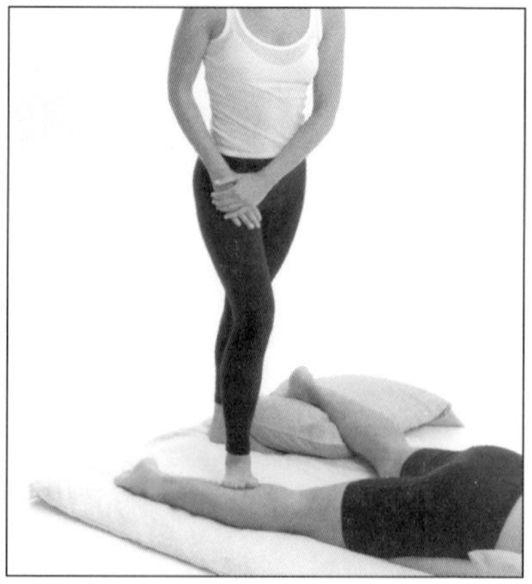

16. Patience - hold for 10-15 seconds.

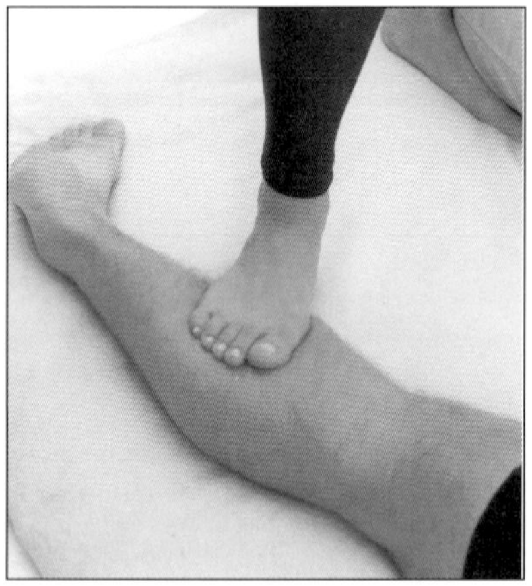

17. Just right.

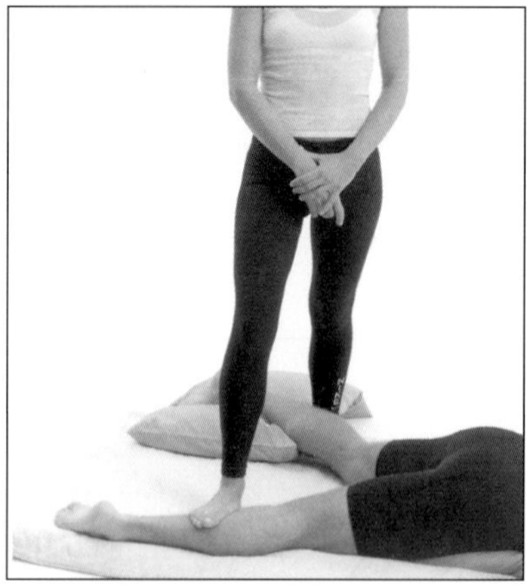

18. Change of angle.

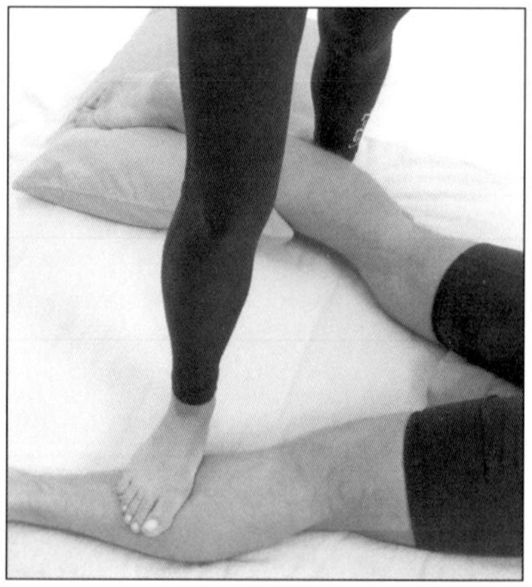

19. Sink.

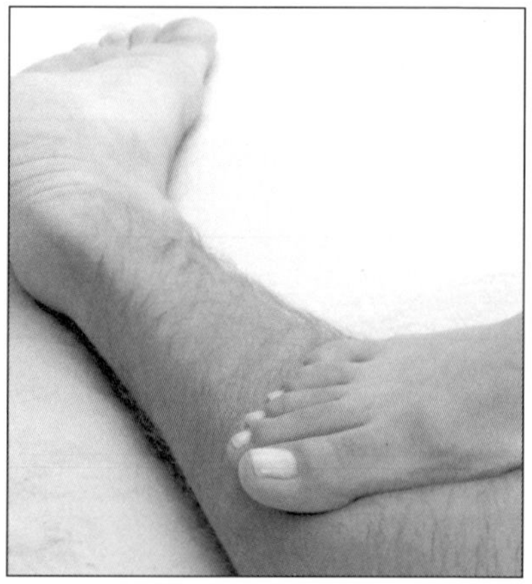

20. Wait.

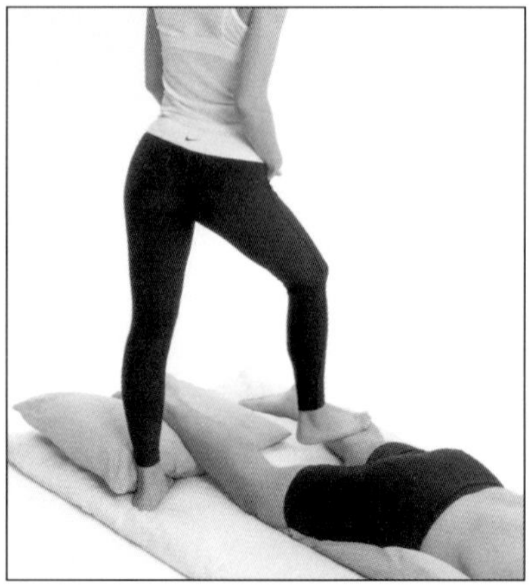

21. Gentle from the opposite side.

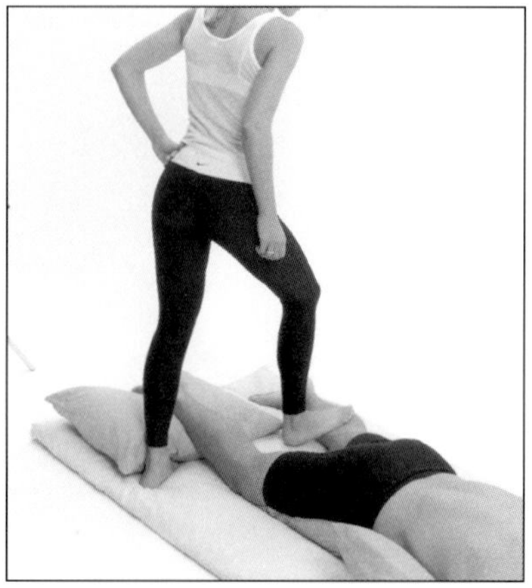

22. Supported heel = depth control.

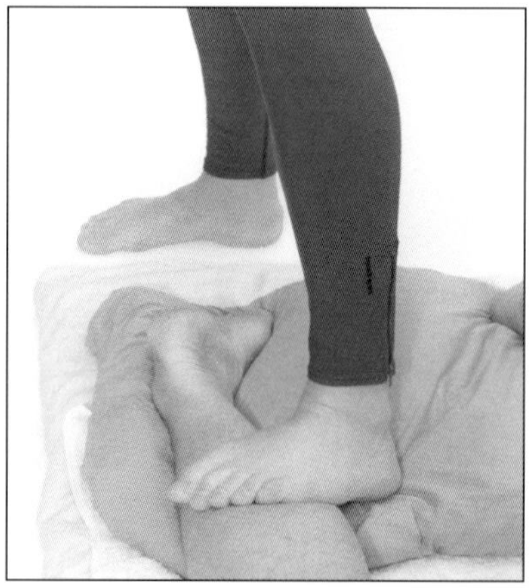

23. Stretch & compress.

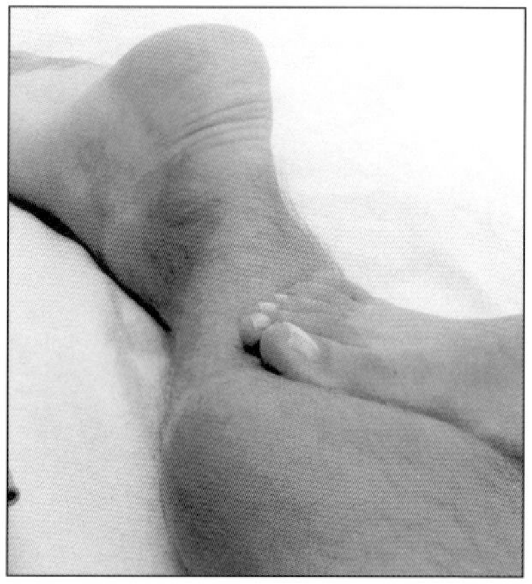

24. Pull & compress.

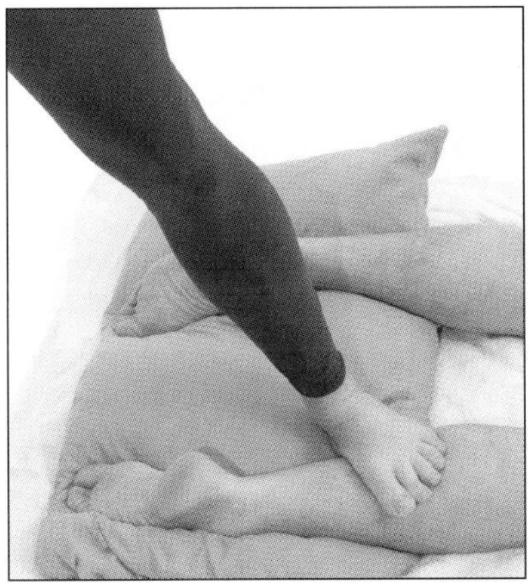

25. Musculotendinous juncture stretch & compress.

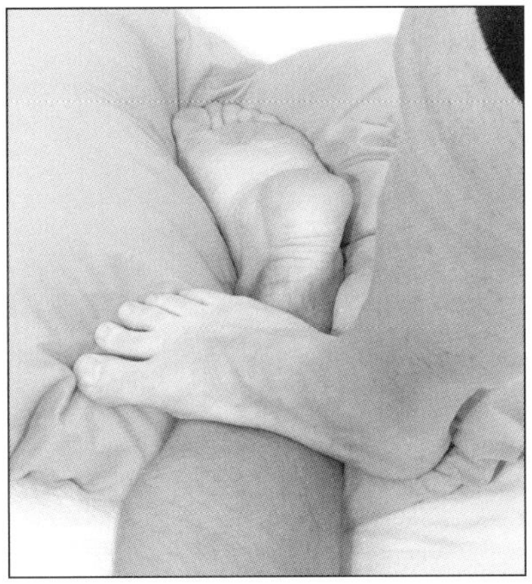

26. Enter slowly.

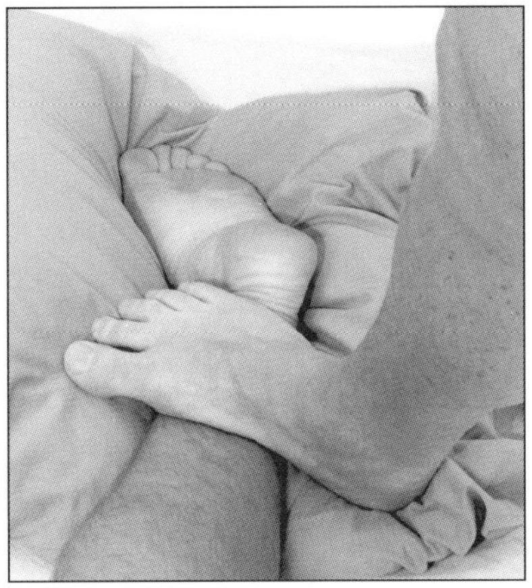

27. Pull & compress.

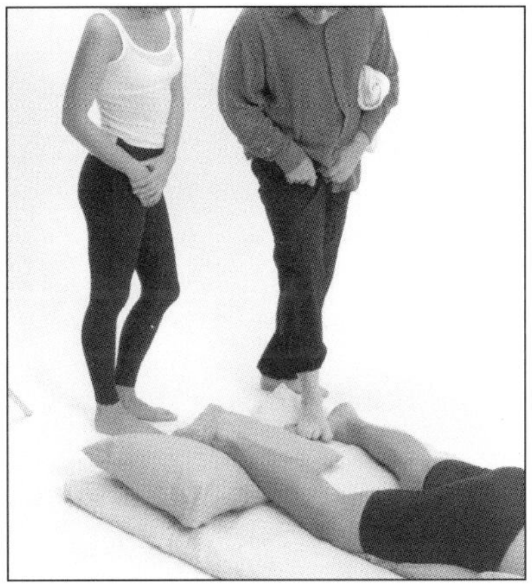

28. Foot to foot.

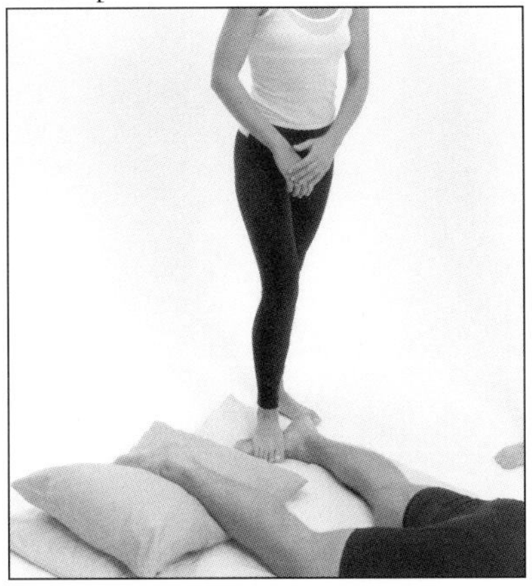

29. Look up occasionally - relax.

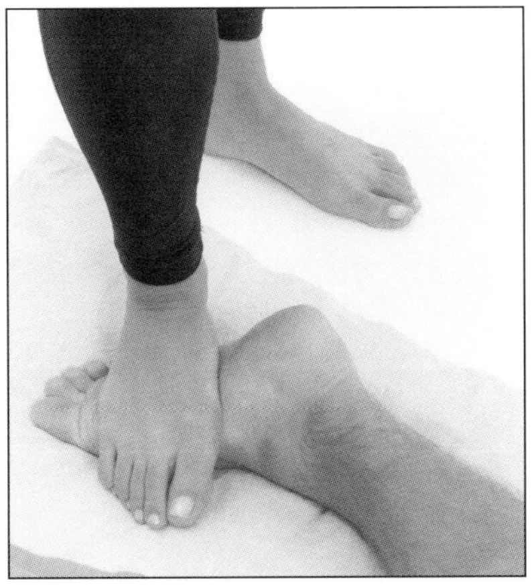

30. Ahh.

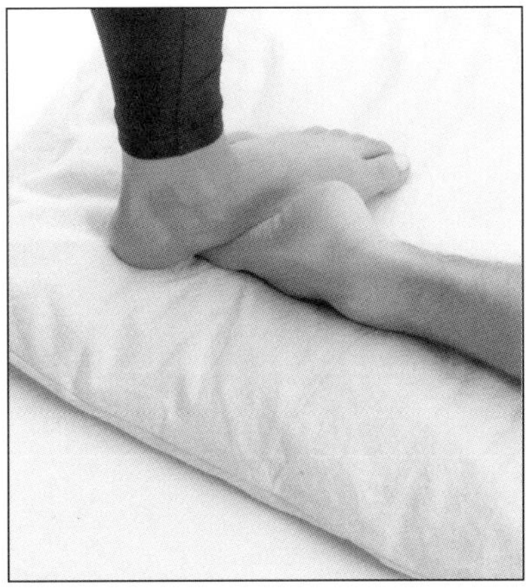

31. Change of feet.

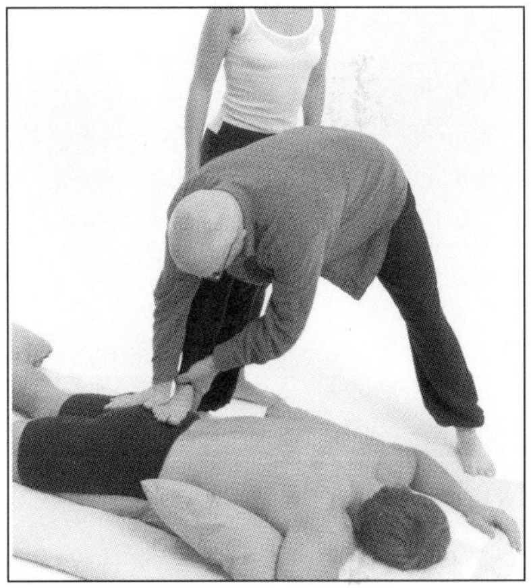

32. Back up to the glutes - just right.

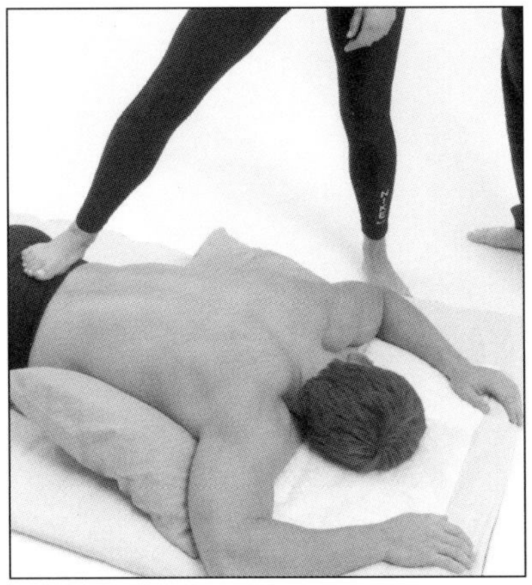

33. With ease.

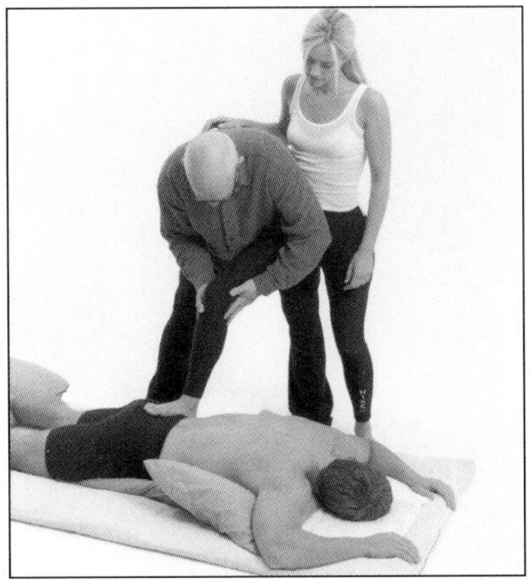

34. Varied attack.

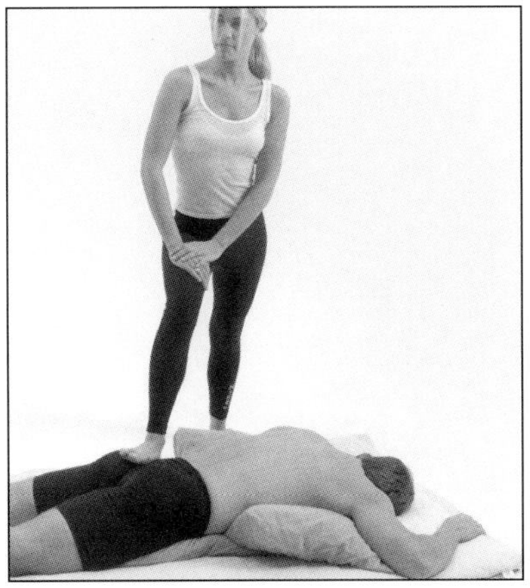

35. Looking up.

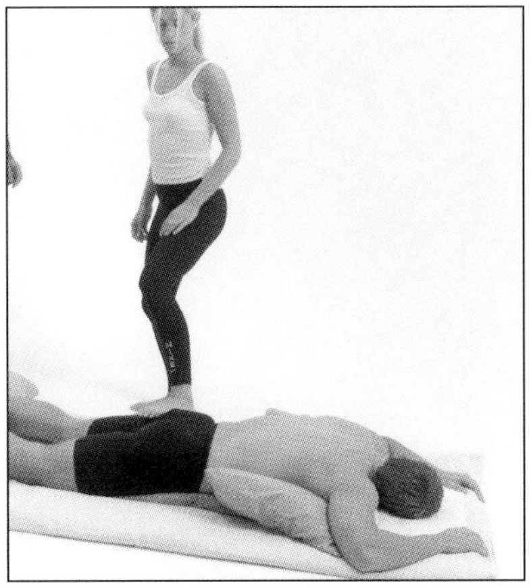

36. Get feedback.

POSTERIOR – PRONE

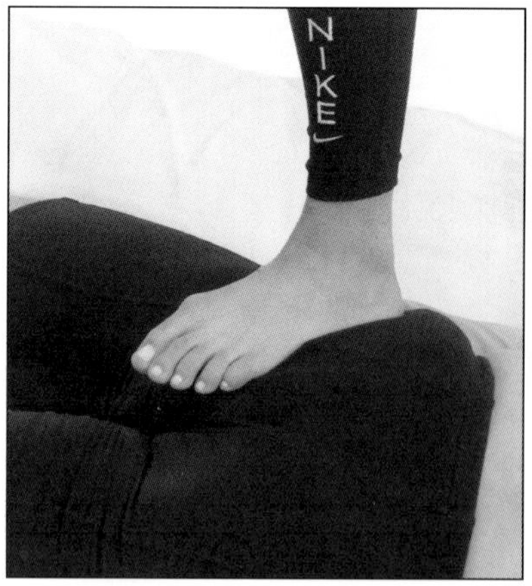

37. Better.

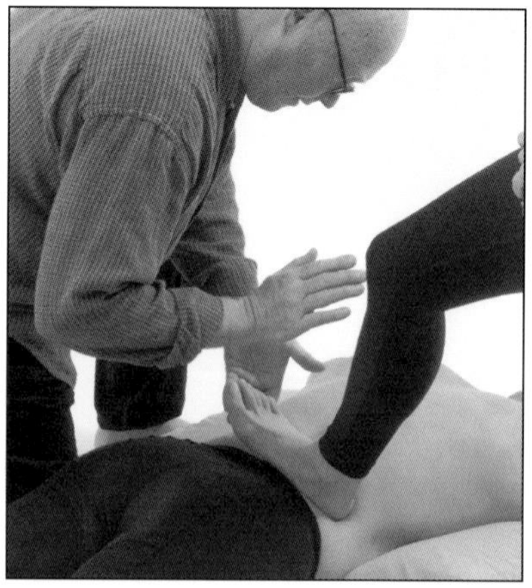

38. Slow.

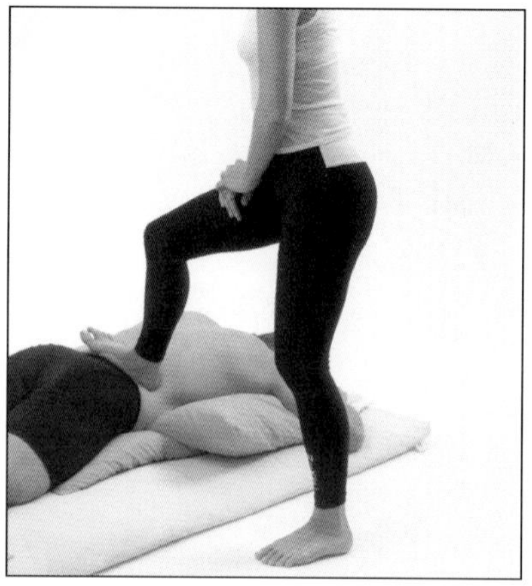

39. Hangin' out.

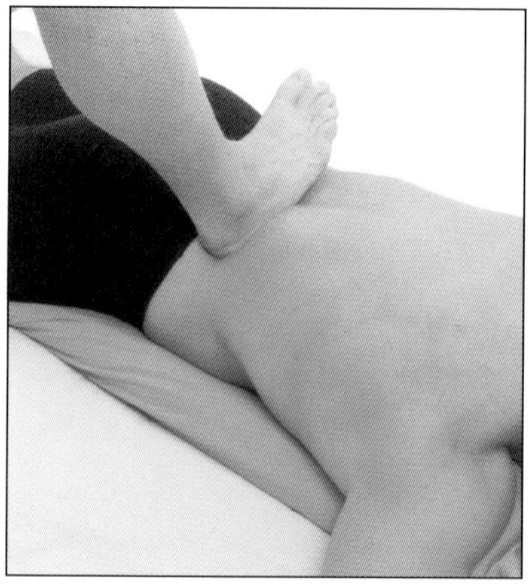

40. Use gentle paraspinal approach.

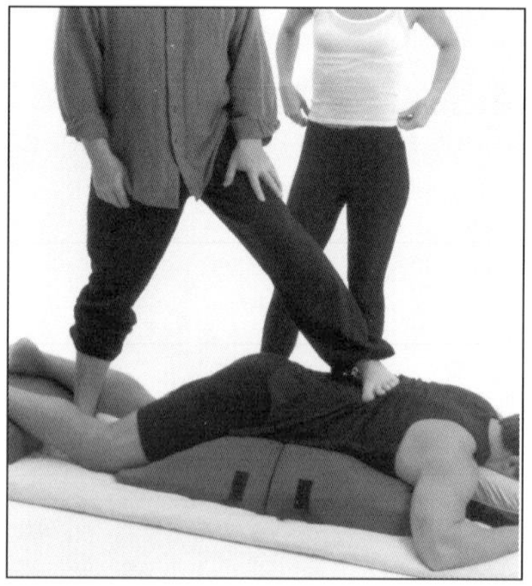

41. Solid on the support leg.

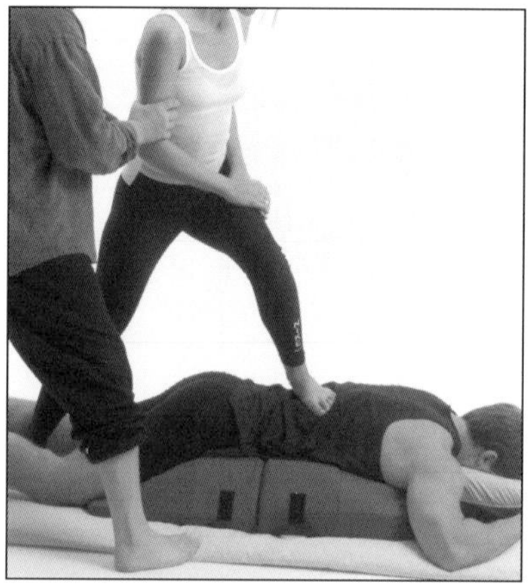

42. Unsteady? Use a balance aid.

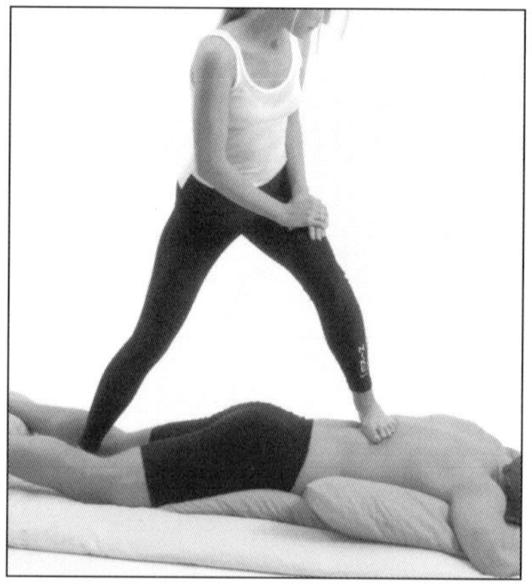

43. Press & stretch.

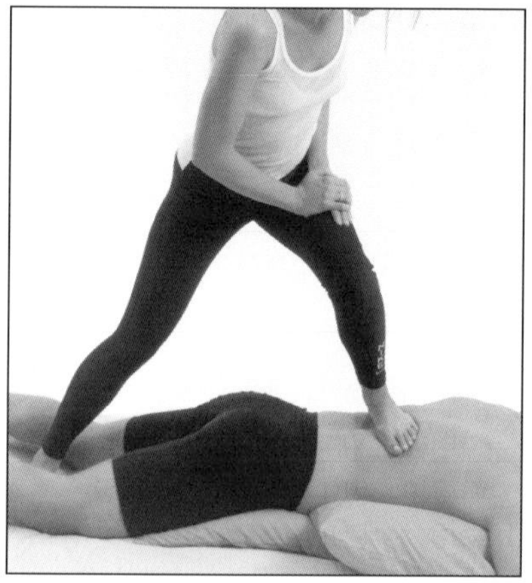

44. Powerful.

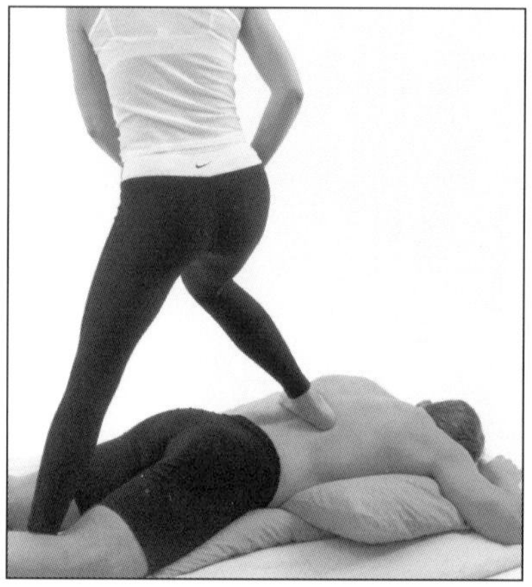

45. Protect your knee – watch angles.

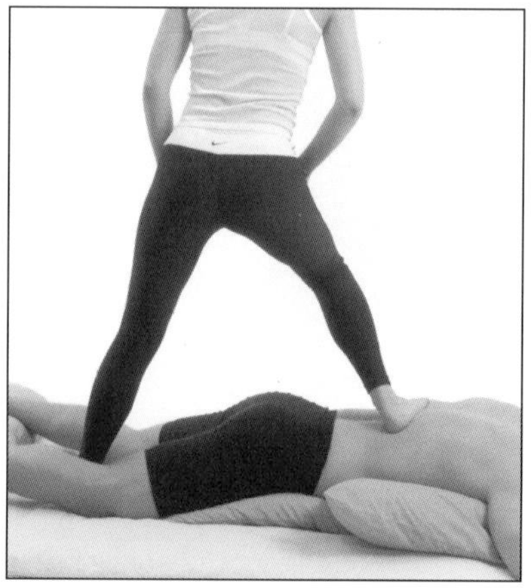

46. Better.

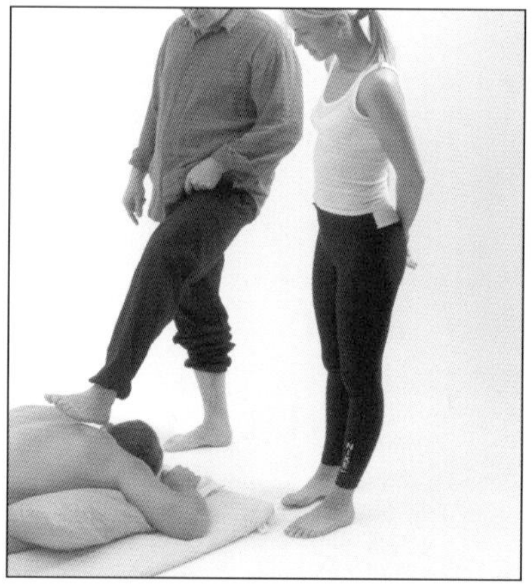

47. For mid-traps & rhomboids…

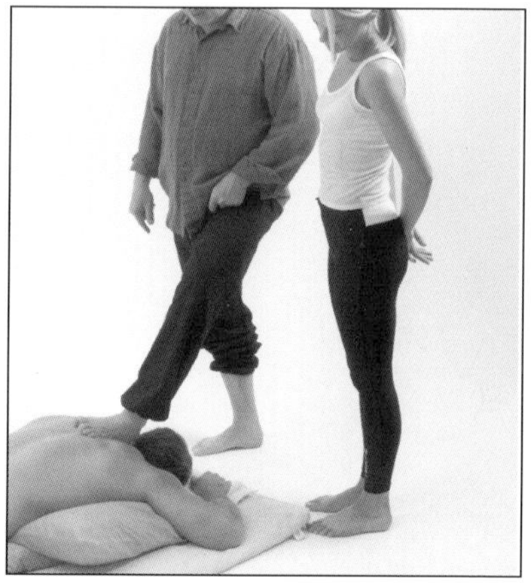

48. …use the lateral edge of your foot.

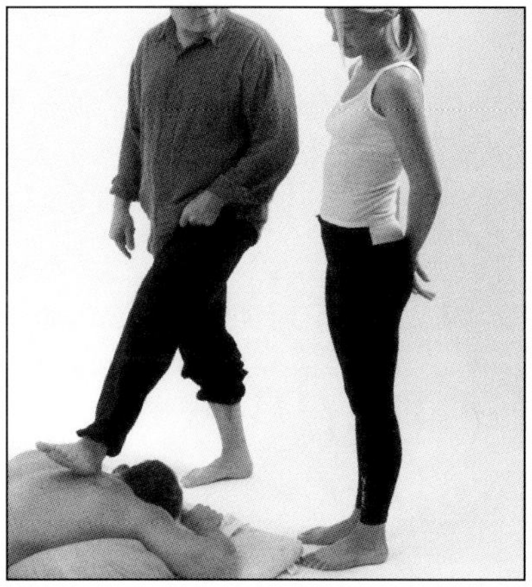

49. …or deeper with your heel.

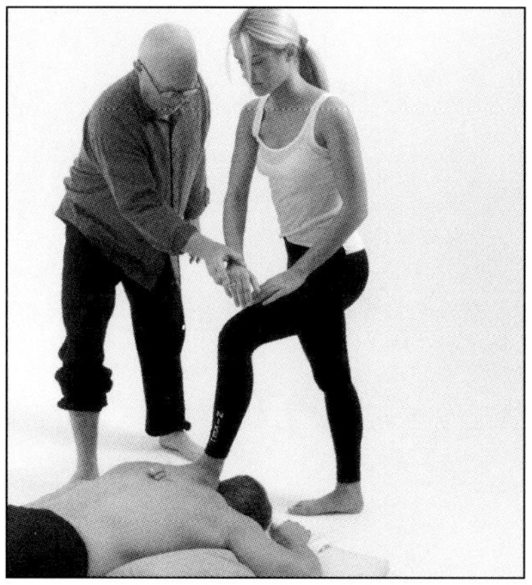

50. Compress up to veterbral border.

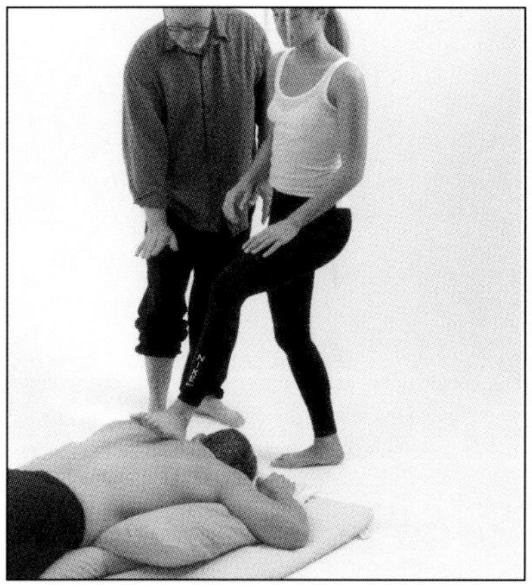

51. Use heel for larger clients.

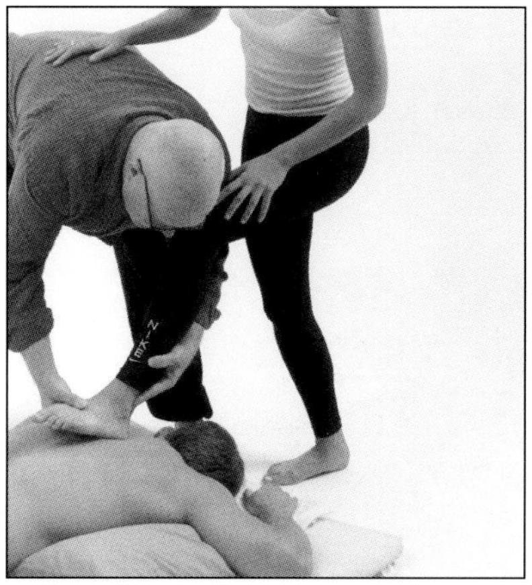

52. Sink slowly.

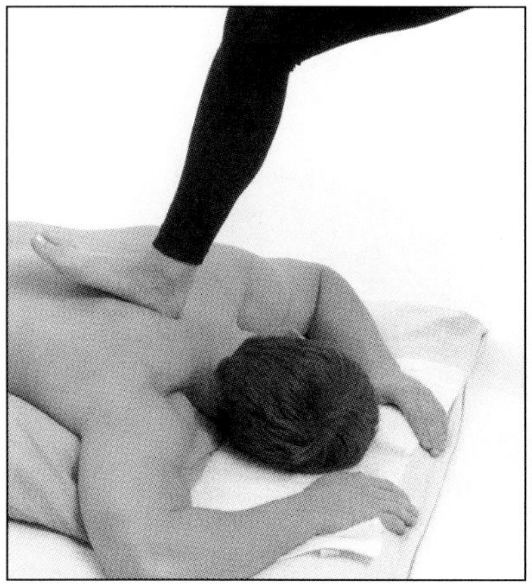

53. Weight…

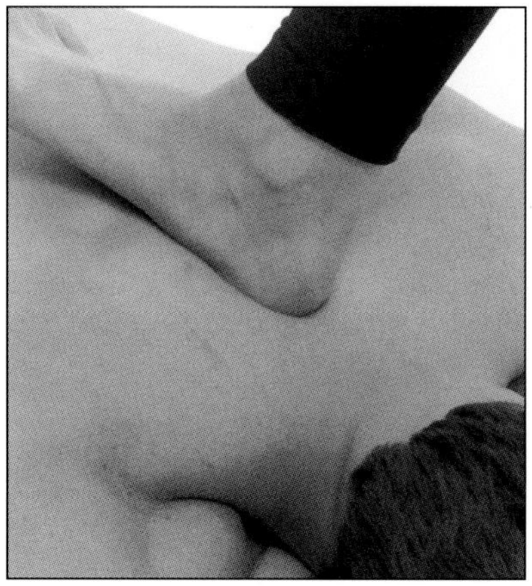

54. …and wait.

SIDELYING – LATERAL

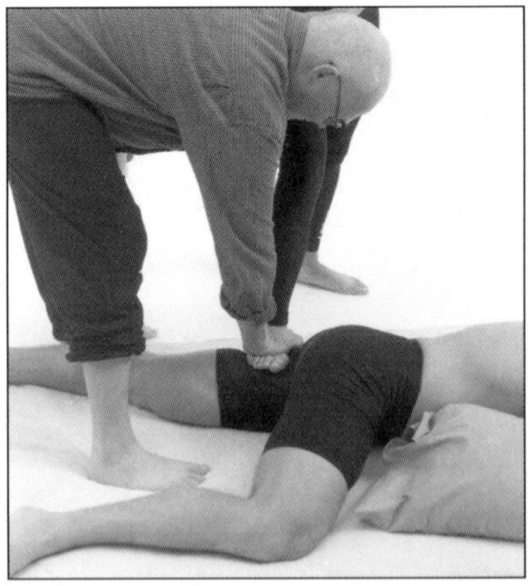

1. Remember to use a soft foot.

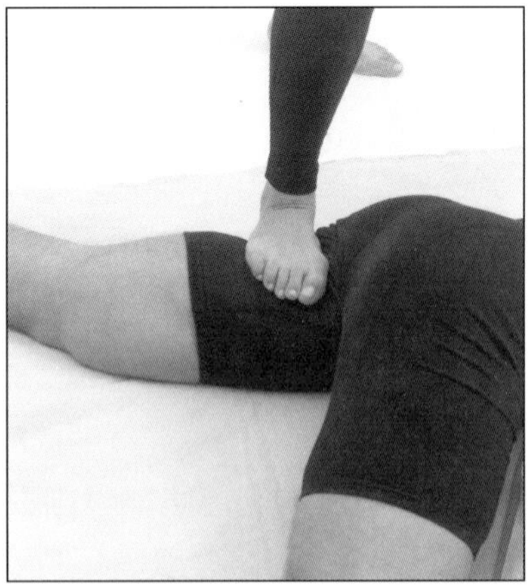

2. Adductor magnus & medial hams.

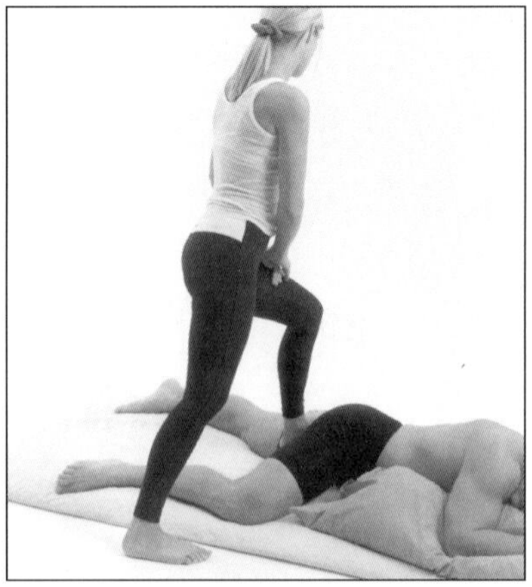

3. Change of angle of attack.

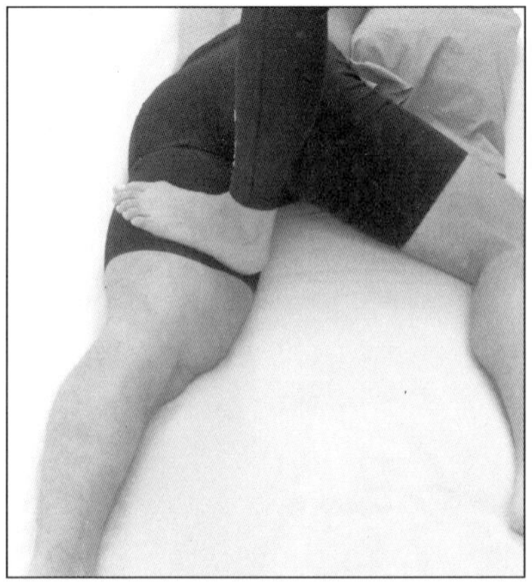

4. Adductor Longus, adductor brevis, gracilis & vastus medialis.

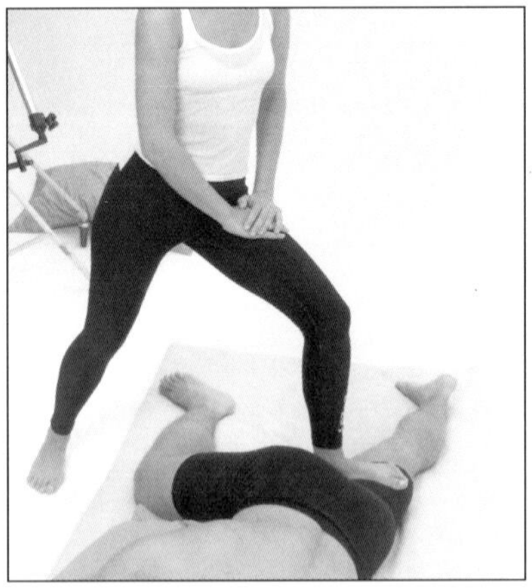

5. 15 seconds for each compression.

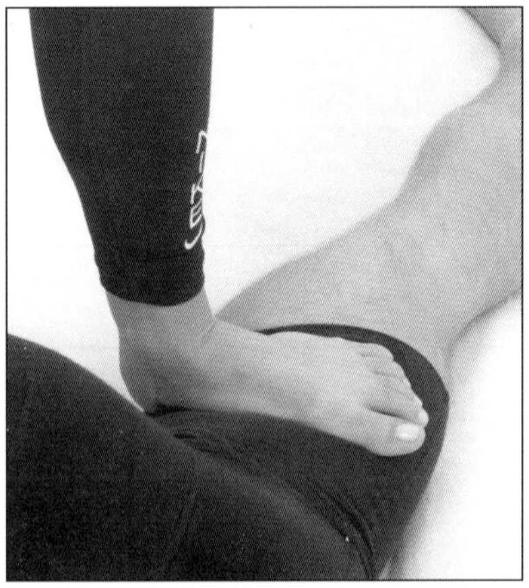

6. Moving towards an endangerment site – Hunters canal.

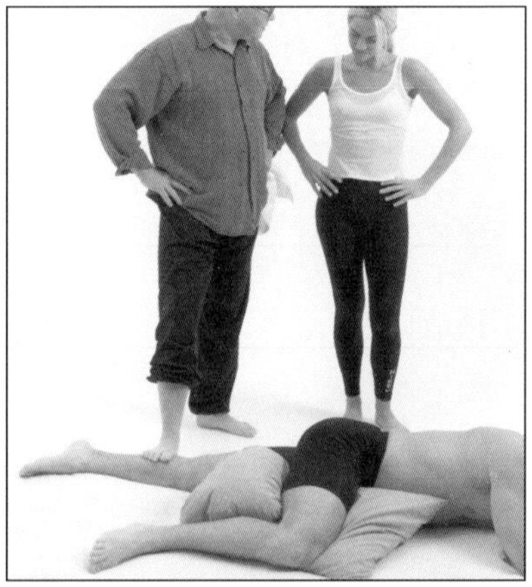

7. If you find a tender area, hold it.

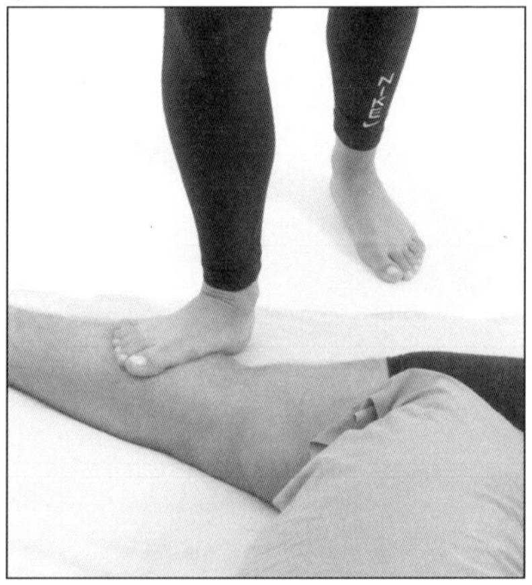

8. Pull & sink.

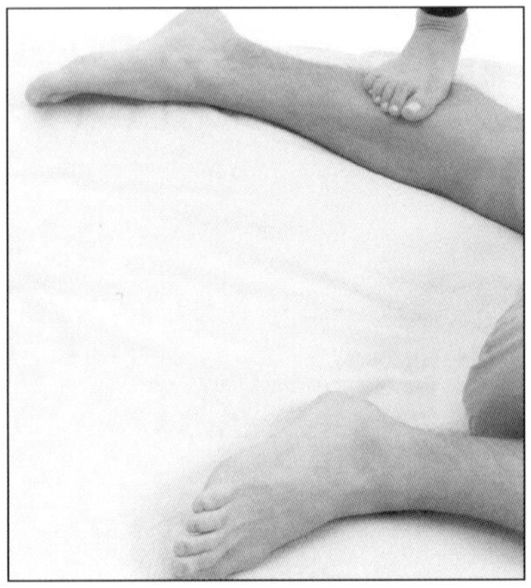

9. Distal.

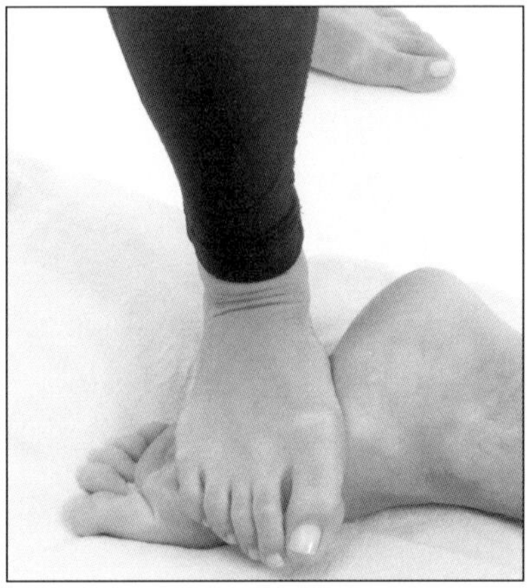

10. Pressure goes to all 4 layers.

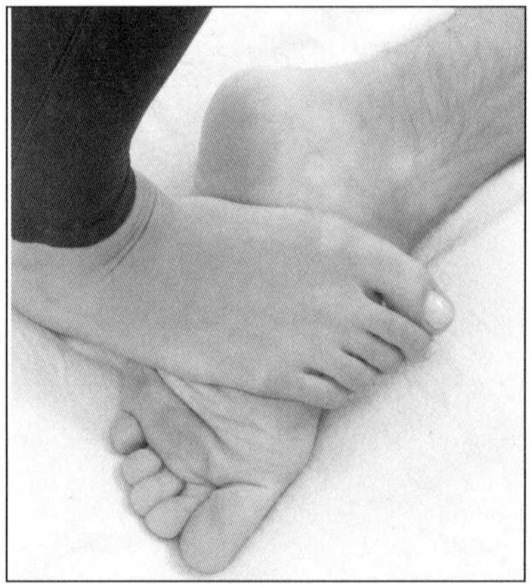

11. … it's a stretch, too.

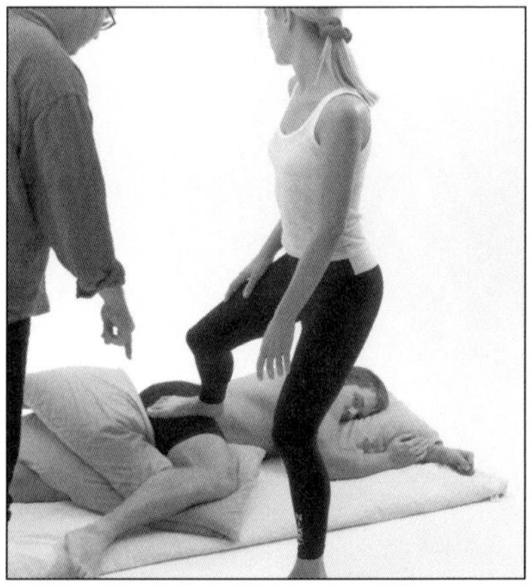

12. Watch posture, too many pillows...

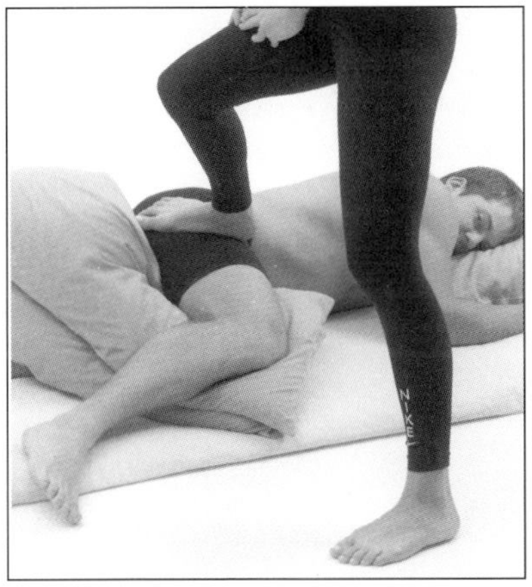

13. ... puts therapist at risk.

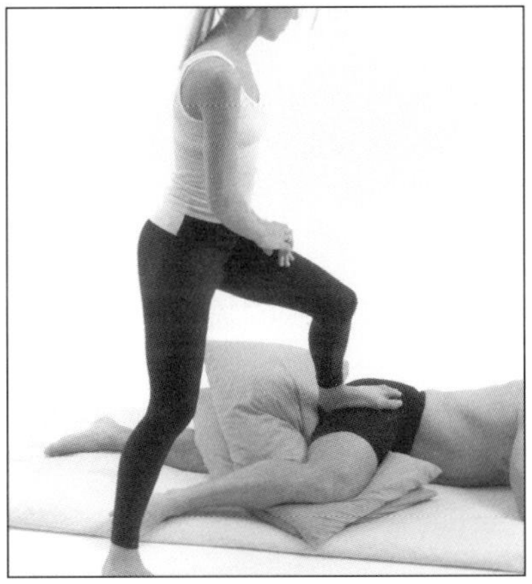

14. Change of approach protects you.

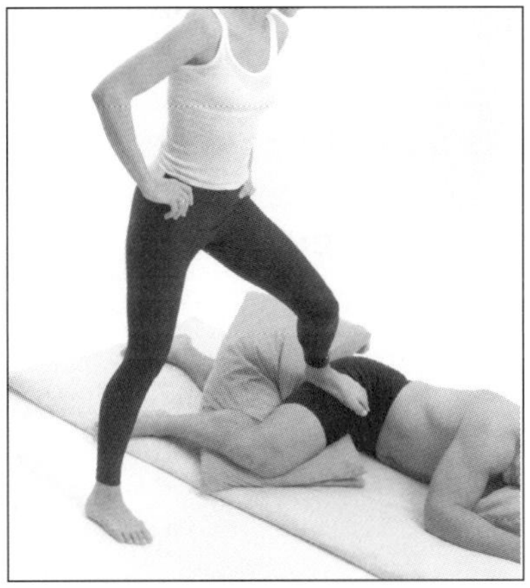

15. Bingo.

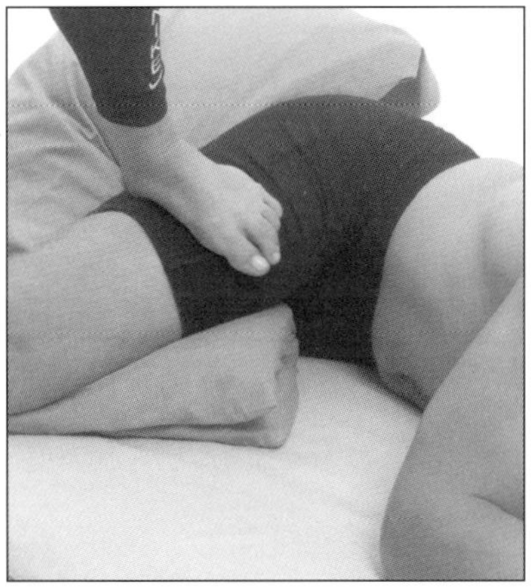

16. Rolling foot forward shifts muscle.

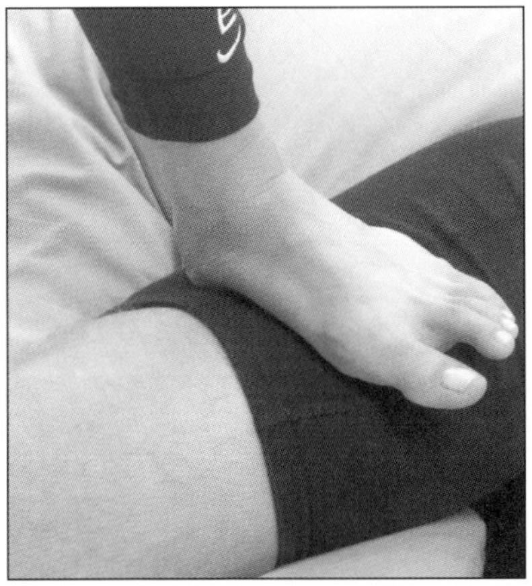

17. Roll it back & sink.

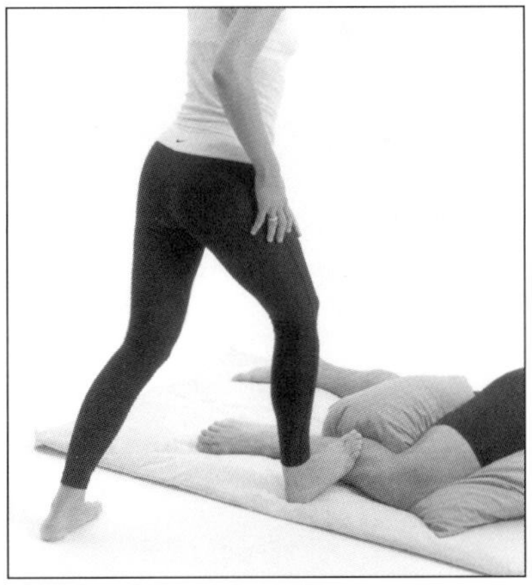

18. Continue to anterior compartment.

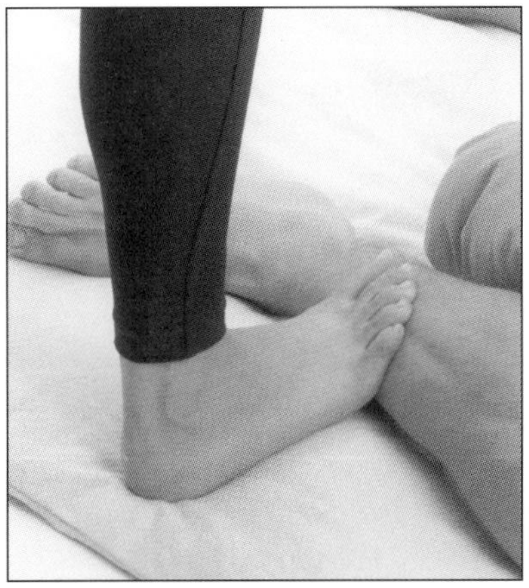

19. Musculotendinous juncture, tib anterior.

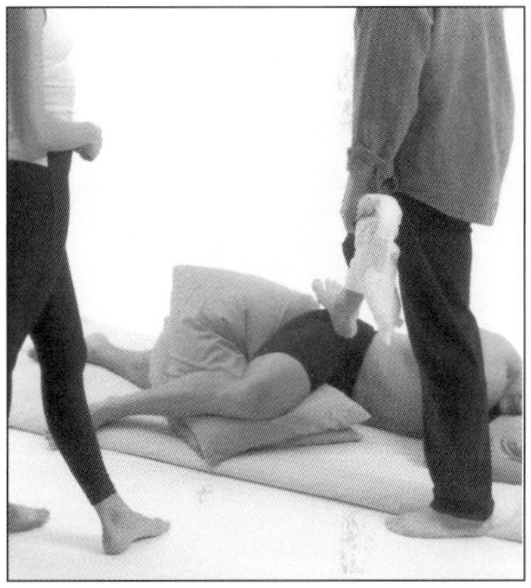

20. Tensor fascia latae is often tender.

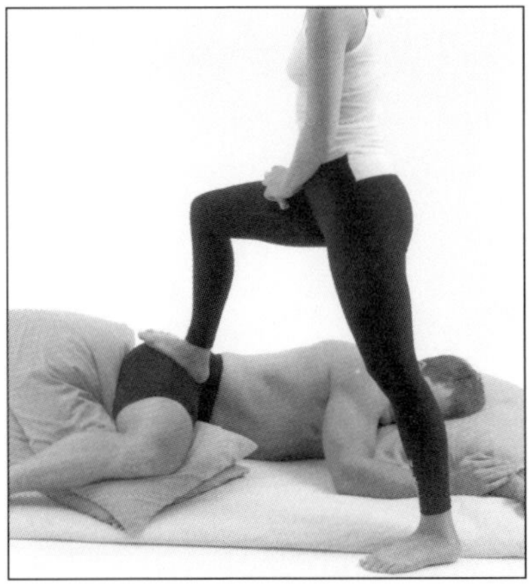

21. Warm it.

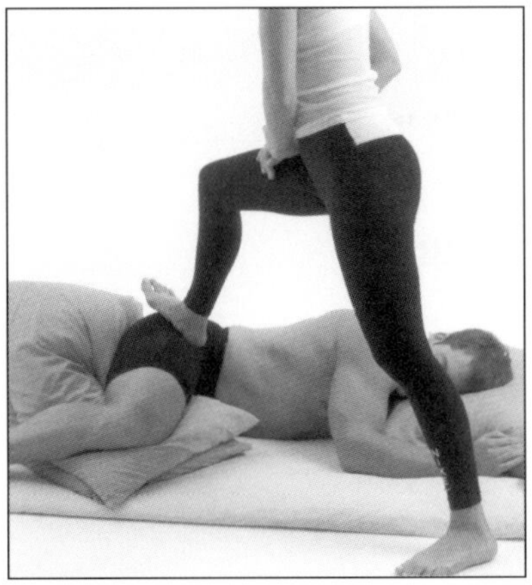

22. Melt it.

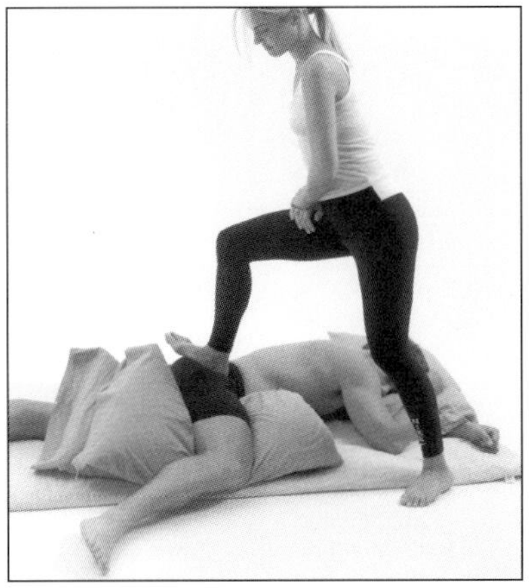

23. Posterior portion, TFL.

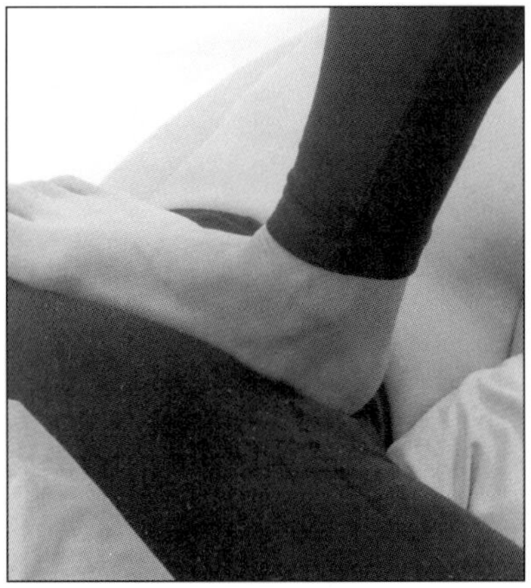

24. Broad surface, firm pressure, relaxed client.

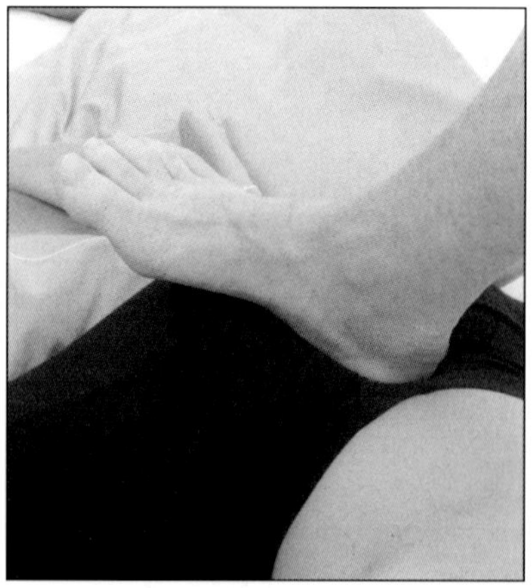

25. Change angle of attack.

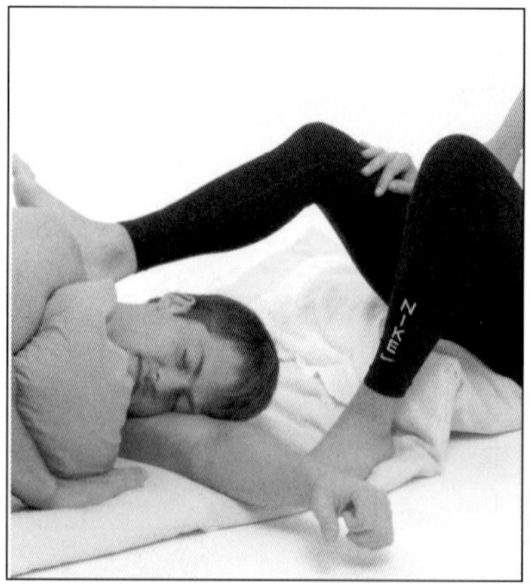

26. Move to upper trap.

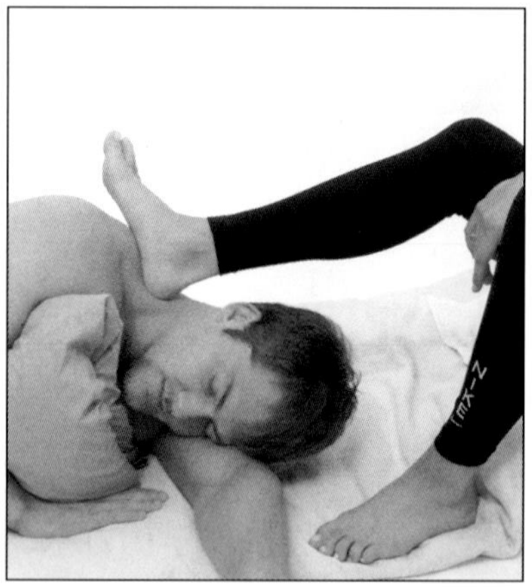

27. Moderate pressure, long duration = letting go.

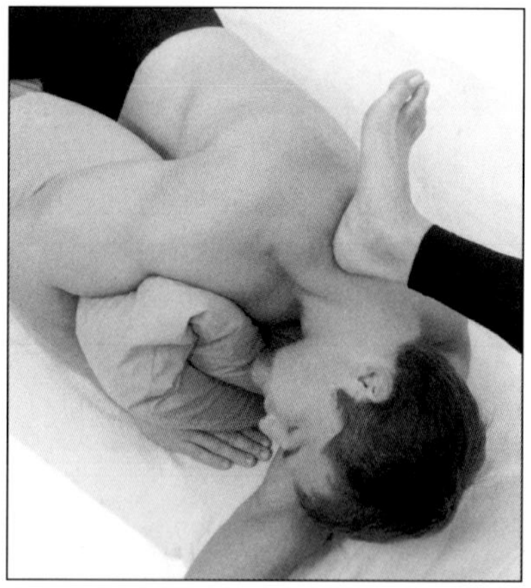

28. Supraspinatus.

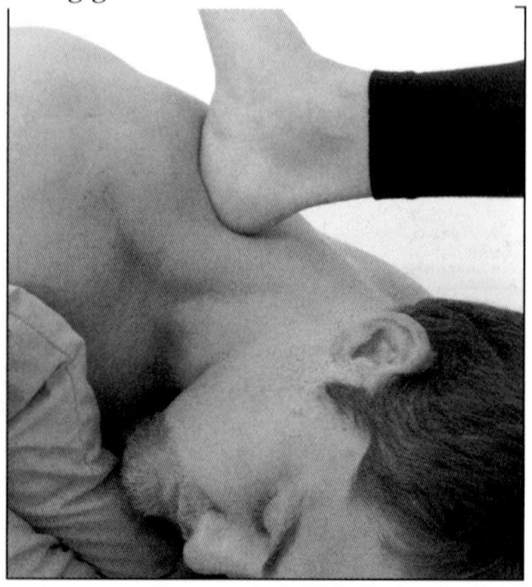

29. Levator.

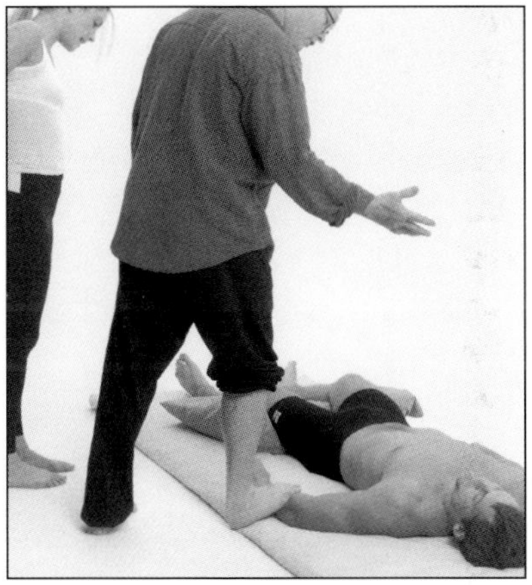

1. Wrist & finger extensors.

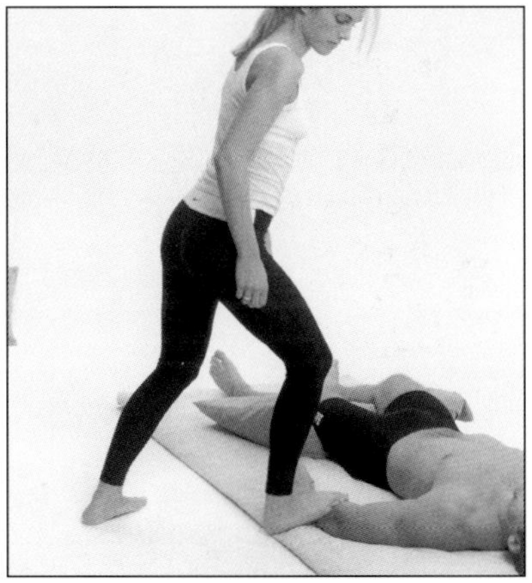

2. Support heel to moderate pressure.

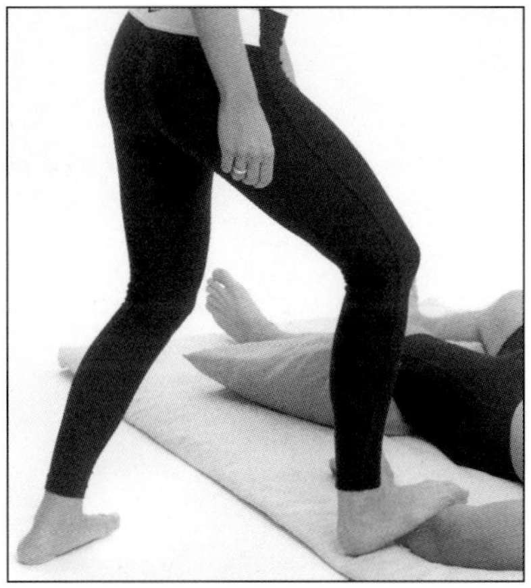

3. Stay below the elbow joint.

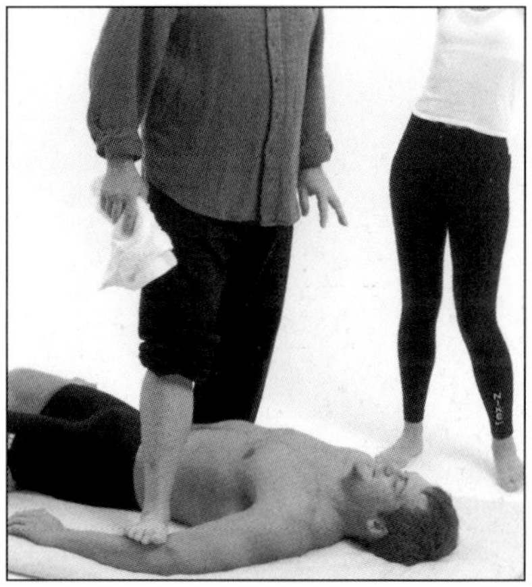

4. Maintain your balance.

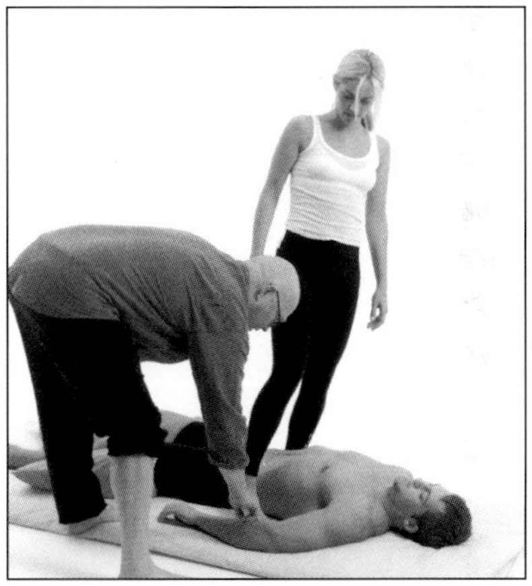

5. Leaning away = no pressure.

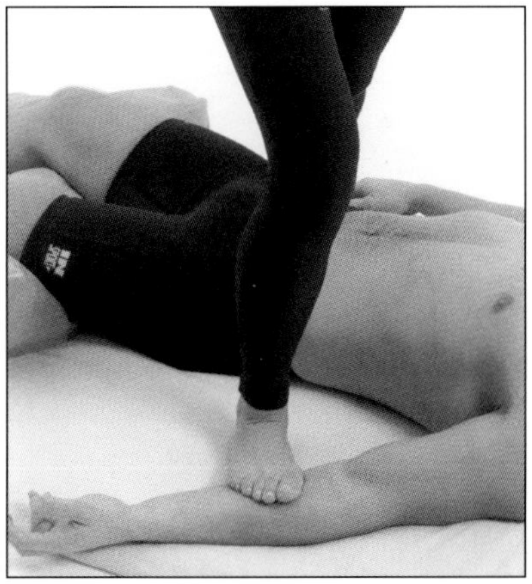

6. Leaning in = lots of pressure.

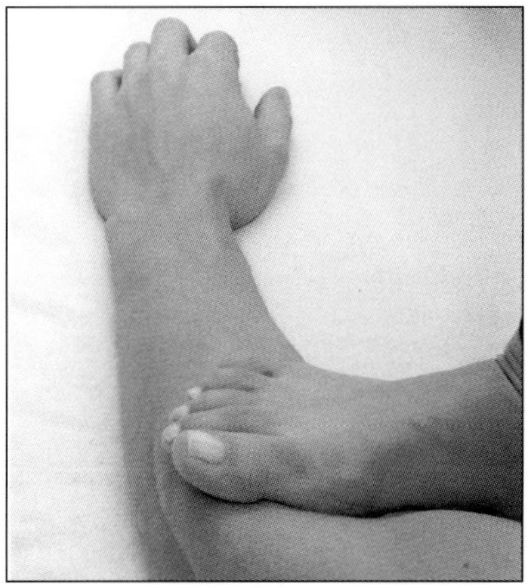

7. Medial approach…

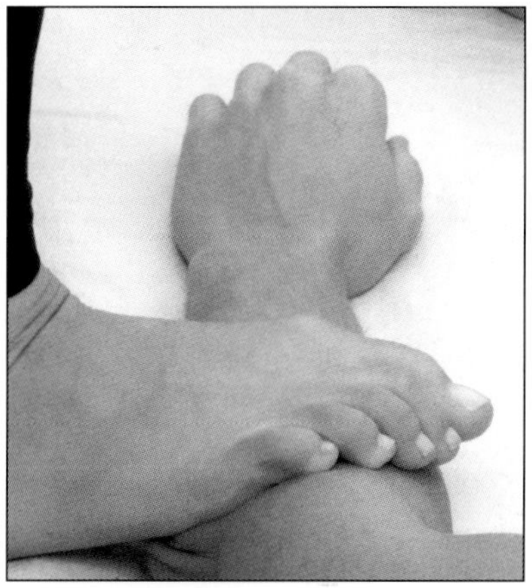

8.…& lateral approach to WAD.

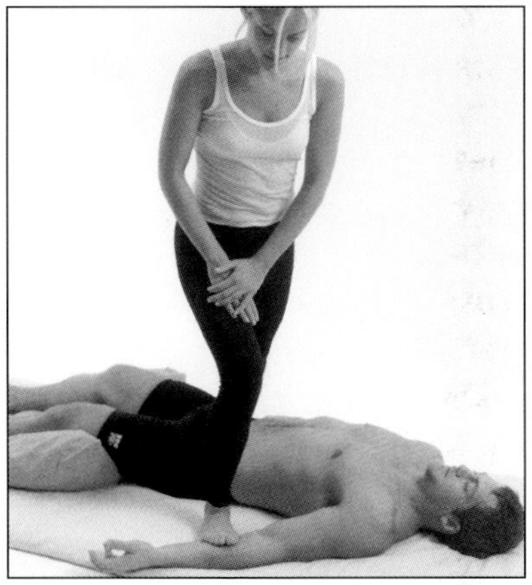

9. This stance is unstable…

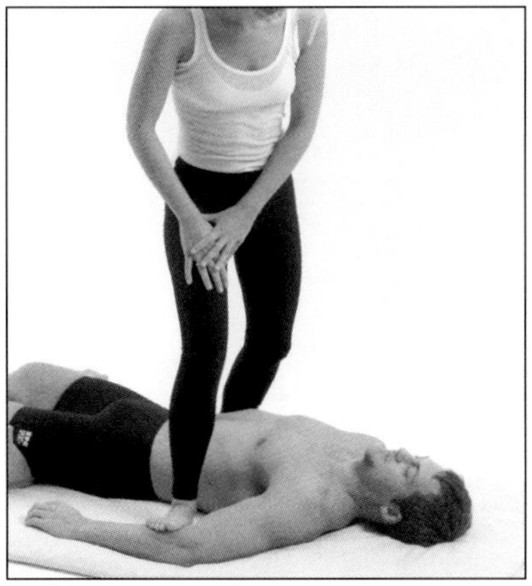

10. …shift your suport leg.

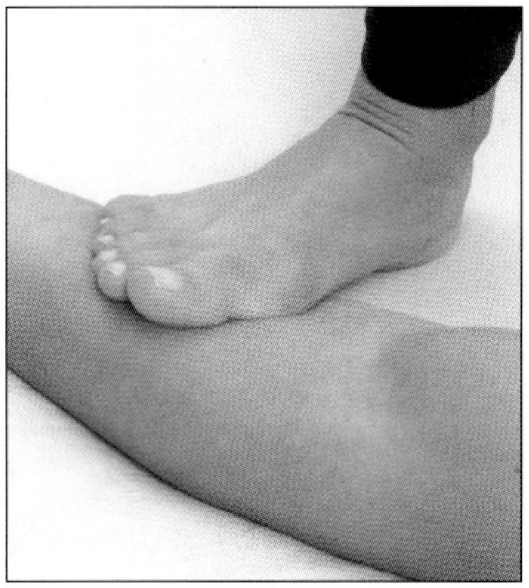

11. Superficial & deep finger flexors.

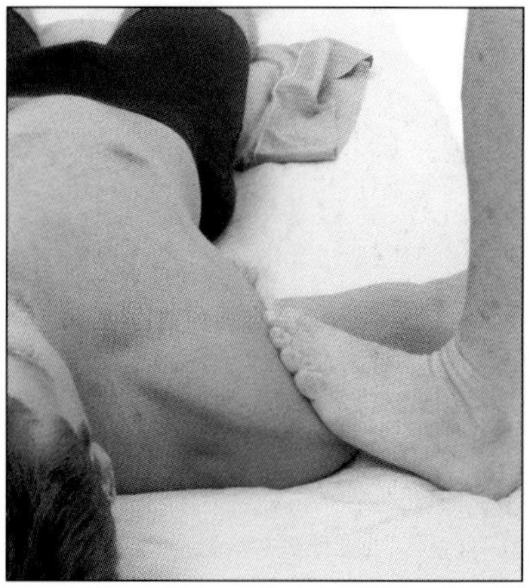

12. Delts.

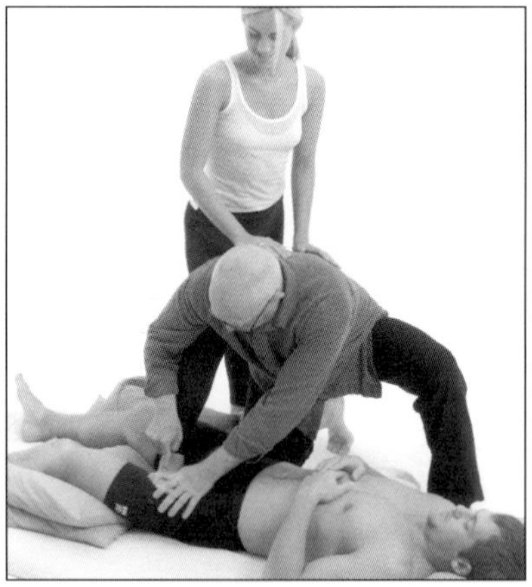

13. A subtle angle change shifts results.

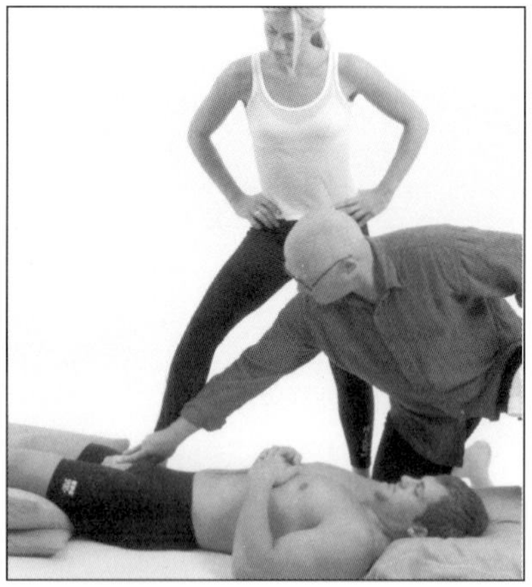

14. Slide & sink.

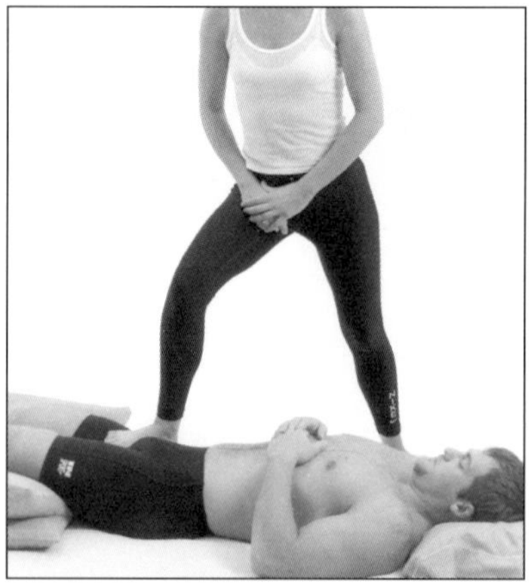

15. Roll outward & sink.

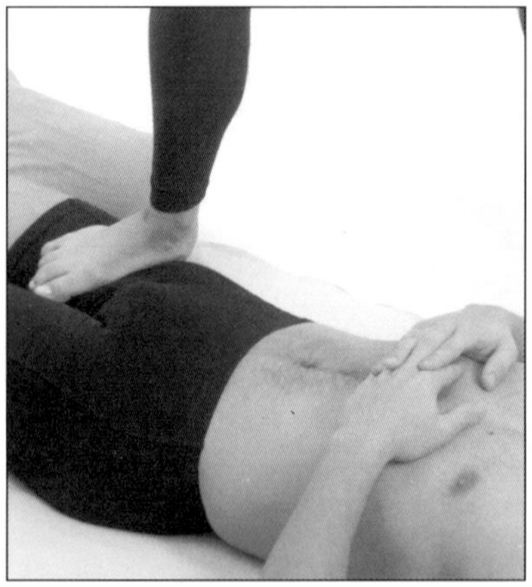

16. Use a soft foot.

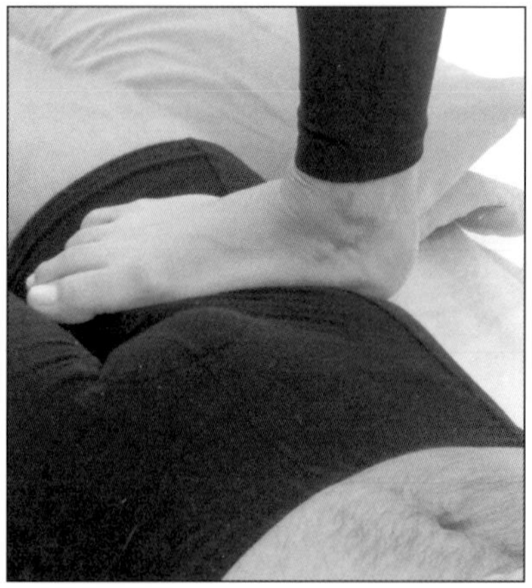

17. Compress at 90 degrees.

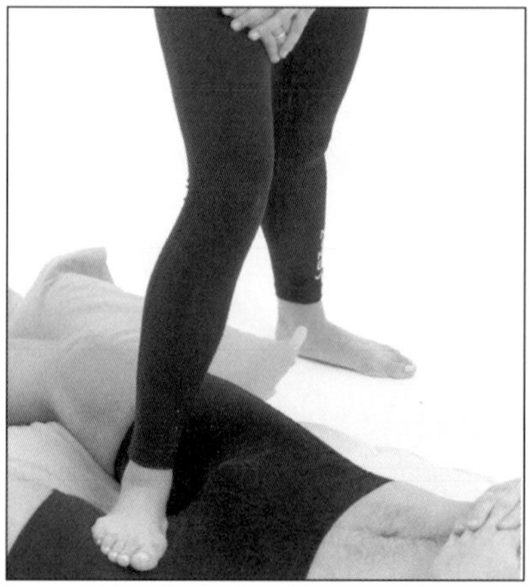

18. Work across to adductors.

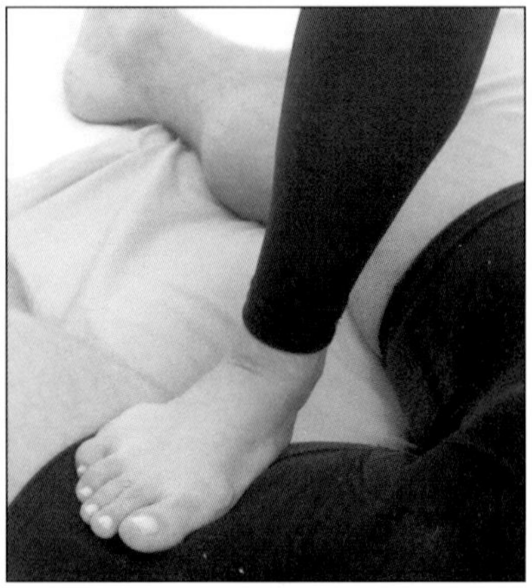

19. End with a slight stretch.

PART 3

Therapeutic Protocols

CHAPTER 7

Prolonged Direct Pressure As A Trigger Point Treatment

Overview

MYOFASCIAL TRIGGER POINTS are the cause of most chronic muscular pain. Direct pressure to the trigger point, by heel or hand, provides a way to alleviate or end this pernicious source of human misery. The following section will provide you an understanding of the basic nature of trigger points and ways to eliminate them. Understanding these procedures prepares you to take optimal advantage of the safe, effective and specific treatment plans presented in the five Regional Protocols.

Trigger points are hypersensitive areas primarily found in muscle, but also in skin, fascia, tendon, periosteum and joint capsules. Trigger points are locally tender to the touch and, when sufficiently irritated, cause or increase referred pain. Most of our work is done on trigger points found in muscle bellies (often at motor nerve endplates located near the center point of a muscle fiber) or at musculotendinous junctures.

> **INTEGRATED HYPOTHESIS**
>
> "Our current understanding of trigger points results from the convergence of two independent lines of investigation, one electrodiagnostic and the other histopathological. Fitting together the lessons from each leads to an INTEGRATED HYPOTHESIS that appears to explain the nature of trigger points. It is now becoming clear that the region we are accustomed to calling a trigger point or a tender nodule is a cluster of numerous microscopic loci of intense abnormality that are scattered throughout the nodule. The trigger point is like a nest of hornets that contains multiple minute sources of intense trouble. The critical trigger point abnormality now appears to be a neuromuscular dysfunction at the motor endplate of an extrafusal skeletal muscle fiber, in which case myofascial pain caused by trigger points would be a neuromuscular disease."
>
> –*Travell and Simons, Myofascial Pain and Dysfunction,* Vol. I, 2nd ed. pg. 57

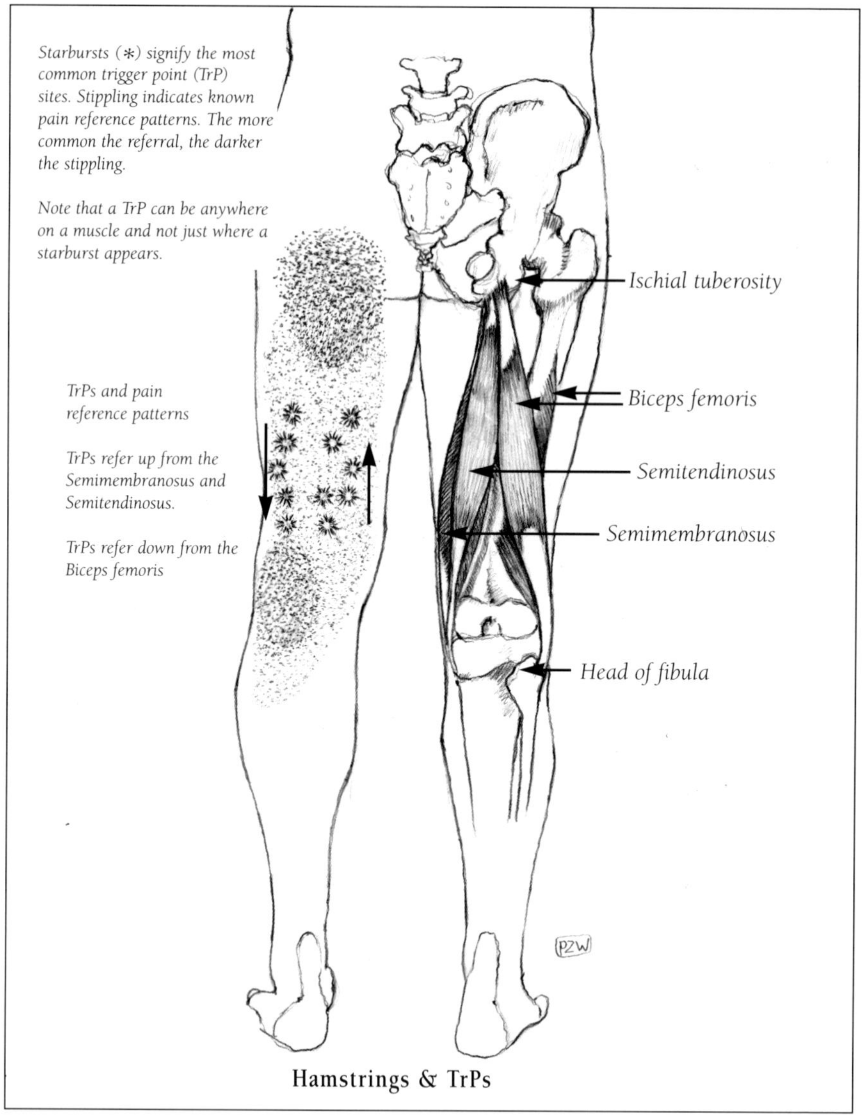

All trigger points present predictable pain referral patterns.

Major Causes of Trigger Points

Acute trauma and muscular overload, overuse, or muscular strain resulting from excessive activity or postural anomalies and asymmetries cause most trigger points to form. When these locally tender points are sufficiently irritated, they generally cause pain at a site distant from the initiating trigger point itself. This referred pain is your clients' usual presenting symptom.

Most insults (injuries) to muscle heal spontaneously and completely in 4 to 6 weeks. Trigger points, however, become chronic and can cause pain, weakness and restricted range-of-motion for decades. They can change their status from active (currently referring pain) to latent (not currently referring pain). When sufficiently irritated, latent trigger points become active and resume their pain referrals. Clients can be plagued with numerous and often confusing changes into and out of pain.

For most of the more than 20 years we've worked with trigger points, the exact pathophysiology has been uncertain. Speculation on causation has ranged from chemical to electrical to mechanical, or a combination of all three. More is understood now, and current theory suggests calcium leakage from damaged sarcomeres plays a key role. However, regardless of the physiologic mechanisms involved, you will be able to alleviate or end chronic pain in many of your clients.

> There is an "… energy crisis hypothesis which postulates a vicious cycle of events that appears to contribute significantly to myofascial trigger points. The function of the sarcoplasmic reticulum (SR) is to restore and release ionized calcium that induces activity of the contractile elements, which causes sarcomere shortening. An initiating event such as trauma or a marked increase in the release in the end-plate release of acetylcholine can result in excessive release of calcium from the SR. This calcium produces maximal contracture of a segment of muscle which creates a maximal energy demand and chokes off local circulation. The ischemia interrupts energy supply which causes failure of the calcium pump of the sarcoplasmic reticulum, completing the cycle."
>
> —Travell & Simons *Myofascial Pain and Dysfunction – The Trigger Point Manual,* Vol. I, 2nd ed., 1999, Pg. 71 fig. 2.26

The direct pressure you apply to trigger points will end this cycle of ischemia-induced dysfunction.

Perpetuating Factors

Even with treatment, perpetuating factors often keep trigger points from healing. These factors include postural distortions such as an anatomically short leg or short hemipelvis, restrictive clothing, prolonged periods of inactivity, poor posture, or simply holding awkward positions while working. Client awareness can eliminate many of the mechanical stress factors. Elimination of other perpetuating factors can require orthotics or ergonomically designed furniture and workstations.

Depression, anxiety and the labile (ever-changing) emotional states of posttraumatic stress disorder can slow or prevent the healing of myofascial pain syndromes. Chronic infections, parasites, and other medical conditions can also inhibit or prolong recovery. Viral infections, which are generally myotoxic, sometimes extremely so, perpetuate trigger points.

Nutritional deficiencies also keep clients from responding to treatment. Drs. Travell and Simons found that nearly half of their patients needed resolution of nutritional inadequacies for lasting pain relief (see Appendix – ***When Clients Won't Stay Better***). We refer clients for medical evaluation if vitamin deficiencies are suspected.

If clients don't make substantial progress in 3 or 4 visits, we refer. They may have perpetuating factors or metabolic problems that require diagnostic skills we don't possess.

Early Treatment

The sooner trigger points are located and treated, the better. Vasoconstriction, a narrowing of blood vessels caused by high intensity nerve impulses from an active trigger point can reduce blood supply to the brain, spinal cord and peripheral nervous system. Headaches, indigestion, diminished cognition and a wide range of other symptoms can result. When allowed to become chronic, they become increasingly difficult to rectify and often lead to a panoply of associated problems. If trigger points are treated early on, they are much easier to eliminate. A complete clearing of trauma-induced trigger points can occur in just one to three visits.

In some cases, your client will present with unusual symptoms, perhaps without pain. This interesting phenomenon of trigger points is their capacity to initiate bodily reactions through the autonomic nervous system. Secondary autonomic phenomena include: vasoconstriction, vasodilation, coldness, sweating, pilomotor response and hyper-secretion. Referred pain may or may not be concomitant with these phenomena. We've witnessed tinnitus (single ear only as ringing in both ears usually indicates a nerve problem), goose flesh, tissue blanching, sweating, runny nose, tearing eyes, flushing and proprioceptive distortion – all resulting from "triggers." These distressing symptoms often respond favorably when trigger points are eliminated.

Types of Treatment

Physicians inject trigger points with procaine and saline. This approach, while often effective, can prove painful, invasive and frightening to many. However, injection is a particularly useful method for trigger points that can't be reached by hand or foot. Dry needling, as in acupuncture, is also effective.

Physical therapists can employ ultrasound and electro-stimulation to treat trigger points, but more often trained therapists will use "spray & stretch," a modality in which vapo-coolants are sprayed along the involved muscle and pain referral pattern. They then stretch the involved muscle(s). The quick cooling of the skin provides a distraction, overriding the pain, and allows a stretch (the treatment) of the affected muscles. However, deep or prolonged cooling will exacerbate the problem as cold (and chills) intensify trigger point pain. Passive stretching of a muscle with trigger points can increase pain unless the muscle is cooled. Current emphasis is to use the more ecologically friendly ice-massage in lieu of ozone depleting vapo-coolants.

Client self-treatment can be an important adjunct to your work. Teach your client to use direct pressure on their own trigger points by using a tennis ball or other trigger point tool. Self-treatment should also utilize light exercise, gentle passive stretching in a hot shower or tub, applying moist heat directly to the pain source and avoidance of prolonged immobility.

Massage therapists and other bodyworkers generally use direct pressure to the trigger point followed by stretching. This potent tool has helped thousands of clients return to active, pain-free lives.

Developing a Treatment Plan

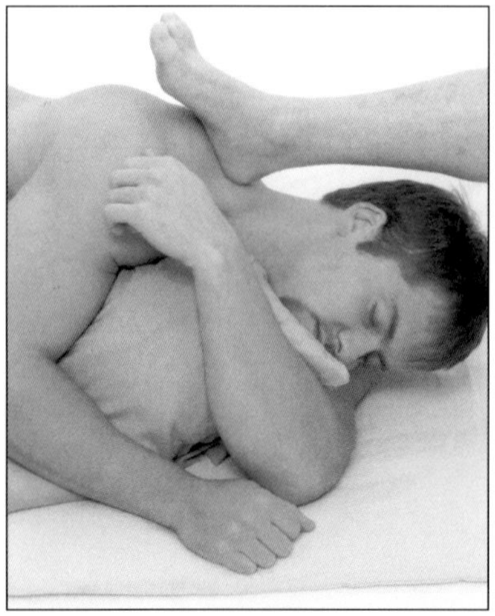

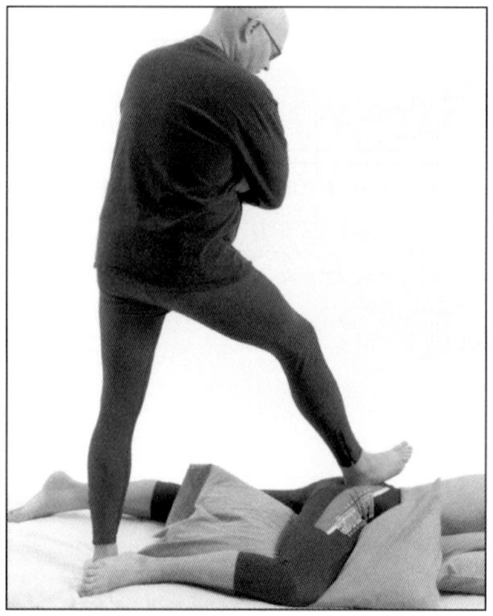

Direct pressure applications.

Single muscle trigger points are generally easy to locate and treat. Client pain patterns give clear indications of the trigger point location. Each area of pain has one or more possible causatory trigger points. Several muscles can refer to the same area, but one will usually be the primary source of the pain. Trigger point pain usually presents as an ache that is intensified with direct pressure. When your therapeutic pressure elicits any sort of nervy (tingling, buzzing, banged-funny-bone-like) feelings, you are most likely pressing on a major nerve. Move off the nerve or diminish your pressure. Trigger points located near a nerve plexus require moderate pressure to avoid temporary nerve damage.

Reference to pain referral charts indicate the most likely origins of trigger point pain. Travell and Simon's tomes have done an excellent job of mapping the entire body. For additional, seminal information, we can't recommend these manuals highly enough. They represent a profound source of knowledge for bodyworkers.

Begin the palpatory search of a suspect muscle using direct pressure. Clients will pull away in pain (a jump response) when you palpate a trigger point. Stroking ALONG the muscle fibers, you'll sometimes feel a small nodule. If you stroke ACROSS the fibers, you'll often find a small area of taut fibers. Either of these findings generally indicate the presence of a trigger point.

If you sufficiently irritate a latent trigger point, it will become active and begin to refer pain. Some latent trigger points can take up 10 seconds of direct pressure before beginning to refer pain. Experience will teach you which muscle groups are slower to respond. Use sustained direct pressure (10 or 15 seconds) during your assessment of those muscles.

Pain from active trigger points intensifies when you apply direct pressure. Clients will report increased pain in their reference zone (the region at a distance from the trigger point where pain or other autonomic phenomena are noted).

Sufficient palpatory irritation of a trigger point will often cause a transient firing (contraction) of its muscle fibers. This local twitch response is evinced by a flutter (think stressed-eye twitch) that can be felt and sometimes seen by the therapist. A twitch response strongly suggests you are pressing on a trigger point.

PETE'S STORY

Pete walked through the door carrying only pain where an arm had once hung. While riding his bike, he was forced off the road by a drunk driver. The impact launched him over the guardrail and into a sharp, upright metal sign. Ensuing complications forced an arm amputation at the shoulder joint.

Unbelievably, following the surgery, he found unrelenting pain where the arm used to be! Pete consulted many medical authorities. They offered mind-numbing pain medications and a helpful term defining the problem, "phantom limb pain."

The initial consultation indicated we were (most likely) talking about referred pain. A check of Travell and Simon's *Trigger Point Manual* indicated trigger points in *scaleni* muscles could be the cause of his phantom limb pain. After three trigger point sessions focused on Pete's *scalenes*, the arm pain vanished, and a true believer in the wonders of trigger point therapy was found. Years of practice have stood the test of time.

Intensity and Pressure

Travell and Simon's most recent edition of *Myofascial Pain and Dysfunction*, Volume I, recommends a gentler protocol, "trigger point pressure release." This treatment approach replaces the deeper ischemic pressure found in their previous edition. In their most recent text, they suggest "only enough pressure to melt the taut band(s)." While both approaches work, you can have the best of both. Strong pressure, effortless duration (with a simultaneous stretch) and less pain for your client result when using direct pressure from you heel.

For most clients we suggest a 7 or 8 pressure/pain rating on a 10 scale. This feedback technique is thoroughly briefed in the "Deep Compressive Massage" section. Briefly, 10 is where your clients tighten-up or armor against the work – in other words, it really hurts. Go just deep enough to get the job done. Too much pressure is less effective and almost always increases post-treatment soreness.

Duration

The experts propose very different guidelines for the duration of direct pressure treatment time. Raymond Nimmo, D.C., indicated 5 seconds of pressure was adequate to interrupt the pain cycle and allow the body to self-heal. Drs. Travell and Simons originally suggested 60 to 90 seconds of gradually increasing pressure.

Our preference is based on client receptivity to pressure and pain; we normally use direct pressure for a minimum of 15 to 30 seconds. There is an optimum pressure and treatment time for each muscle and these factors vary with each client. You'll learn to observe client response and trust your own good sense.

Endorphins and enkephalins are released in response to the irritation of direct pressure during trigger point treatment. These endogenous morphines block pain, help eliminate reflex arc activity and allow muscles to relax.

Trigger Point (TrP) Protocol

1. Take a thorough medical history from your client. Be alert to contraindications and cautions.

2. Have client draw their pain pattern onto a pain chart. This optional task forces them to focus enough to add specificity to their often vague description of where they hurt.

3. Ask client to describe the duration, level, precipitating cause (if known), nature of their pain (sharp, deep, dull aching, pulsating, etc.) and factors that exacerbate it.

4. Determine which TrPs can cause the client's pain.

Each of the 5 Regional Protocols describes pain in different areas of the body. For example, when a client presents with a leg pain, you will refer to the regional protocols for the leg that will indicate, via illustration, likely TrP locations for referring pain to the leg.

Composite patterns (caused by multiple TrPs) are more difficult to decipher and require a methodical approach. Treat the most obvious TrP first. Sometimes the pain patterns of previously obscured TrPs become apparent as eliminated TrPs stops referring. On occasion, TrPs can refer pain for up to 24 hours after they've been treated. There may be 1, 2, 3 or 4 significant TrPs that need treating in any particular muscle.

5. Position the client to give you good access to the involved muscle. A TrP in a slack muscle is often difficult to locate and to treat. Trigger point treatments generally work best with the involved muscle on a moderate

stretch. However, deep stretching of the muscle can fire the TrP and create unnecessary pain.

6. Warm the muscle with compressions and/or light or dry kneading prior to treatment. Gentle passive stretches soften the tissues and reduce local tenderness. Bruising and severe jump signs are less likely to occur.

7. Palpate likely muscles for taut palpable bands, twitch responses and jump signs that signify TrPs.

8. Gradually sink into the locally tender area. STOP pushing as soon as a change in resistance (a tissue barrier) is felt, or when you reach a 7 in the therapeutic range. If you push hard or abruptly, you may elicit a 15 pain range. Not good.

9. If direct pressure to the taut band intensifies the referred pain, you've likely verified a major TrP. Be patient - you may have to wait up to 10 seconds for some latent TrP s to begin or intensify their referred pain.

10. Begin treatment with direct pressure (by hand or foot) to the trigger point. Stay within the client's therapeutic range – 6 to 8 on the 10 scale.

11. Apply gradually increasing pressure directly to TrPs from 15 to 30 seconds. One application of direct pressure on each major TrP is usually a good first treatment. Pain will generally subside within minutes. Inform client that occasionally TrP pain can continue (even intensify) for up to 24 hours after your treatment.

12. Search surrounding muscles (agonist, antagonist, synergists and stabilizers) for other TrPs. If not treated, satellite TrPs (associated TrPs formed in the pain reference area of the primary TrP) and secondary TrPs (associated TrPs formed in fatigued muscles that are overused or ill-used by assuming compensatory roles) sometimes perpetuate primary trigger points. However, the good news is elimination of primary TrPs will often deactivate the "associated" ones.

13. Have client actively stretch the treated muscle. Follow with a pain free range-of-motion (ROM) to encourage normal muscle function (strength, stretch and ROM). Treated muscles that aren't stretched and contracted will retain diminished function.

14. Apply moist heat to the treated muscles to prevent or reduce post-treatment soreness.

15. Inform your client that a continuing program of stretching and strengthening are needed to maintain optimum muscle health.

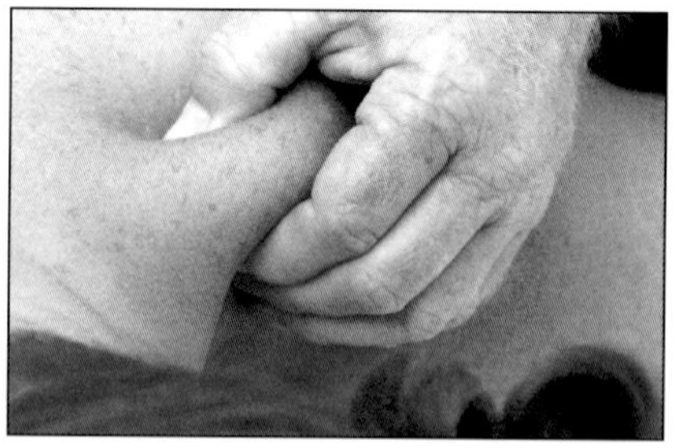

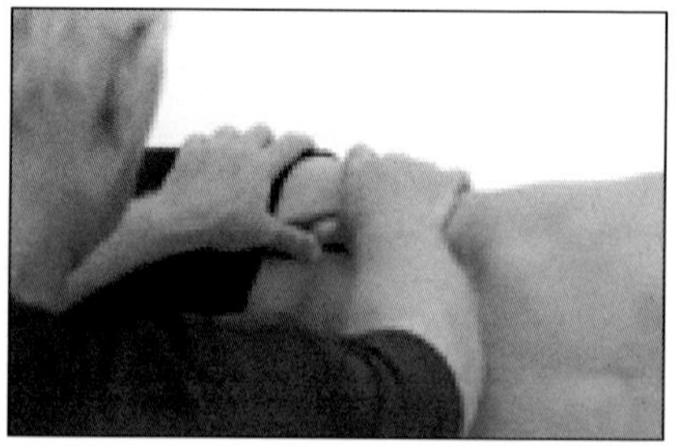

Special Caution – Dissociation

Dissociative states are potential client responses to trigger point work. They generally occur in clients suffering from posttraumatic syndromes. Dissociation (leaving one's body) is a mental mechanism used to avoid fear, overwhelming feelings or physical pain. We sense this in our clients as a "nobody's home" feeling that is quite different from a client in deep relaxation or actively spacing-out. Following the session, these clients will often feel violated by your treatment regardless of how careful you are.

One practical approach for the dissociative client is to interrupt the treatment and help the client gently return to their body, e.g., ask them, in a relaxed manner, about pressure, speed or discomfort. The interruption will refocus their attention on you and their body. You may decide to discontinue the massage. If you are unable to keep the client present, they can be further traumatized by your well-intentioned treatment. For added information, see PTSD in the "When Clients Won't Stay Better" appendix.

CHAPTER 8

Cross-fiber Friction for Sub-acute or Chronic Tendonitis, Tenosynovitis and Painfully Scarred Muscle Bellies

Overview

CROSS-FIBER is a primary tool for treating chronic tendon and muscle lesions. The following protocols reduce pain and address underlying pathology while simultaneously creating pain-free movement. Gentle cross-fiber friction promotes adhesion-free scars while firmer cross-fiber friction teases open adhesions in poorly formed scars. Used in conjunction with non-weight bearing, non-resisted movement, friction massage speeds injury recovery and increases a scar's resiliency to reinflammation.

The probable outcomes of cross-fiber treatment include reduced pain, enhanced range-of-motion, fewer compensatory mechanisms and enhanced ability to rebuild strength. Although the physiologic and mechanical mechanisms of cross-fiber friction may not be fully understood, thousands of therapists witness the curative results daily. This section presents guidelines for specific cross-fiber treatments found in the five Regional Protocols (page 60 – 104).

Cross-fiber's Salutary Results

A counter-irritant effect is produced when cross-fiber friction stimulates fast-firing, small diameter nerve impulses. These fast, acute pain impulses block chronic pain transmitted by slower firing, larger diameter nerve fibers. In bodywork parlance, "noxious stimuli from cross-fiber friction suppress chronic nociceptive (pain) impulses."

Increased secretion of cortisol (a natural anti-inflammatory) is initiated in response to the irritant friction massage. Cross-fiber friction's tissue irritation also evokes histamine release that dilates capillaries and increases blood flow. The improved blood flow helps flush muscle tissues of metabolites and inflammatory byproducts. Tissue healing is enhanced by increased blood and lymph circulation. Therapeutic movement becomes easier and less painful as friction massage breaks up adhesions, supports pain-free fiber alignment and mobilizes tissue.

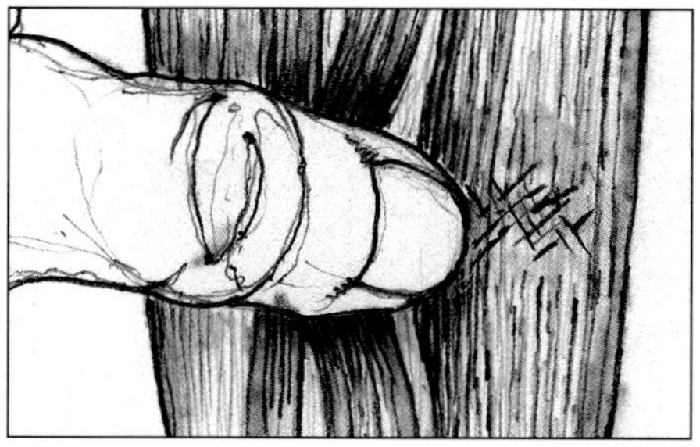

A few minutes of moderate cross-fiber friction across the belly of the muscle eliminates unwanted adhesions and restores normal, pain-free function.

Drawing by P. West based on Dr. Cyriax's ILLUSTRATED MANUAL OF ORTHOPAEDIC MEDICINE.

ABOUT CROSS-FIBER FRICTION I

Cross-fiber Friction for Tendonitis

Friction massage mechanically loosens the superficial scars from a tendon's surface. This destruction of the scar helps keep it from re-inflaming.

Cross-friction administered slowly purportedly re-hydrates the tendon's dense connective tissue, increases collagen production by fibroblasts, attracts collagen cells from surrounding tissue and helps to orient them. Heat, pressure, stretch and bioelectric energy change the chemical nature of collagen fibers.

A controlled trauma results from cross-fiber friction. Counter-inflammatory responses and pain inhibition are initiated. Cortisol, the body's own anti-inflammatory, is secreted in response to the irritation.

Friction, a noxious stimulus, suppresses nociceptive pain impulses by flooding the "gate" with faster nerve impulses that block the slower, chronic pain impulses. Endogenous morphines that suppress peripheral nerve signals are also released in response to cross-friction. Lewitt's P-factor, a neurotransmitter of pain conduction, is depleted or inhibited by cross-fiber friction.

ABOUT CROSS-FIBER FRICTION II

Cross-fiber for Tenosynovitis (inflamed sheathed tendons)

Tendons that rub across bony surfaces (primarily at the wrist and ankle) are encased in a synovial sheath to prevent them from wearing against bone or other tissues.

Cross-fiber friction is administered to a stretched sheathed tendon. It creates a rolling, to-and-fro movement of the sheath against the underlying taut tendon. The friction grinds the sheath against the tendon, smoothing both while rupturing adhesions.

A counter-inflammatory response (cortisol secretion) is also initiated by the cross-fiber friction.

ABOUT CROSS-FIBER FRICTION III

Cross-fiber Friction for Ligament Sprains

Cross-fiber friction moves sprained ligaments in imitation of their natural movement to prevent or break up adhesions from the ligament to surrounding tissues.

Friction to the ligament is administered with the joint in flexion and in extension.

A joint swollen with traumatic arthritis will have limited range of motion. Don't force a temporarily restricted joint into flexion or extension as a temporary traumatic arthritis can be made permanent by "forced" flexion or extension.

Dr. Cyriax

Dr. James Cyriax, a British orthopedic physician, popularized the use of deep transverse friction, manipulation and injections for the treatment of musculoskeletal problems He treated over 70,000 patients throughout his career, achieving significant results without surgery.

"It follows that for soft-tissue lesions the non-specific remedies such as heat, cold, water, exercises, ointment, bandages, diffuse massage, and analgesics are, with insignificant exceptions, palliative rather than curative. The object of scientific treatment is recovery and accordingly the criterion is not whether the patient has received a course of therapy, but whether the treatment has yielded any amelioration. Thus the patient is continually reassessed to see if range is improved and pain diminished. If not, either the diagnosis or the treatment has been misconceived."

—Dr. J. H. Cyriax
Illustrated Manual of Orthopaedic Medicine

As an initial tool for treating chronic tendonitis and adherent scars, we adopted Cyriax's methods as presented in his exceptional text, *Illustrated Manual of Orthopaedic Medicine*. Although his 20 minute treatments on each lesion were the norm, we were concerned with the likelihood of excessive post-treatment trauma. We also found the 20 minute sessions physically demanding and tedious. We apparently weren't alone. Since Dr. Cyriax's death, gossip has it that trainers of his work shortened the standard 20 minute deep transverse friction protocol to 10. Our guess is that the shorter treatment was requested by the physiotherapists who administer Dr. Cyriax's work.

Our Approach to Cross-fiber Friction

We have used some form of friction massage for the past 20 odd years. We adapted Cyriax's work to suit the needs of our clients and ourselves. Using Dr. Cyriax's basic principles, our cross-fiber approach has shorter treatment sessions, fewer total treatments and friendlier biomechanics for the therapist. Client range-of-motion, pain level (during and post-treatment) and self-assessment determine the intensity and duration of subsequent treatments. Cross-fiber treatments are progressive. Generally both the intensity and duration of cross-fiber friction increases from session to session. Evaluation takes place at the beginning and end of each session. If a client complains of excessive post-treatment soreness, back off in the next treatment.

Sedentary people can go through their entire lives without latent tendon problems reaching clinical levels. If the client is sedentary, elderly, or pain intolerant, it's often best to decide (mutually, with client input) not to treat their microtrauma with friction massage.

Session Duration

Brief sessions have proven effective and generally provide satisfactory results in treating tendonitis, tenosynovitis and adherent scars in muscle bellies. Initially we were puzzled by good results with sessions as short as 15 or 20 seconds. Did our clientele of strong, healthy, well-hydrated and well-nourished athletes heal faster? Not necessarily. Good results continued when we worked with a more diverse population.

Perhaps a tendon could become habitually inflamed and require very little therapist input to achieve healing? It seemed to us that chronic tendon problems (those not caused by poor biomechanics and over-use) could be "habits" of inflammation. We found that clients often came to us with what appeared to be a partial healing with a chronic low-level inflammation remaining. When we administered cross-fiber friction, a fairly strong, painful stimuli, it seemed to serve as a reminder to the body – a reminder to rekindle the healing process. Hence our understanding changed in scope, moving from a strictly mechanical process to a combined mechanical and chemical/neurologic one.

With friction, as with remedies in homeopathy, LIKE SEEMS TO CURE LIKE – that to some chronically painful tendons, an application of moderately painful friction reinitiates healing. It's as though the body forgets to completely heal these niggling tendon problems and simply needs a reminder to complete the process.

Painful Scars

Some scars cause pain. Some cause pain because of trigger points, others cause pain because of adhesions. Whether caused by adhesions or trigger points, some scar pain referral patterns are random to the point of confusion. Direct pressure for trigger points or gentle fascial stretching for adhesions occasionally clears problems in scars found in skin and/or the underlying superficial fascia. Adherent scars in muscle bellies are treated with cross-fiber friction.

Client exercise in the form of non-weight-bearing, non-resisted movement is the easiest way to assist nature in the formation of a pliable, flexible, pain-free scar. Most scars, given the above, will heal properly even though it takes up to a year for a scar to assume its final fiber configuration. This process is called "remodeling." Muscle use determines collagen fiber alignment in the scar, so remodeled scars have these fibers aligned in the direction of muscle pull. Painful adhesions form if weight bearing exercise, overuse, immobility, or in some cases, stretching or deep massage are initiated too soon.

The value of non-weight-bearing, non-resisted movement for proper scar formation can't be overstressed. Methods therefore must provide a satisfactory compromise between healing and training. For instance, many runners with painful hamstring scars won't quit running long enough to complete the remodeling process. To avoid overloading the newly forming scar, they can achieve both training and healing by "running in harness" at the deep end of the swimming pool.

Tendons, Muscles and Treatment Timing

Chronic injuries are treated sooner than acute ones, with tendons treated earlier than muscle bellies. Generally treat a chronic injury immediately. Treat an acute tendonitis within a few days and a torn muscle belly with cross-fiber (lightly) after five or 6 days. Increase treatment pressure progressively as the scar matures.

Have your clients commit to 3 or 4 visits. If they don't show substantial improvement, it's time for a change of plan or a referral. Relieving pain may not address the source of the pain. Overuse, poor biomechanics, structural anomalies, or pathology are potential causes for tendonitis that will need to be addressed if their pain recurs.

> Anti-inflammatories taken orally or injected will reduce inflammation in a scar, but they will leave the superficial scar with a rough surface. This rough superficial scarring is easily irritated. Strenuous movement or continuous load (chronic muscle tightness) predisposes the scar to future tendonitis.

Anatomy and Cross-fiber

You must know where your parts are. Manual therapies require precision. We highly recommend Stanley Hoppenfeld's *Physical Examination of the Spine and Extremities* to teach you these skills. An on-going study of surface and palpatory anatomy will increase your cure rate.

Cross-fiber Friction and Tendons

About Tendons – Overview

The musculotendinous juncture (that point at which muscle becomes tendon) is highly susceptible to soft tissue injury. It is less vascular than the muscle belly, tends to heal slower and has less movement during muscular contraction. The tissue is less extensible and more susceptible to micro-trauma (overuse injury) and ultimately, to macro-trauma (clinical-level acute injury).

Occasionally you will find an apparently healthy tendon that hurts when frictioned. Consider this microtrauma a prodrome or indicator of future clinical-level problems. Several brief cross-fiber friction treatments will often abort this incipient injury.

Dr. Cyriax suggested that 8 to 12 treatments with deep transverse friction would heal most tendon injuries. We've found 3 or 4 sessions of cross-fiber friction often put an end to the pain of tendonitis. We use 1 to 3 minute sessions instead of the 10 to 20 minute friction sessions Dr. Cyriax usually recommended.

JANE'S STORY

Jane, an accomplished marathoner, took up yoga to stay flexible. Over-training had created a hamstring tendonitis at her ischial tuberosity. When she asked her yoga instructor what to do, he told her daily hamstring stretches would be best. When we saw her, a year later, she had stretched daily and could hardly walk. Her hamstring attachment was one big, painful scar. This should not have happened! Her compliance with questionable advice resulted in a disaster. In bodywork, lack of progress demands re-evaluation or referral.

Tendon/Ligament Protocols

Cross-fiber Friction for Subacute or Chronic Tendonitis and Tenosynovitis

Clients present complaining of intermittent or continuous pain in the region of a tendon. The pain often comes on over time. Clients will generally wait for soft tissue pain to heal spontaneously. You will generally see them after they've exacerbated their problem by overuse. Clients demonstrate what hurts and what doesn't.

1. Take a history to ascertain whether the tendon problem is acute or chronic:

• If the tendon injury is acute, wait 3 or 4 days (sometimes even longer) before treating. Beginning treatment too soon can prolong or exacerbate the natural process of inflammation. Heat over the site of the lesion plus swelling and tenderness help define the acute stage. Acute stage pain will be relatively constant and diffuse and cause some clients difficulty with falling or staying asleep.

• If the tendon injury is chronic, begin work immediately. Pain is generally considered chronic if it exists longer than 3 months. Most chronic tendon injuries exhibit pain that intensifies with overuse and subsides with rest. Chronic pain is felt in the general region of the lesion with seldom any temperature increase over the lesion. Sleep interference is generally not reported with chronic pain except in cases of shoulder or hip tendonitis or bursitis.

• Give your clients full disclosure of the effects of cross-fiber friction and ask them to commit for 3 visits over 7 to 10 days. Be sure to note the treatment is often painful when administered and can result in residual soreness. There can be bruising on rare occasion. Icing may be necessary to relieve discomfort – teach your client how to ice to relieve pain. (See Appendix.)

2. Assess the suspect tendon with gentle friction. Use your thumb or braced fingers to friction on dry skin (no oils) or friction through clothing. If it hurts, a tendonitis likely exists. The most painful area on the tendon identifies the exact site of the lesion.

3. Treat at the exact site of the lesion, be it a sprain, strain, adhesion or microtrauma:

• Begin with moderate friction perpendicular to the tendon's fibers. Tendon fibers are aligned with the muscle's direction of pull. Friction sheathed tendons (found primarily at the ankle and wrist) on a stretch. This stretch gives a firm base to friction the sheath against.

• Start below a therapeutic level and progressively increase your pressure to 7 on a 10 scale. If your client tenses, you're above a therapeutic level.

• Using equal pressure in both directions, friction back and forth across the tendon. Move the client's skin and subcutaneous tissues over the lesion being treated. Never glide over the client's skin surface as painful blisters can result.

• Use sufficient sweep and duration with a stroke broad enough to access the whole lesion. Friction slowly. Friction works best when administered at a slow pace, about 2 sweeps per second. Rapid friction is irritating with paltry therapeutic results.

• Friction for 1 minute or less on first visits – long enough to make a mechanical impact. Client response to the previous visit determines future treatment length and pressures. Subsequent treatments may last as long as 5 minutes on the thickest and densest tendons.

• Treat on alternate days to allow the tissue to recover and become less tender. We recommend a minimum of 2 treatments per week. Consider using ice to ameliorate post-treatment soreness.

CAVEAT

Stop treating if the pain from the friction massage significantly increases during the treatment. Pain should begin to subside within 2 or 3 minutes. If the pain doesn't subside, suspect either client hypersensitivity (with the possibility of ensuing shock) or that you are treating highly inflamed tissue (acute or infected).

ATHLETES

Cross-fiber friction is not used just prior to training or competition. Soreness created by cross-fiber massage can create compensatory mechanisms resulting in distraction, compromised performance or even injury. Friction massage for athletes is best used during the off season or well in advance of competition.

Cross-fiber Friction and Muscles

About Muscles - Overview

We see muscle belly tears (strains) less frequently than tendon problems, but clients do come to us because of the chronic muscle belly pain resulting from adhesions in scars. These strains respond well to cross-fiber friction in conjunction with therapeutic movement. Direct trauma, usually from a bump or blow, can tear a muscle. Sharp or sudden contractions against resistance can cause tears to both conditioned and deconditioned muscles. Strains also result from a fatigued or chronically shortened muscle subjected to a sudden stretch.

We often see hamstring tears in runners with strong hip flexors and short, weak, fatigued hamstrings. With prolonged contractions during running the quads remain strong with the hams beginning to fail as they fatigue. Tired hams loose their capacity to release during hip flexion. The stronger hip flexors can overwhelm and tear slowly releasing hamstrings. In some cases the hamstrings will become inflamed at their musculotendinous or tenoperiosteal junctions at the ischial tuberosity. (See tendon protocols on previous page.)

Most muscle tears are sports related. In many instances there will be a palpable open gap in the muscle. Don't treat at this point. Any hands-on work at the lesion will add to secondary hypoxic tissue death exacerbating the injury and prolong healing.

CROSS-FIBER FRICTION FOR ADHERENT SCARS

Adhesions can be formed when an injured muscle is immobilized or overused during early healing. The adhesions cause pain when the muscle is contracted and broadened. This broadening pulls on the adhesions that have formed between muscle fibers.

The mechanical effects of deep cross-fiber massage breaks (pulls apart) the painful adhesions formed between muscle fibers during early scar formation. The resultant increase in mobility encourages the scar to re-form without forming further adhesions.

Muscles and Timing

In time, most scar tissue becomes flexible, pliable and pain-free as nature intended. If a muscle belly tear is recent, don't friction or stretch the area since either action can tear the newly forming scar tissue and create a larger lesion. The tearing creates more secondary cell death and prolongs the clearing of tissue debris. Immobilization helps promote proper healing. Excessive stretching of a newly formed scar or loading (using the muscle against resistance) the muscle too early in the healing process will occasionally create thickened, painful scars.

In older, serious runners, we've found many adherent hamstring scars that restrict flexibility and limit range of motion. These adhesions are formed when scar tissue binds muscle fibers together. When the muscle contracts, causing it to shorten and broaden, these adhesions are stretched and cause pain. Use cross-fiber friction on these scars at the exact location of these adhesions to tease them apart. This promotes pain-free, longitudinal (aligned with the muscle fibers) scar formation. The new adhesion-free scar allows pain-free, normal muscle use. Runners will increase their stride and take fewer steps per mile. This makes running easier and faster.

Remember that newly formed scars are vulnerable to re-tearing through active or passive stretches and weight-bearing contractions. Non-weight-bearing, non-resisted movement (of which cross-fiber friction is a component) creates strong, flexible, pliable, pain-free scars.

MYOSITIS OSSIFICANS

A hard blow from sports or other trauma to the anterior thigh resulting in a hematoma must not be massaged. A long-term bony growth within the muscle (myositis ossificans) can result.

Muscle Protocol

Cross-fiber Friction andTrigger Point Therapy for Painful Muscle Bellies

Clients with chronic muscle belly adhesions will present with intermittent pain predominately felt during prolonged or strenuous work or exercise. The scar in the belly of the involved muscle will be painful. Advise your client that the frictioned scar will have post-treatment tenderness. They should not engage the involved area in overly strenuous activity following treatment.

1. Take a history to ascertain whether the problem is acute or chronic:

• Acute muscle belly problems aren't frictioned. Generally wait 7 to 10 days so that you don't interfere with or prolong the early process of scar formation.

• Heat, swelling, tenderness and bruising over the site of the lesion identify the acute stage. Bruising may not become visible until the second day, but the muscle will be very tender at the site of the tear. Pain during the acute stage will be relatively constant and diffuse. Sleep problems are usually concomitant with acute muscle tears.

• Chronic muscle belly scars, though painful, can be worked immediately except when post treatment soreness will interfere with important physical activities. Chronic muscle injury pain is generally exacerbated by overuse and relieved by rest. Chronic pain (muscle pain is generally considered chronic if it exists longer than a few months) is felt in the general region of the lesion, seldom with any temperature increase.

• Give your clients full disclosure of the effects of cross-fiber friction and ask them to commit for 3 visits over 7 to 10 days. Advise them that the treatment is often painful when administered and can result in residual soreness. There can be bruising on rare occasion. It may be necessary to review icing procedures with your client (see appendix) since residual soreness can result.

2. Identify the suspected muscle lesion with gentle friction. The most painful portion of the muscle identifies the exact site of the lesion. Discontinuity (a gap or hole) in muscle tissue will occasionally be felt. A bulge followed by a gap will indicate a completely torn muscle. Typically we see this in the rectus femoris muscle. Some clients with this torn and rolled-up muscle may not realize what has happened. If acute, don't treat. Refer.

3. Apply the treatment protocol to the exact site of the lesion:

• Administer friction massage to dry skin or through clothing. Use the thumb or braced fingers to move the client's skin and subcutaneous tissues over the lesion being treated. Use no oils. If a client has oil on their skin, friction through a towel.

• Begin with moderate friction. Start below a therapeutic level and progressively increase your pressure during the treatment to 6 or 7 on a 10 scale. If your client tenses, you're above a therapeutic level. Friction perpendicular to the muscle fibers. Muscle fibers are generally aligned with the direction of pull of the muscle. Work a muscle on a moderate slack in order to gain access to its deeper portions.

• Using equal pressure in both directions, friction back and forth across the lesion. Move the client's skin and subcutaneous tissues over the lesion being treated. Never glide over the client's skin surface as painful blisters can result.

• Friction slowly. Friction works best when administered at a slower pace, about 2 sweeps per second. Rapid friction is irritating with paltry therapeutic results. Use sufficient sweep and duration with a stroke broad enough to access the entire lesion.

• Treat for 1 minute or less on first visits. This is usually long enough to make a chemical/mechanical impact. Client response to the previous visit determines future treatment length and pressures. Our maximum treatment of 4 or 5 minutes is reserved for lesions deep within the belly in thick, dense muscles, e.g., hamstrings.

• Treat on alternate days. A 48 hour rest period allows the treatment-induced inflammation to subside. Consider using ice to ameliorate post-treatment soreness. We recommend a minimum of 2 treatments per week at the exact site of the lesion (strain, adhesion or microtrauma).

IN A NUTSHELL
Cross-fiber Friction for Tendons & Muscles

1. History – ascertain whether the problem is chronic or acute.

2. Assessment – use friction to determine the exact site of the lesion.

3. Treatment – apply friction massage on alternate days.

Trigger Points – a Reminder

In some cases what appeared to be a tendonitis was, in fact, a painful trigger point site. Trigger points are a more common source of muscle pain than adherent scars. Clients present complaining of pain. The problem (if a trigger point) will need to be treated at the trigger point – the SOURCE of the pain, but usually not the SITE of the pain. Trigger points refer pain. This referral pattern may be immediate to the trigger point or distant – as far as from the neck to the hand or the calf to the sacrum. Your knowledge of referral patterns gives you a likely spot to begin palpating for the trigger point. Friction massage has a similar physiologic effect as direct pressure and can occasionally provide a quick-cure. Refer to "Trigger Points" (page 40) for a complete protocol.

JOE'S STORY

Joe the painter took a class on friction massage for tendon injuries, mainly because his own shoulder hurt. Joe self-diagnosed a tendonitis of the tenoperiosteal juncture of the supraspinatus tendon. He dutifully put his arm into a hammerlock and rubbed the tendon daily for months with no noticeable improvement. Why did friction massage fail? The pain - while in the exact site of a supraspinatus tendonitis - was actually a subscapularis trigger point that referred pain into the tendon and mimicked a tendonitis.

In a class six months later, Joe complained of a lack of improvement. Cleverly, we decided that since the tendon pain didn't respond to cross-fiber, its source could be referred pain from a trigger point. It took two 30 second treatments of direct pressure to end his problem. Joe had simply forgotten to change approaches after no improvement in three tries.

Treatment

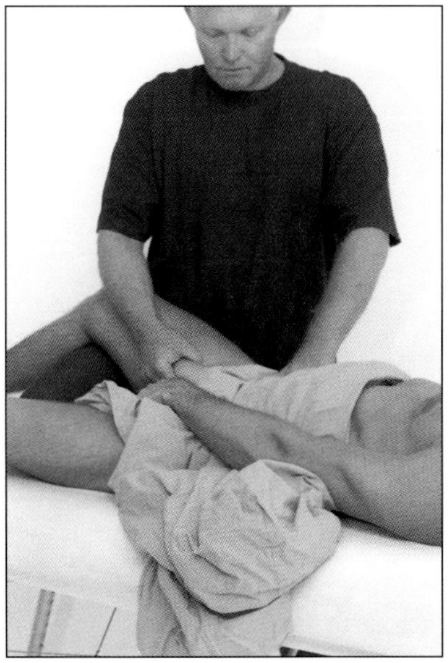

Cross-fiber to the adductor longus using pincer palpation

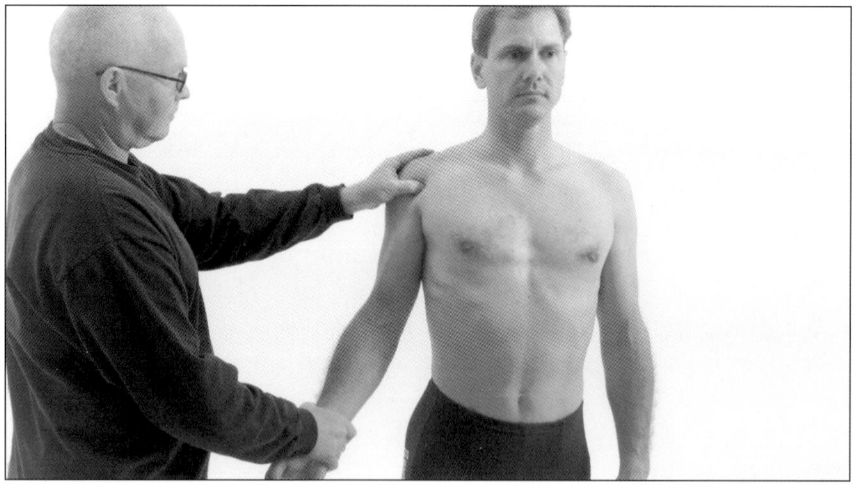

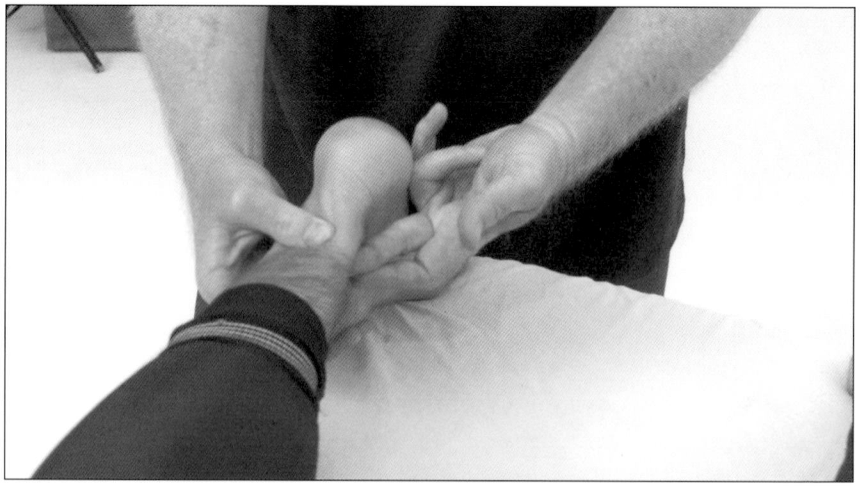

Frictioning the subscapularis tendon attachment into the tubercle of the lesser head of the humerus.

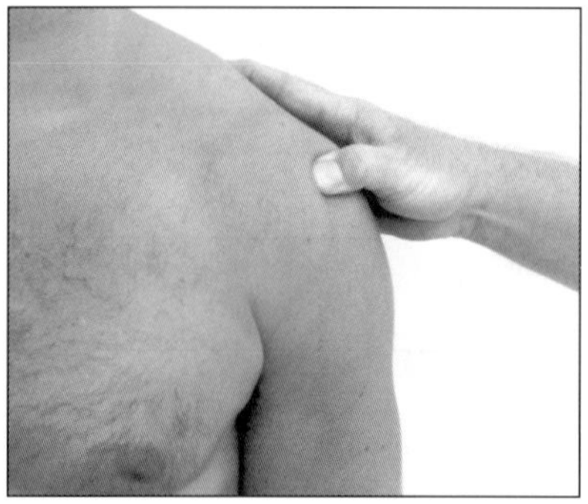

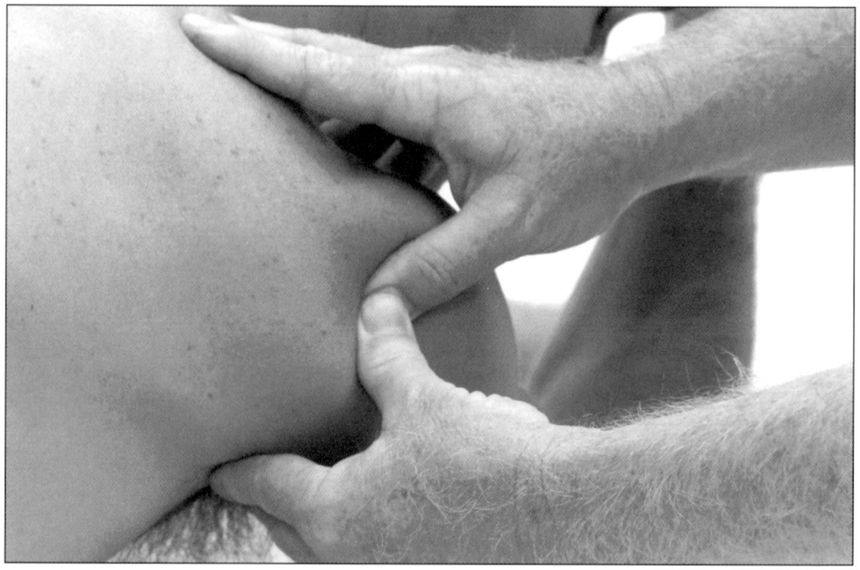

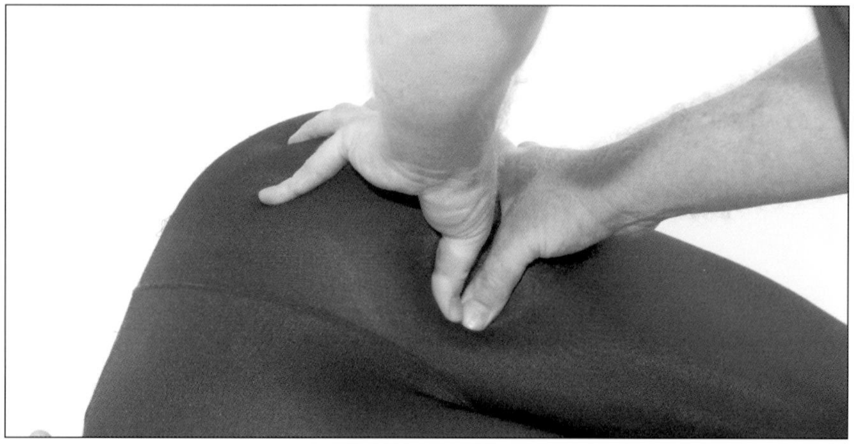

Thumb on thumb cross-fiber to the infraspinatus tendon.

CHAPTER 9

Fascial Stretching and Release

Overview

Fascial stretches are accomplished by hand or foot. Restricted fascia's location and the size and type of body you're working with determine which method is used to maximize therapeutic benefit. This overview provides a basic understanding the nature of fascia (connective tissue), identifies some of the problems associated with fascial restrictions, and presents procedures for safe fascial releases.

Composition

Fascia exists on three levels – superficial, deep and subserous. Its structural composition varies according to functional requirements. Fascia permeates your entire body on a three dimensional grid (a sort of web) and is so omnipresent that with all your other structural body components removed, you would still be recognizable as you.

Fascia is comprised of three primary components – collagen, elastin, and a ground substance.

1. Collagen, the fibrous component, contributes strength comparable to steel. Tendons and ligaments consist primarily of collagen.

2. Elastin supplies flexibility and elasticity to skin and arterial fascia. This component won't tear until stretched one and one-half times its normal length.

3. Ground substance primarily provides lubrication and absorbs shock. Cartilage is good example of a shock absorbing tissue composed primarily of ground substance.

Compressive deep massage changes fascia by providing heat, pressure, gentle stretch and bio-electric/bio-energetic energy to shift the ground substance from gel (an aged, semi-solid state) towards sol (a more fluid form). Rejuvenated connective tissue allows increased pain-free movement.

Problems

Restrictions in fascia usually result from trauma, inflammation or infection. Restrictions are often caused by prolonged muscle tension associated with repetitive use syndromes, postural distortions or chronic emotional stress. "Burning" pain is the most common symptom or presenting complaint.

Prolonged muscle contractions encourage fascial shortening. Fascia, if not released when hypertonic muscle fibers are stretched, soon pulls muscle tissue back (fascia has an elastic memory) to restrictive, shortened positions. Pain, restricted movement and resultant postural distortion (e.g., improper gait patterns) continue until the contracted fascial tissue is released and lengthened.

Shortened (shrunken) superficial fascia can exert considerable pressure on underlying tissues. Functioning of nerve, lymph and blood vessels is impaired when they pass through fascial restrictions. Fascial release work lengthens and softens connective tissue and results in healthy, efficient and pain-free movement.

How, When and Where

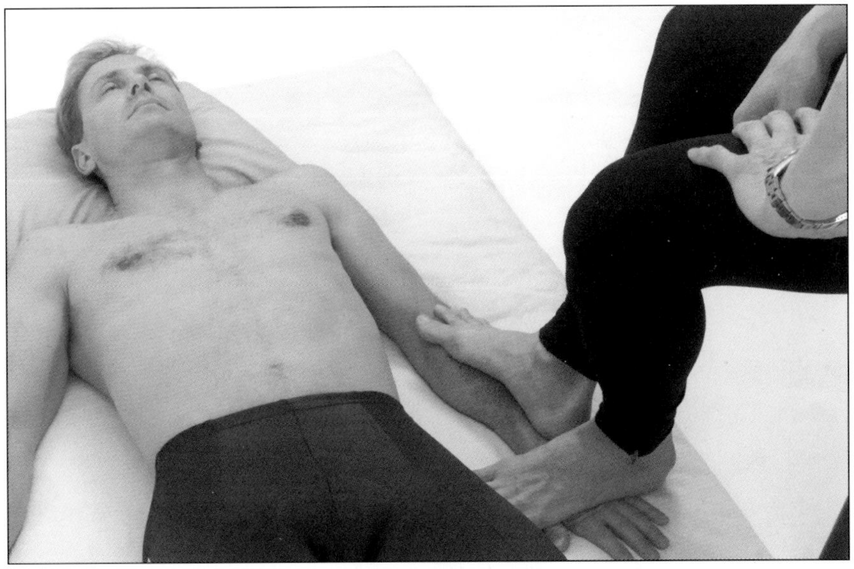

Both hands and feet are used to release bound, contracted or adherent fascial layers found in over-stressed, restricted areas. The iliotibial bands, the lumbosacral area, paraspinals, and forearm extensors are common locations of some major fascial restrictions.

We use fascial release when deep compressions, direct pressure to trigger points or cross-fiber friction fail to provide lasting cures. It is an especially beneficial protocol for headache sufferers when utilized to relax and release restrictions at the sub-occipital region (base of the skull). We find fascial releases melt tension found in the tight jaw muscles of clients suffering from bruxism (grinding of the teeth when sleeping) and TMD (temporomandibular joint dysfunction). We find that some shoulder problems also respond well, especially where a client's primary, relaxed structural character has been replaced by second nature holding patterns.

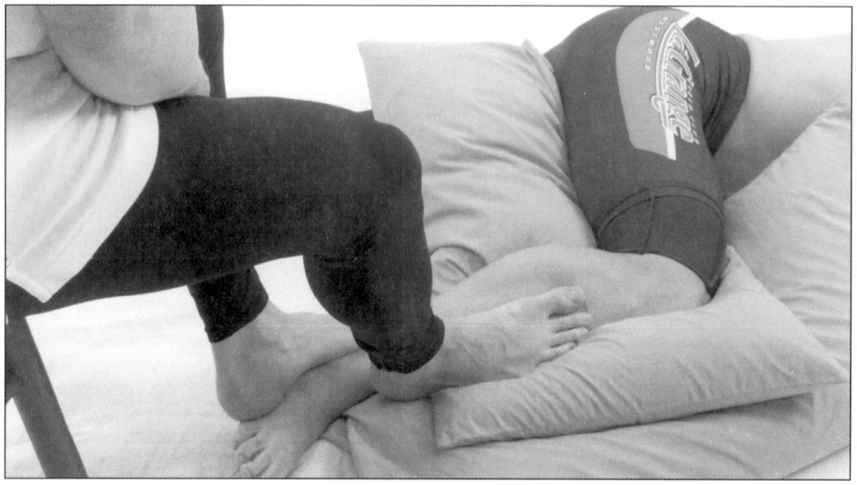

Fascial stretching is a gentle, lengthy process. The work is very deep due to its three-dimensional nature. Success demands therapists stay relaxed. To promote the required sensitivity and protect ourselves, we pay close attention to body mechanics and often use a stool.

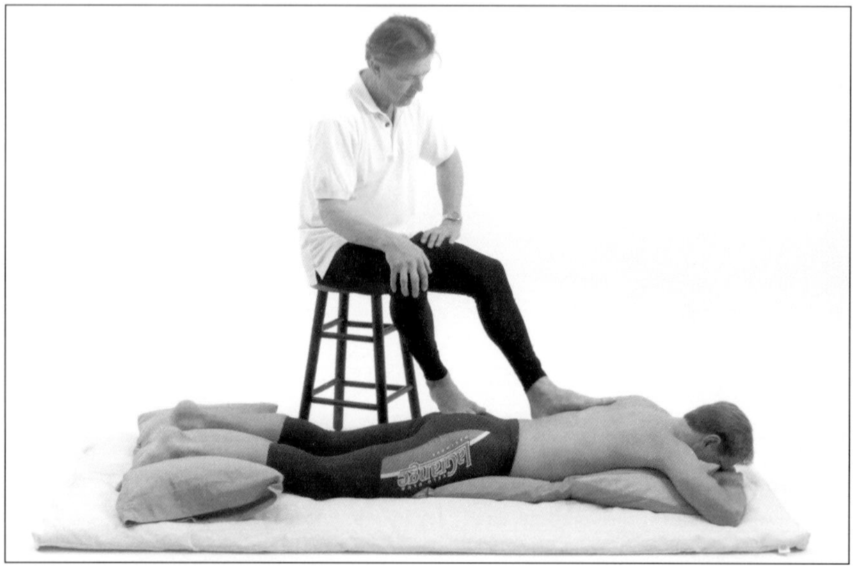

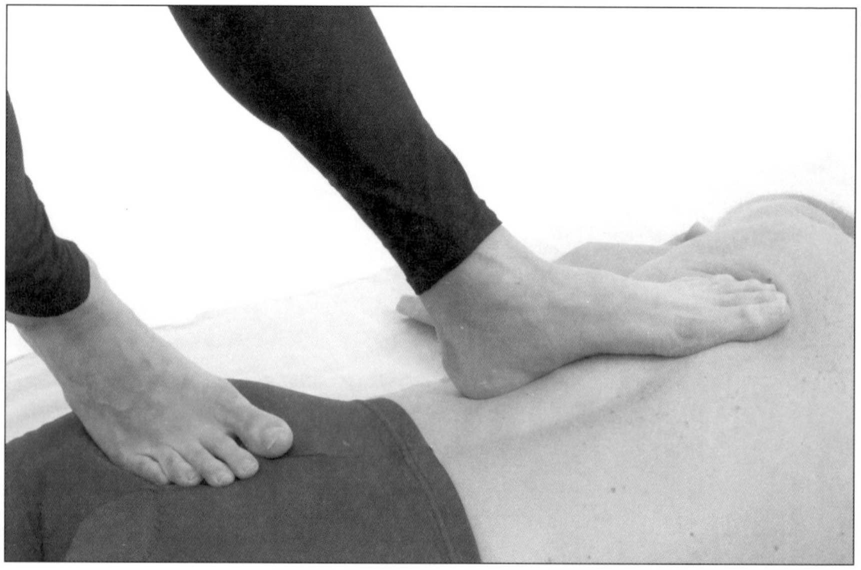

Fascial release work must be done with hands and feet applied directly to skin. Feel for the tight spots – those caved-in or restricted areas. Trust your senses. Shortened fascial fibers feel thick, ropy and lumpy. Restrictions limit both normal movement and circulation. Chronic tissues needing fascial release feel cooler than healthier surrounding tissue. Restricted areas are revitalized after fascial release frees compressed nerves and allows normal blood and lymph flow to resume.

Warm the affected area with the gentle compressions first. Wipe oily and slippery skin with a hot, wet towel or alcohol so you do not slip over the skin. Place your hand/foot on the restricted area. Your opposite hand/foot is occasionally best used to anchor one end of tissues being released. Gently push until you reach the colloidal restriction or barrier found at the end of the initial elastic stretch. Hang-out, wait. Patience is required to get best results. Give your heat and energy time to work.

Release work is analogous to force applied to a block of taffy, that stuff you see at the beach wrapped in little wax paper as Candy Kisses. The taffy block is impervious to a blow, but a soft, resting and warm hand soon melts it.

Fascial behavior follows laws governing viscous flow like a shock absorber on your car. The harder and quicker you push, the more it fights back. Use less force and it gives. Colloids' resistance increases proportionally to the velocity of the force applied. A gentle touch becomes an absolute necessity in order to avoid viscous drag in fascial tissue.

It takes time for the energy contained in your gentle stretch to melt the resistance found at the colloidal barrier. Time is the most critical factor for optimal use of these stretch-release techniques. Rush and you'll

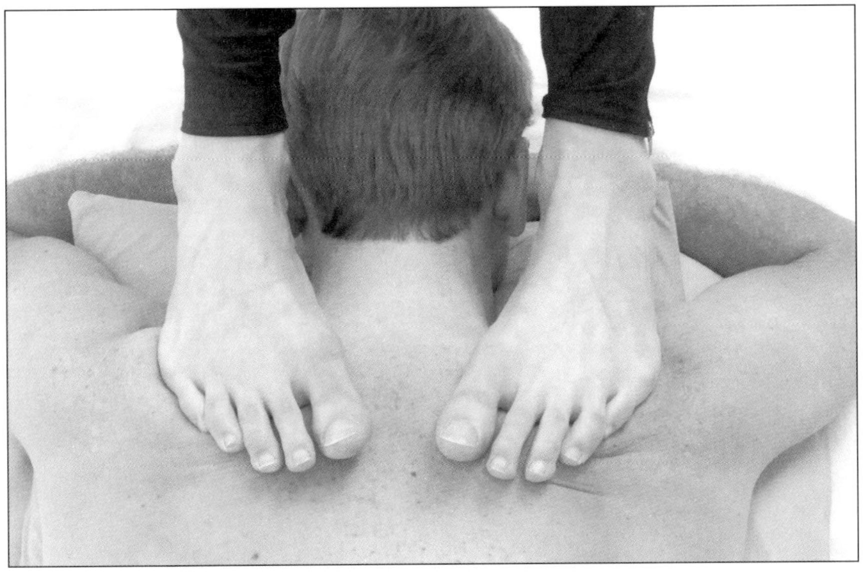

likely fail – you cannot hurry a fascial release. It can take from three to five minutes – sometimes more. Releases almost never occur in less than 90 seconds.

Regardless of what you think or see, put your trust in what you feel. Allow your intuitive, observing mind the time and space to prove itself. Passively observe the flow of tissue and let your client's body dictate the direction of release. Releases are usually tiny – measured in millimeters.

Wait until all release ceases. The nature of a stretching release varies with each client and the location of their restricted tissue. Usually felt as a smooth, continuous flow, releases can also come in waves. Some are gradual and others occur suddenly. Multiple releases are sometimes experienced, but usually there is one flowing stretch.

Subtleties

Sometimes you will get confused as to whether you are sliding or affecting a release – don't worry, we don't know either. Look for tissue change. That will determine whether or not there was a release. A true release will bring increased warmth and softness. Tissue appearance changes from caved-in or swollen to matching surrounding skin contour. Color changes in skin often result. Additional function and increases in range of motion are evident.

Another complication can result from simultaneous releases of fascial tissue in your own treating hand or foot, especially in the early stages of practice. You, as a beginner, as well as your clients, are advised to drink extra liquids to flush the metabolites released as restrictions are eased.

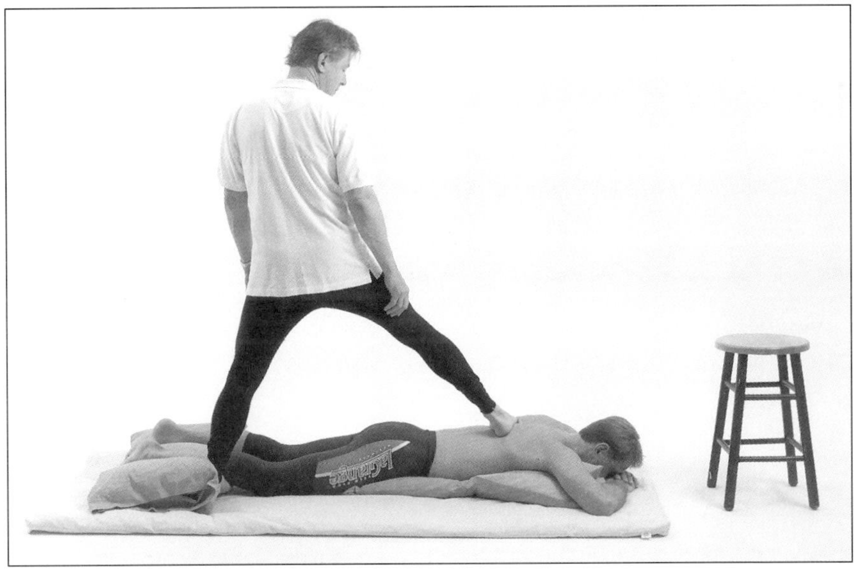

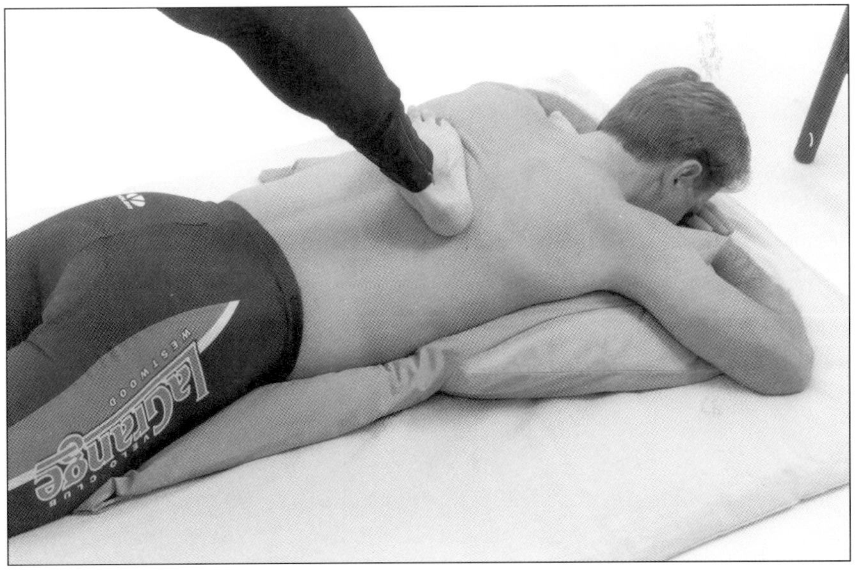

Contraindications

Normal cautions and contraindications to massage apply to fascial stretching and release. When unsure as to the advisability of using any of our protocols, it is best to meet together with your client and their physician.

Pay particular attention to the possibility of malignancy, aneurysm, or rheumatoid arthritis (in acute or flare-up situations). Have your sick or injured clients get permission and specific instructions from their physician regarding fascial release.

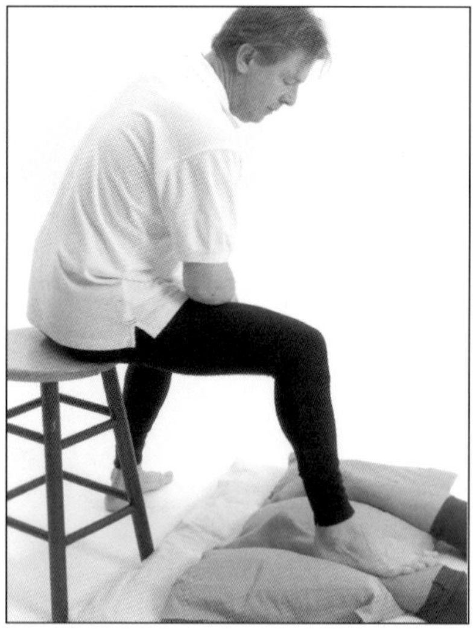

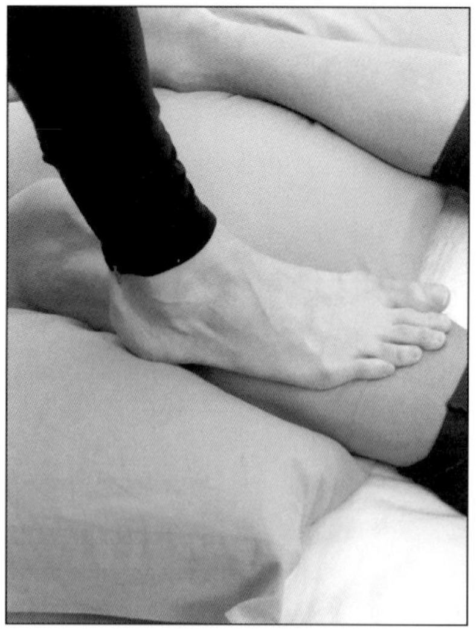

NOTE

Arterial pulses (radial, carotid, femoral, posterior tibial etc.) should be noted. If they vary in intensity from one side of the body to the other, there could be compression, entrapment or a vascular disease worth investigating before performing release procedures.

If you don't feel confident with the answers given by your client to your inquiries, remember your option and our admonition, "When in doubt, refer."

Recommendations for Further Study

Principles of Manual Medicine, 1996, by Philip Greenman, D.O., provides comprehensive descriptions of fascial layers and the three main components of fascia. He also includes instructions for a general treatment protocol.

The Myofascial Release Manual, 1994, by Carol Manheim, MS, MEd, P.T., contains excellent photographic illustrations and instruction for fascial release and various pulse taking procedures.

PART 4

Regional Protocols

Regional Protocols

Most likely pain sources are addressed first.

Illustrations provide basic anatomical information, primary trigger points sites, and pain-reference patterns.

Starbursts (*) signify the most common trigger point sites. Stippling indicates known pain reference patterns. The more common the referral, the darker the stippling. Note that a trigger point (TrP) can be anywhere on a muscle and not just where a starburst appears.

Our protocols have evolved naturally through experience – we give you what has worked for us. This information is a starting point.

CHAPTER 10

Low Back – Lumbar and Gluteal Pain

THIS SECTION ADDRESSES some of the most common problems presented to bodyworkers. Many of the all too common complaints of chronic lumbar pain and stiffness in the low back and hip can be effectively addressed with direct heel pressure. It is relatively easy to deal with client complaints here. You can expect to get some of your best results using DeeperWork protocols in this region.

What we find to be the most troublesome muscles are presented pretty much in the order we address them. We begin with four primary sources of muscularly caused low back pain: the paraspinals, quadratus lumborum, gluteus medius and minimus. Next we work the serratus posterior inferior, gluteus maximus and the hamstrings – all perpetuators of trigger points that affect the low back.

If this work hasn't resolved the pain, we proceed to address the rectus abdominus and iliopsoas. In our experience the rectus abdominus and iliopsoas are involved in muscularly related lumbar pain about 15% of the time. The iliopsoas is also involved in post-laminectomy pain.

We also include an often over-looked source of groin and inguinal pain and early morning back stiffness – the iliolumbar ligament. Our experience suggests that men, more often than women, will experience discomfort from this ligament.

Before You Begin

Safe, effective low back treatments are enhanced by first reading the *Indications, Client Intake, Contraindications, Deep Compressive Massage, Endangerment Sites, Trigger Points, Cross-fiber, Fascial Release, Stretching* and *Hydrotherapy* sections.

Note the specific procedural notes and cautions. They will help you effectively treat your client without harm. Protocols and guidelines are included to help you know when to treat and when to refer.

Lumbar Paraspinals

Look for the simplest solution for every problem, but search widely. Our protocols play the percentages, but intuition and searching "outside the box" are also important.

Once we had become sophisticated as bodyworkers, the lumbar paraspinals received scant attention. Since we knew that most lumbar problems come from the gluteus medius, gluteus minimus and the quadratus lumborum, we gave the paraspinals short shrift.

We almost failed a very treatable client because of this sophistication. After three visits with only paltry success we were ready to refer. Only as an afterthought, after admitting failure, did we examine her lumbar paraspinal musculature and thus locate the crux of her low back pain.

Paraspinal muscles can activate quadratus lumborum trigger points and/or cause pain and stiffness on their own. Tightness that comes from trigger points and the discomfort they generate restricts movement and clients enter a self-perpetuating downward cycle of rigidity. Now that we are less sophisticated, we treat the paraspinals and get better results. We've learned not to be too smart.

The medically-created mythology of the back being weak doesn't hold true in our experience. However, it is true that sedentary people often need to strengthen the back in order to feel strong.

Physical weakness, in general, seems to create unhealthy levels of feeling vulnerable and greatly reduces resiliency to physical and psychological stresses. Humans evolved to be physically vigorous...use it or lose it. Fear of increased back pain often leads to more back pain from the ischemia and muscle acidity that comes from immobility.

Books are written on the subject of how-to-lift. Most claim that back pain is initiated while lifting – with weight of less than a pound often being the initiating culprit. In these texts, the solution is to lift from a squatting position. Fred agrees with the majority, especially when a spinal twist accompanies the lifting motion. John disagrees and thinks this exaggerated care simply perpetuates the vulnerable back myth. He suggests a very slight bend at the knees to avoid hyperextension, and says, "Just bend over and pick it up – whatever." Occasionally experts disagree.

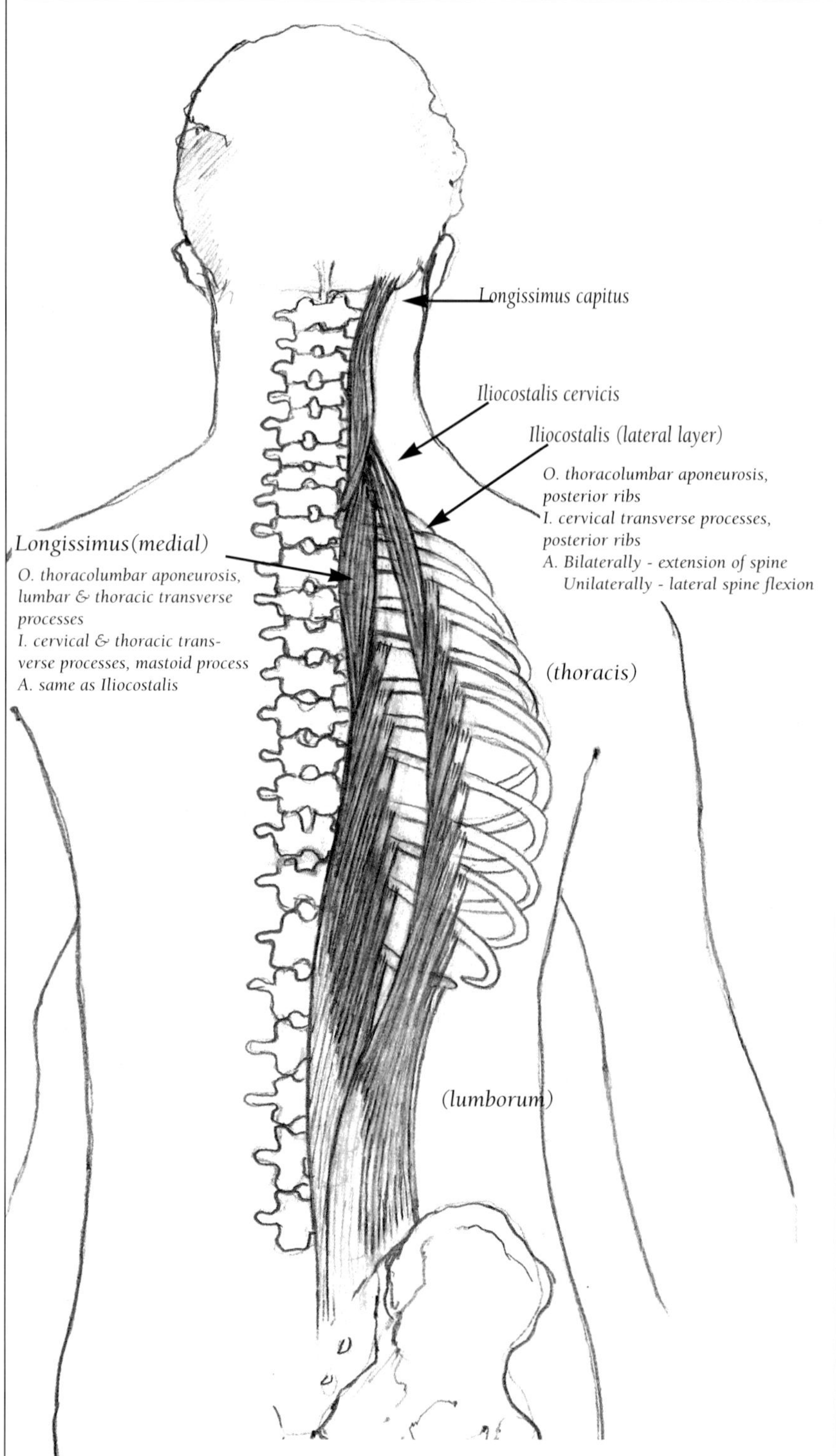

Superficial Paraspinals – Erector Spinae

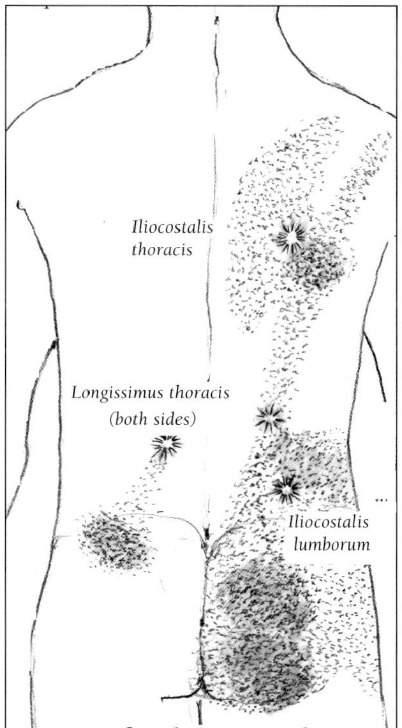

Superficial paraspinal TrPs

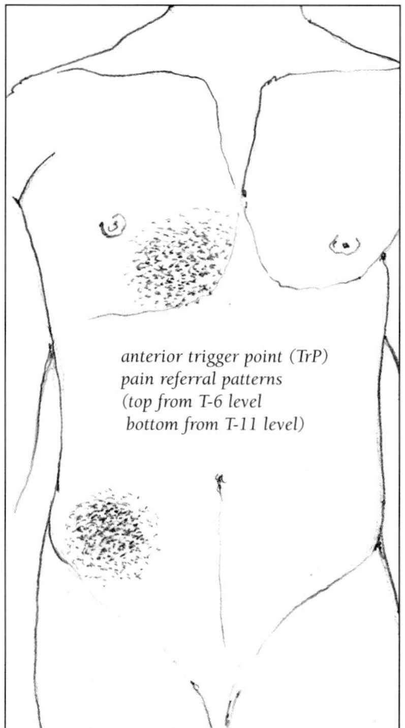

Iliocostalis thoracis TrPs

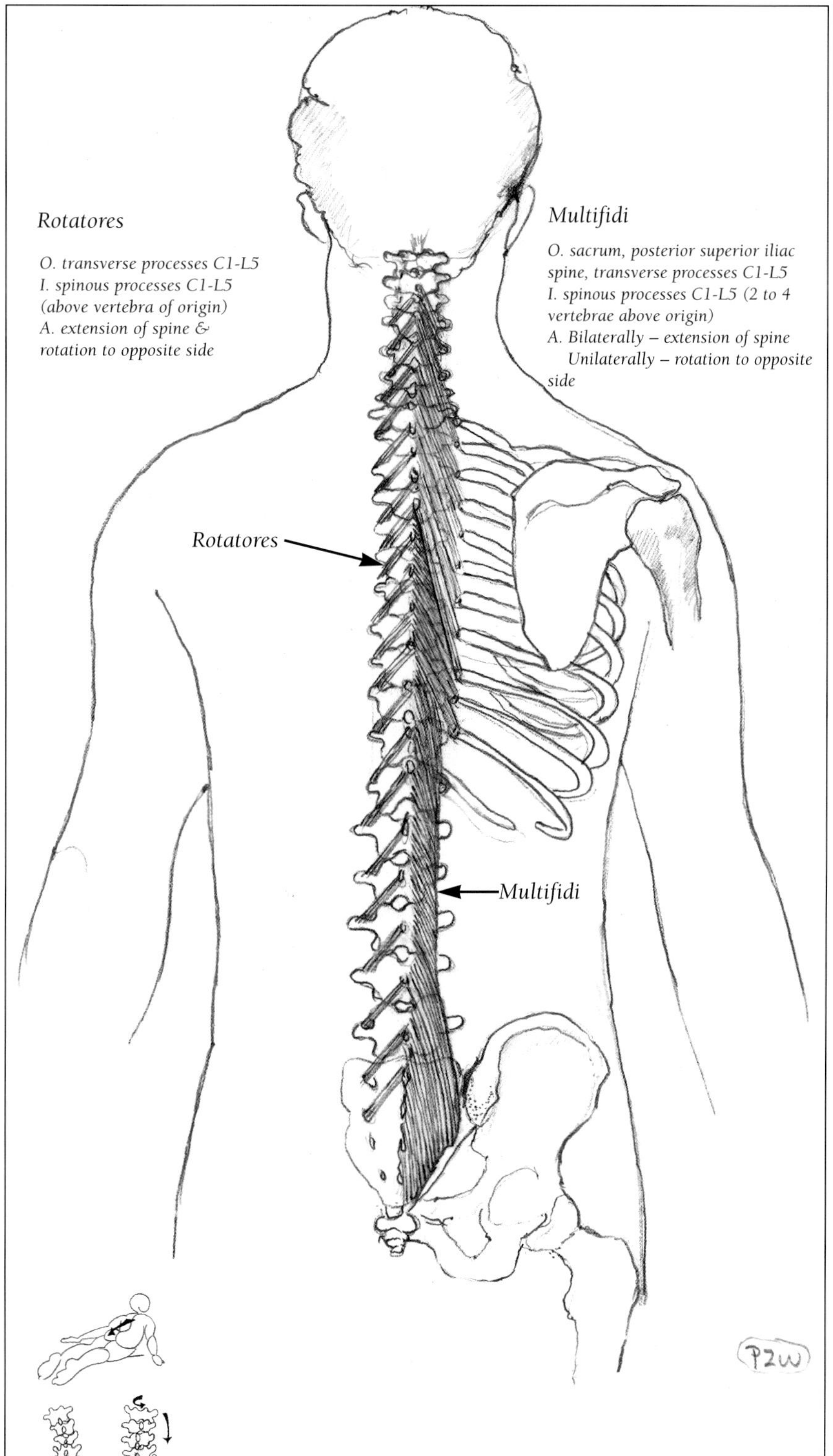

Deep Paraspinals

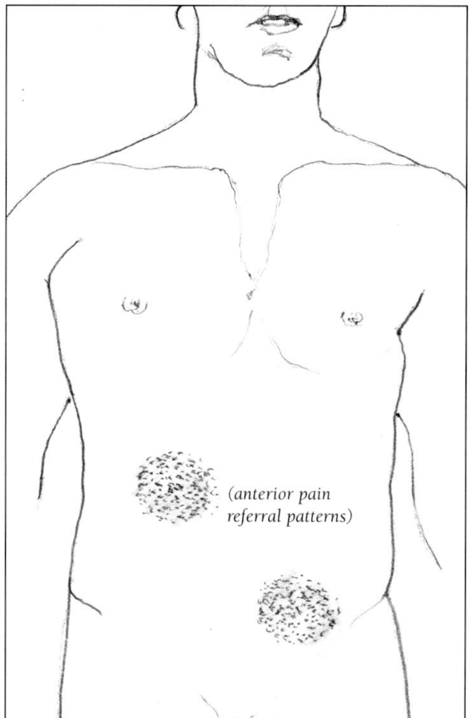

Deep Multifidi TrPs

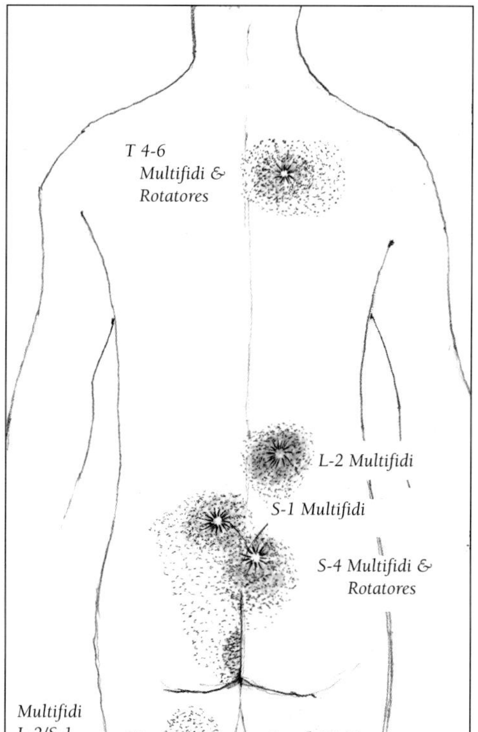

Deep Paraspinal TrPs

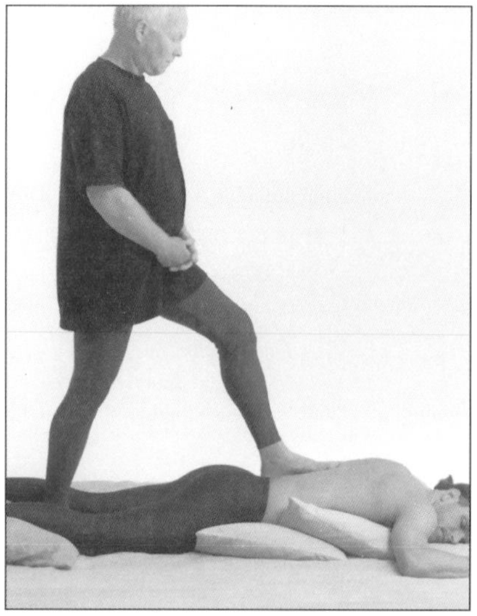

Lumbar paraspinal warm-up – stay off the spinous processes.

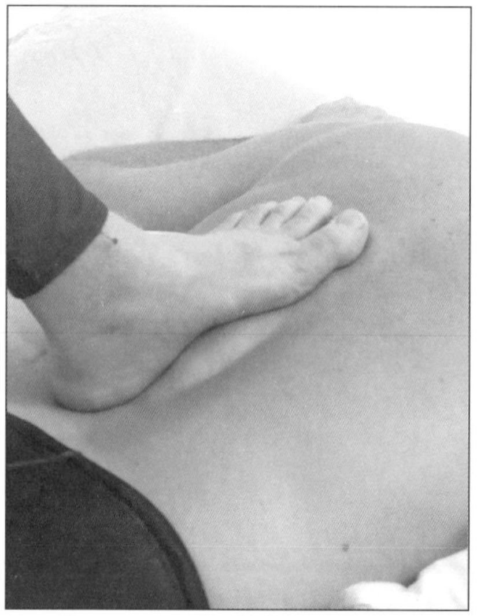

Heel pressure with stretch to superficial lumbar paraspinals.

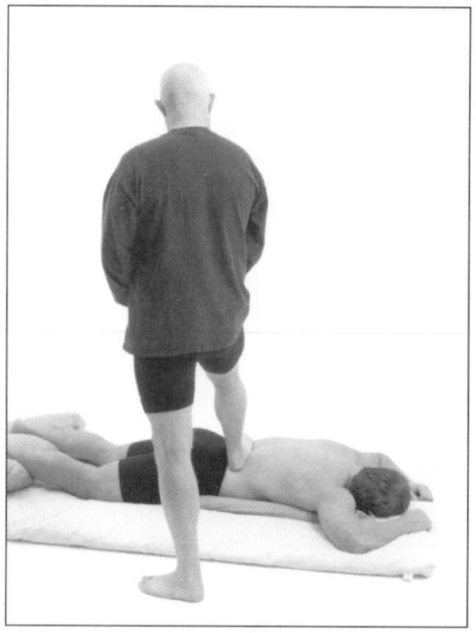

Lateral approach with heel into lumbar paraspinals and quadratus lumborum. Heel is below the 12th rib and above the pelvis.

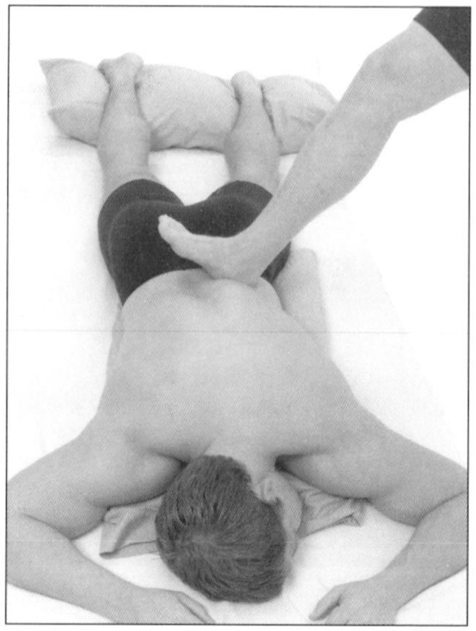

Direct pressure to lumbar paraspinals.

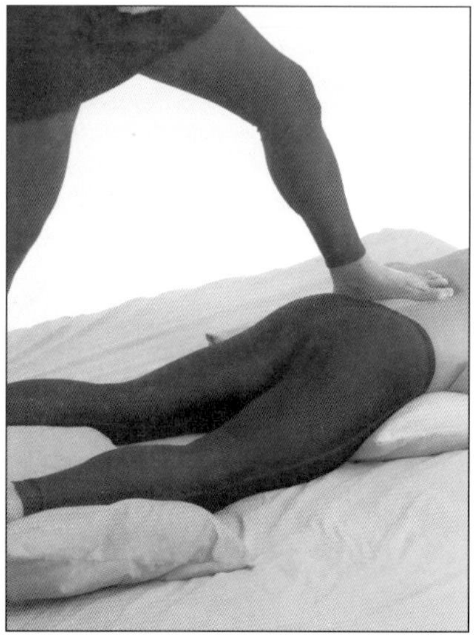

Warm-up and fascial stretch to lumbar paraspinals. Note angle of foot.

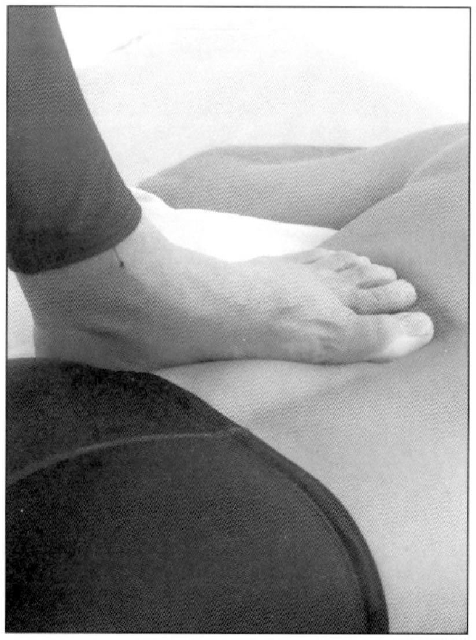

Close-up of warm-up and stretch of lumbar fascia.

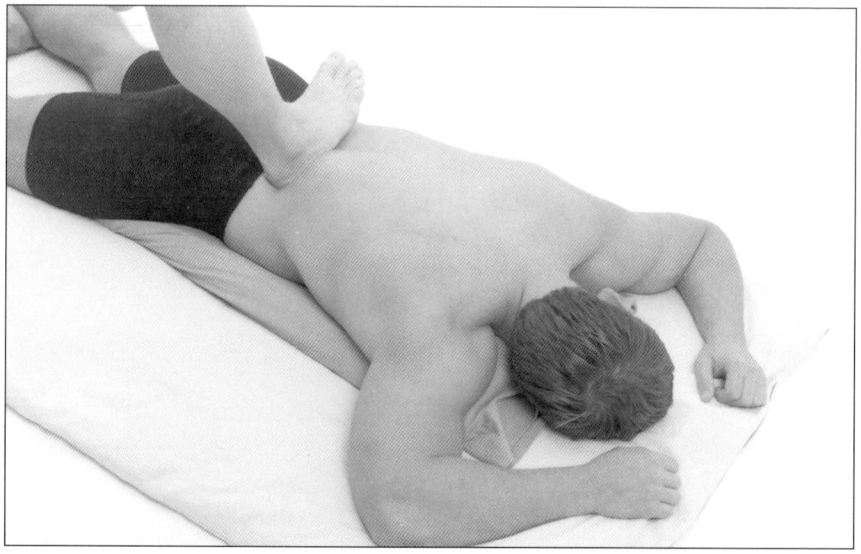

Increase dorsiflexion for stronger direct pressure.

IF YOUR CLIENT walks in the door (barely) and there is an acute angle between the pelvis and torso, check the quadratus lumborum. This muscle is implicated in most functional "C" and "S" curve scoliosis problems. It's also the muscle that Dr. Raymond Nimmo and our experience finds involved in a good 90% of muscularly related lumbar pain.

Some anatomists claim this muscle can't be palpated. We believe differently. With clients side-lying and the twelfth rib separated from the posterior crest, access may be tight, but is possible. Men, with higher pelvic crests and generally tighter lumbar musculature, are particularly suited to the deep compressive massage approach.

The quadratus lumborum is extremely painful if it has trigger points. Our very first experience treating it resulted in a horse-trainer client coming up off the table and spontaneously throwing a roundhouse punch. So enter slowly and build to a therapeutic level rather than having to back off from an invasive one.

Assisted stretches following trigger point inactivation are generally cumbersome and hard on your body. After deactivating the trigger points, get the client up and off the mat or table, and get them to use a side-leaning stretch for the quadratus lumborum and the gluteus medius and gluteus minimus. Caution your client to stretch moderately. The quadratus lumborum may still be highly reactive and can spasm.

We typically work the quadratus lumborum, the gluteus medius and

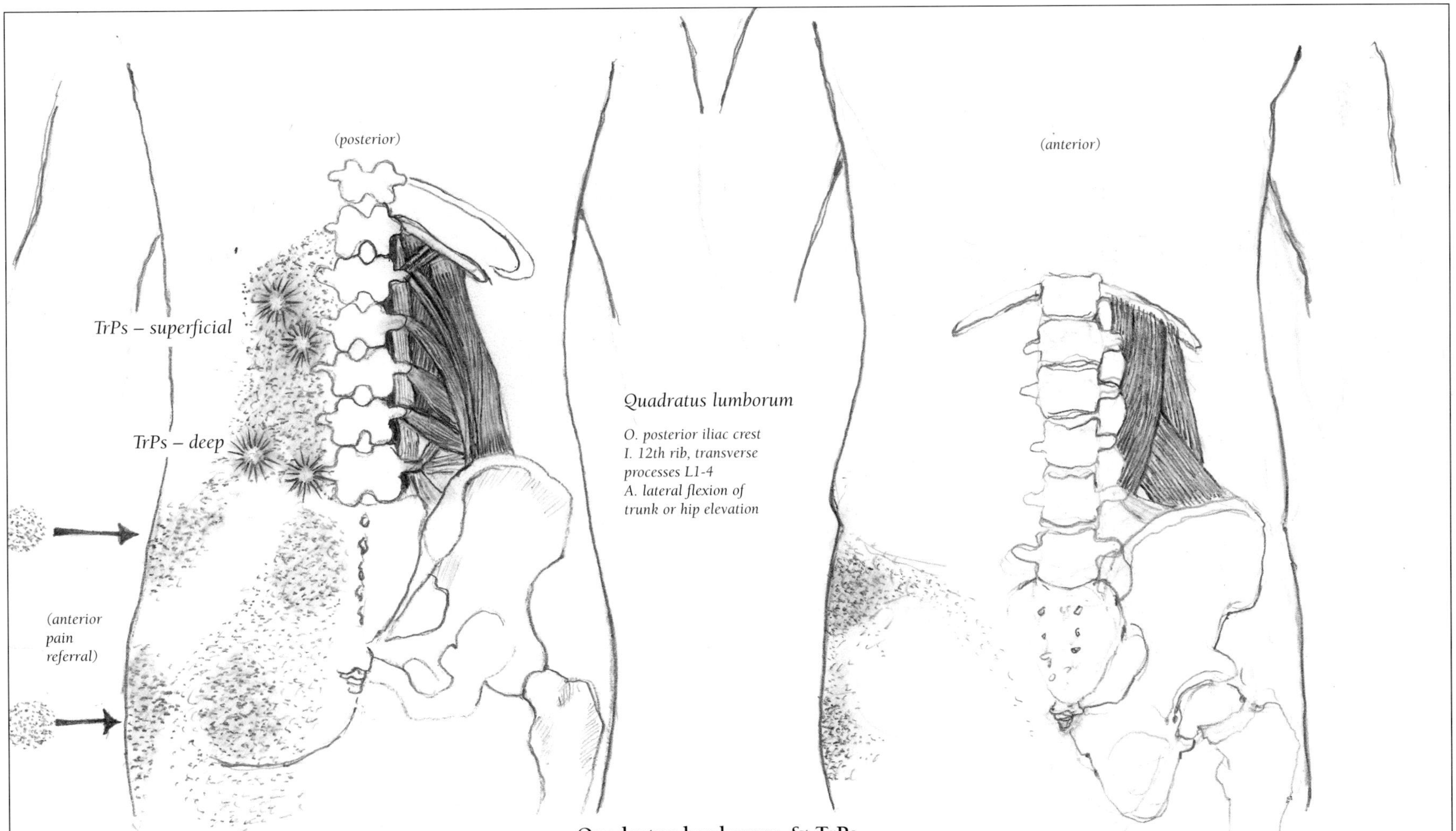

Quadratus lumborum & TrPs

minimus ipsolaterally and then have the client stand and stretch all three muscles with the same side-leaning stretch. Then return to the side-lying position to work the contralateral quadratus lumborum, gluteus medius and minimus.

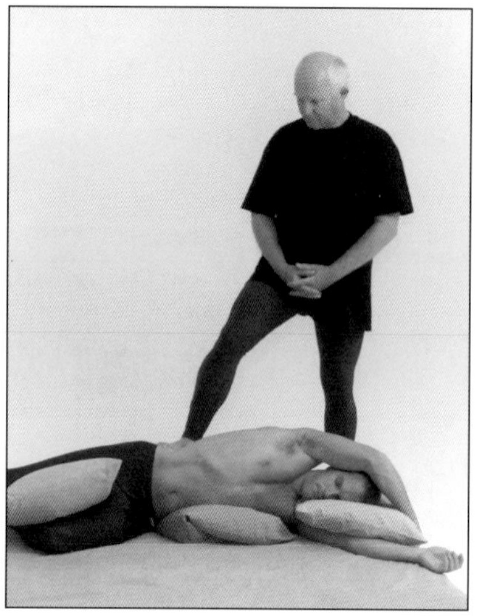

Side-lying approach to quadratus lumborum. Stay off the 12th rib – first ray compresses and stretches belly of quadratus lumborum.

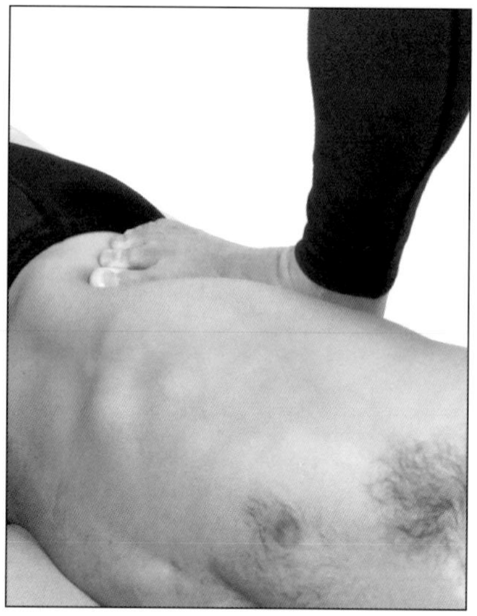

Direct pressure into a quadratus lumborum TrP.

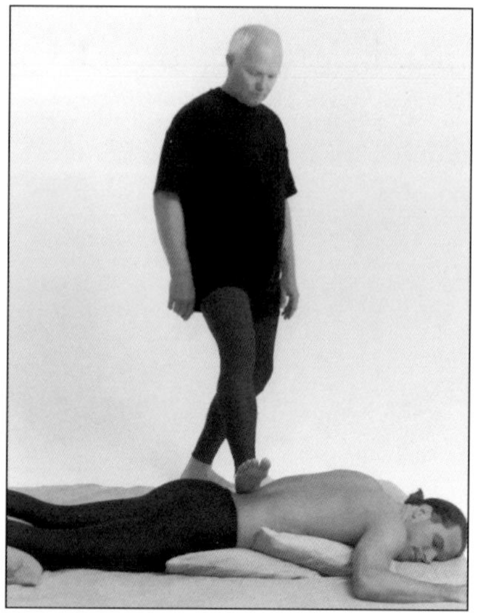

Prone approach to Quadratus lumborum. Avoid strong pressure to the 12th rib. If your client is small, frail (elderly) or has little space between their 12th rib and posterior crest, use your thumbs.

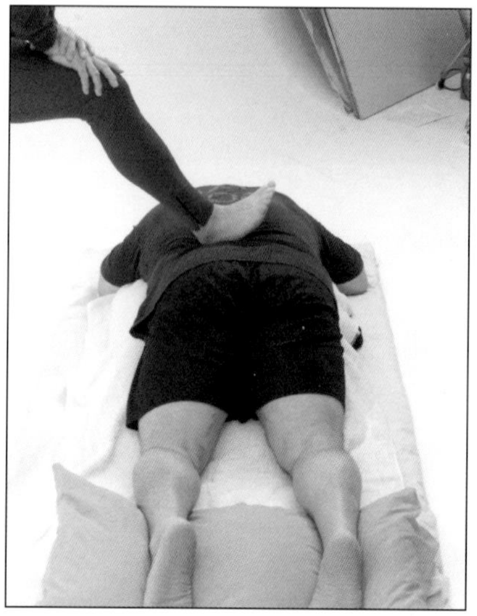

Heel to quadratus lumborum.

If this muscle has trigger points, it is also important to access the iliolumbar ligament that has anatomical attachments to the quadratus lumborum. Use moist heat to prevent post-treatment soreness following work on chronic trigger point pain.

Problems often stem from "deconditioned" lumbar musculature. After the triggers are eliminated, urge your clients to begin a strengthening program to prevent reoccurrence.

> Keep your clients moving (every 5 or 10 minutes) to avoid jelling pain. This action aborts the stiffness often associated with extended immobility during bodywork.

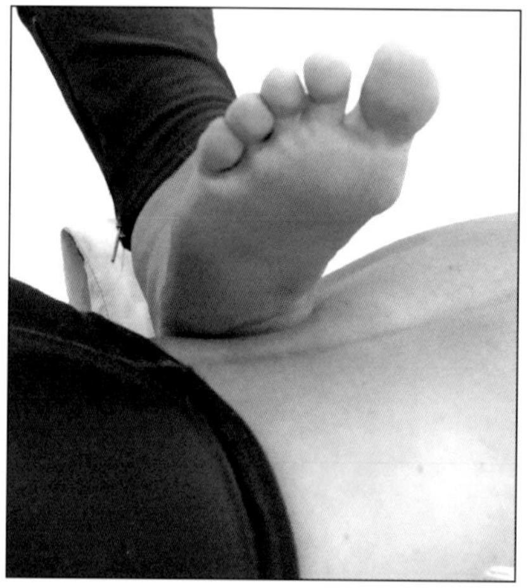

Heel to quadratus lumborum – note angle of approach.

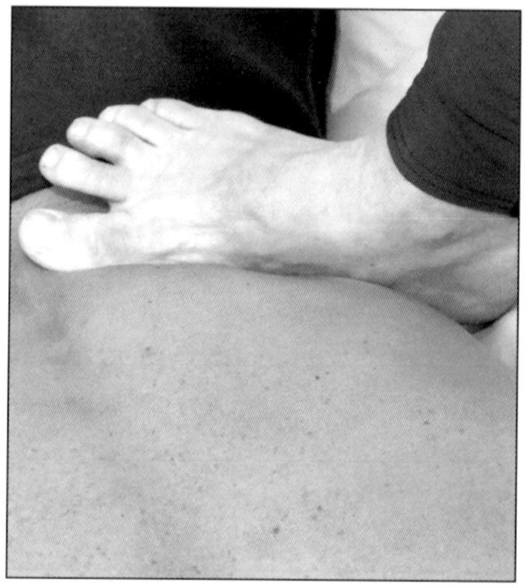

First ray compressing quadratus lumborum at crest attachment.

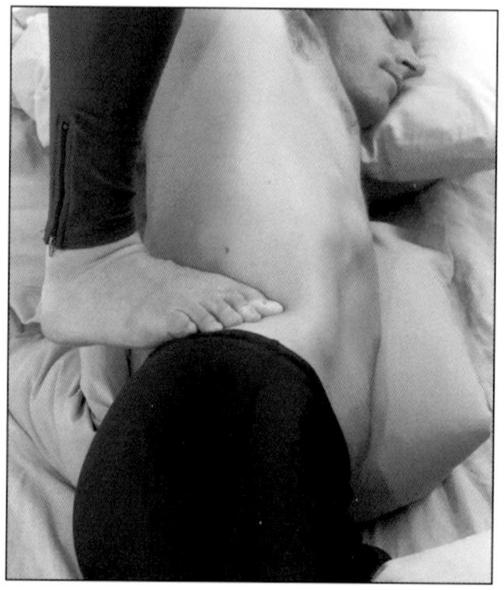

First ray presses TrP.

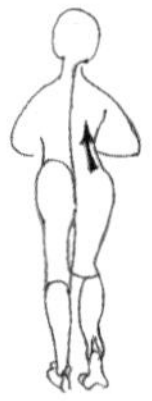

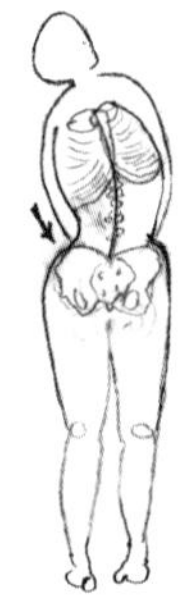

Treatment by Hand

Client is side-lying with a bolster under the lumbar region. Client's top arm should be extended over head with hip extended and back extended slightly. Stand behind client. Divide the client's torso frontally into imaginary thirds. While some authorities have you pushing against the quadratus lumborum at the twelfth rib, we don't.

Push directly into the muscle (posterior to anterior) between the first and second third located above the iliac crest and below the floating rib – just anterior to the bundle of fascially wrapped superficial lumbar paraspinal musculature. This will put you directly into the quadratus lumborum. If you must work by hand, our experience indicates that it is sufficient to push straight down into the belly of the muscle overlying the transverse process.

Then change the angle of entry to 45 degrees toward the posterior crest and slightly anterior to access the second major trigger point located just above the crest.

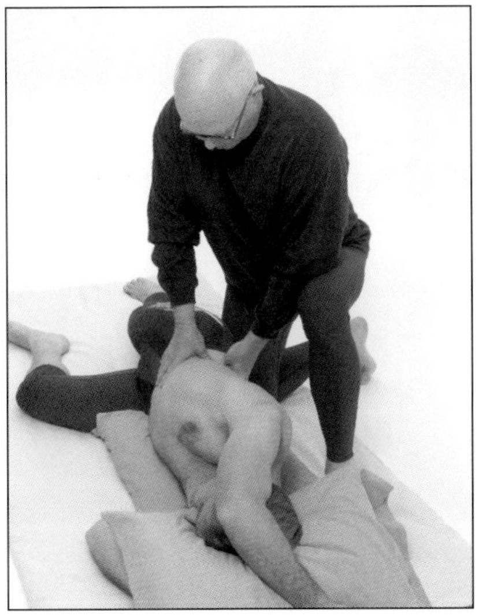

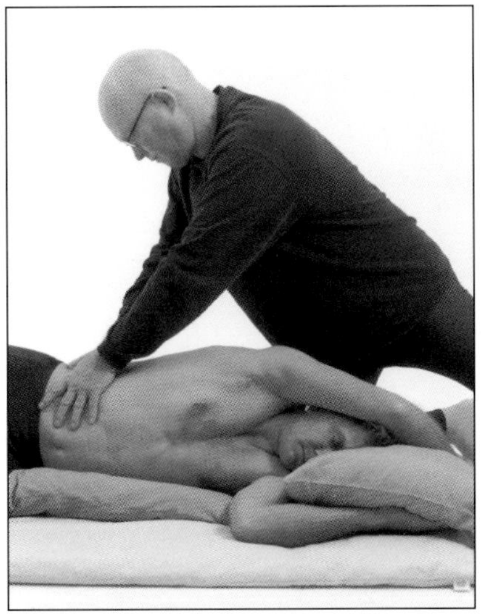

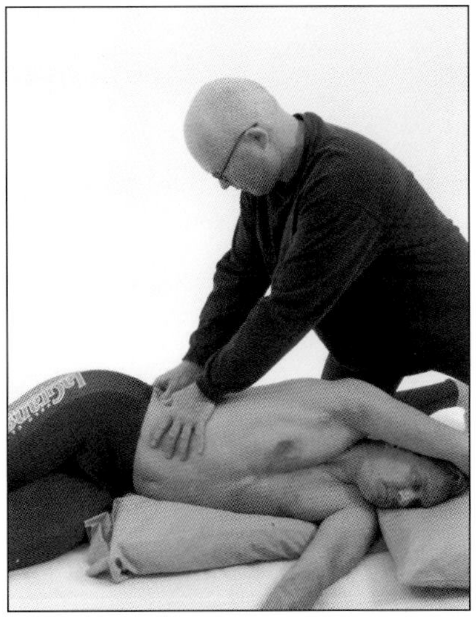

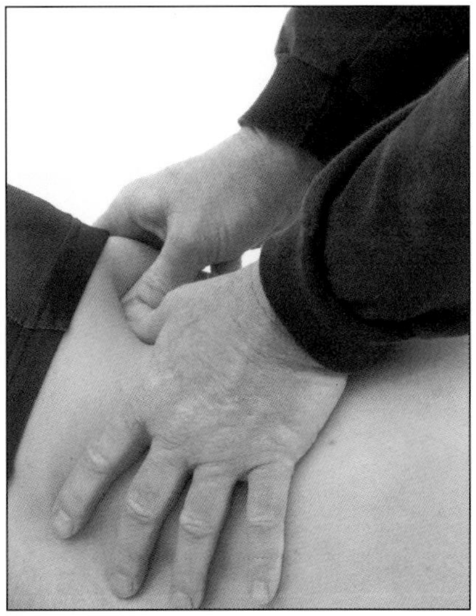

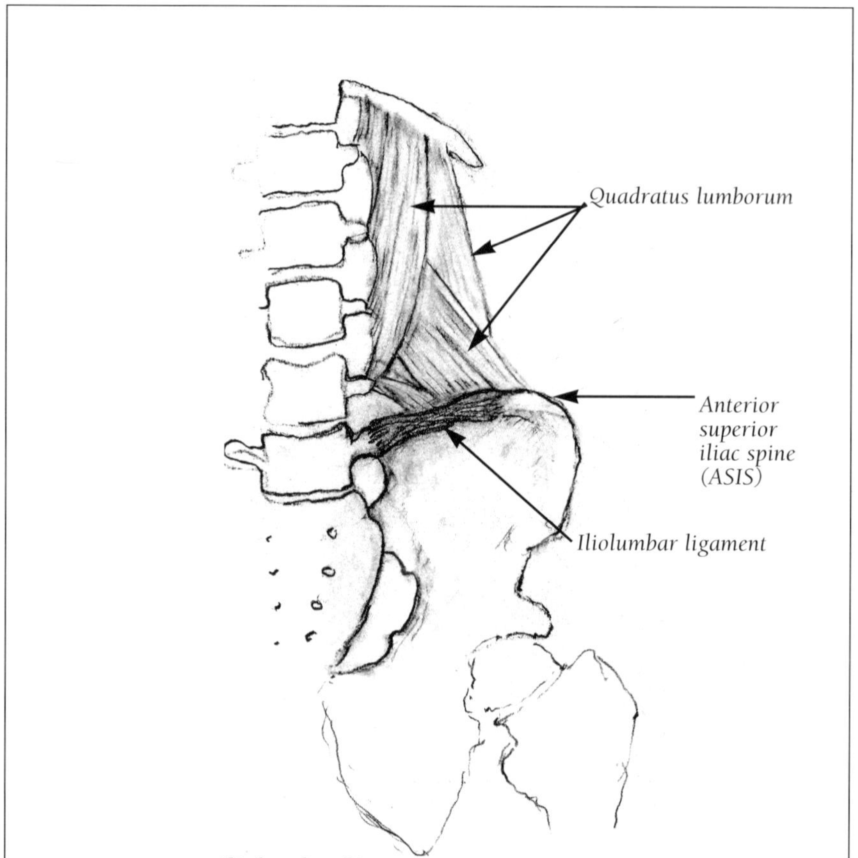

Iliolumbar ligament – anterior

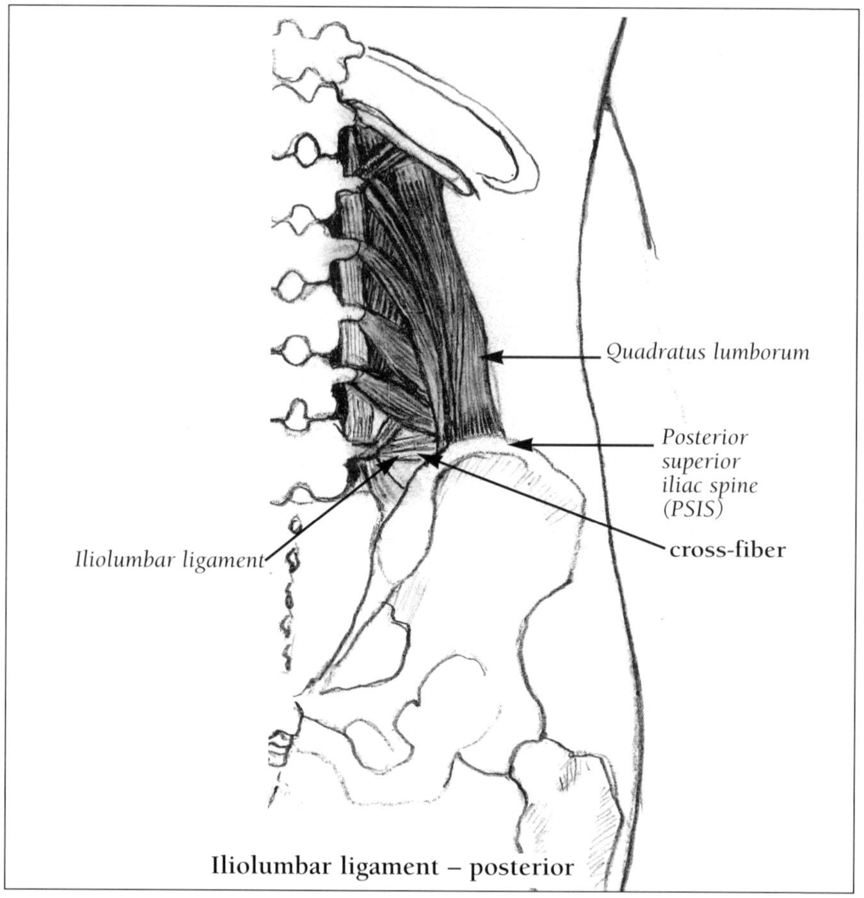

Iliolumbar ligament – posterior

The iliolumbar ligament forms a stabilizing attachment from the anterior surface of the lumbar crest to the transverse processes of L-5 (sometimes L-4). Because it is deep, it is often overlooked as a source of both wake-up, early morning get-out-of-bed lumbar soreness and referred inguinal pain.

Direct thumb pressure, while difficult, only needs to be held for 5 or 6 seconds. Even more effective is cross-fiber friction across the ligament.

To locate the iliolumbar ligament

1. Palpate the posterior superior iliac spine (PSIS) and move slightly medial and then 1 to 1.5 inches up (superior).

2. To confirm the location palpate from the top of the iliac crest straight across to the spine. This is the L4-5 vertebral interspace.

3. Move down to the L-5 spinous process. Now move laterally about an inch to the tip of the L-5 transverse process.

4. The iliolumbar ligament attaches here and sometimes above, at the L-4 transverse process. The other attachment is at the anterior surface of the crest of the posterior ilium.

Treatment

Administer cross-fiber friction or direct pressure.

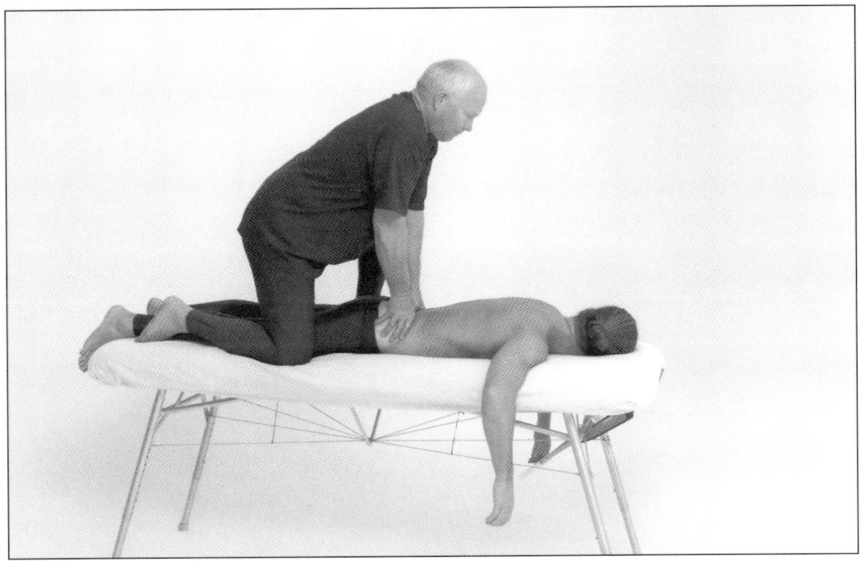

Direct pressure into iliolumbar ligament. On clients with a deep lumbar curve (usually female) work from the head of the table.

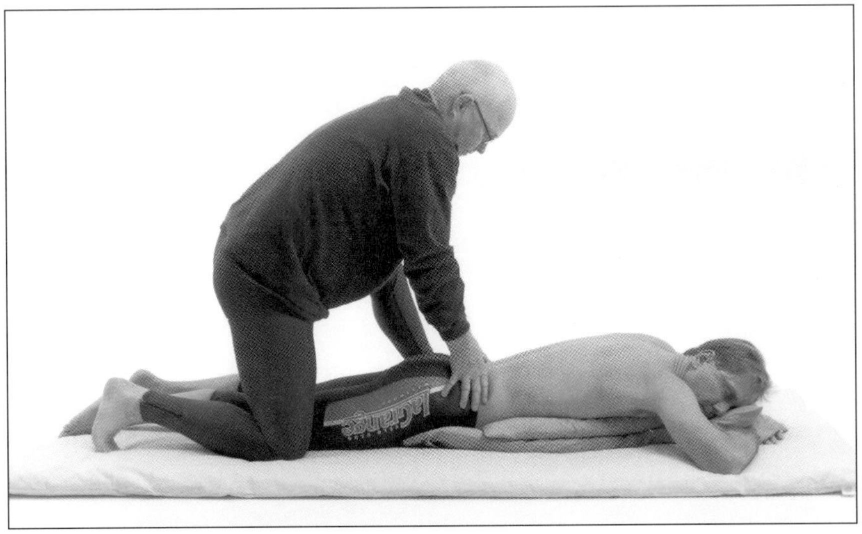

Floor approach.

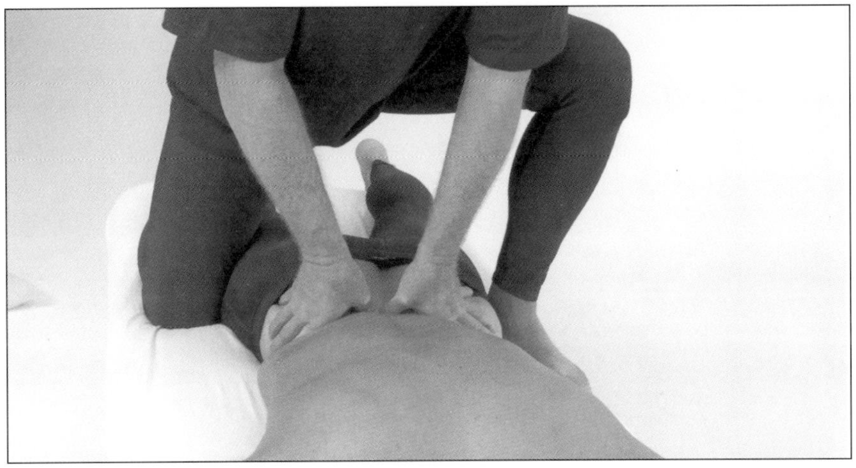

Notice arms are straight but not locked.

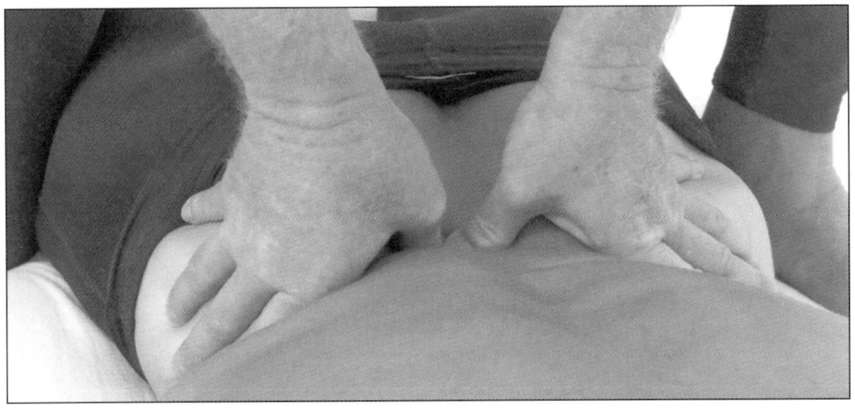

The pressure required is usually strong. Note left thumb pushes on top of right thumb.

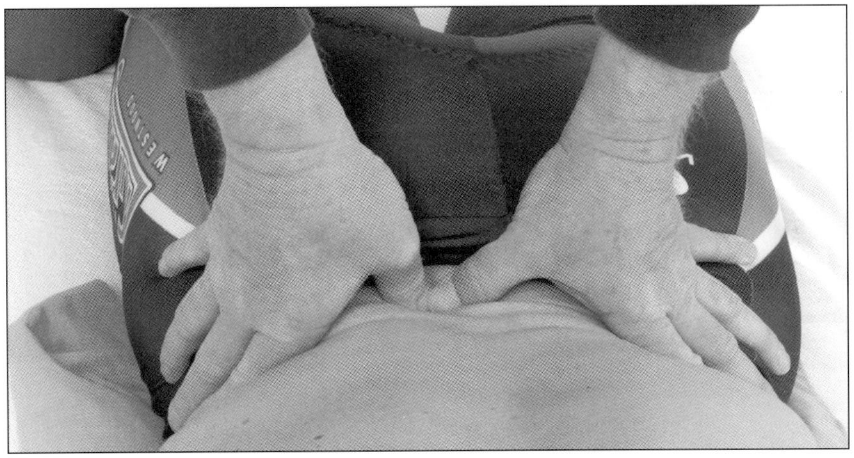

If you have a hypermobile thumb, avoid giving this treatment.

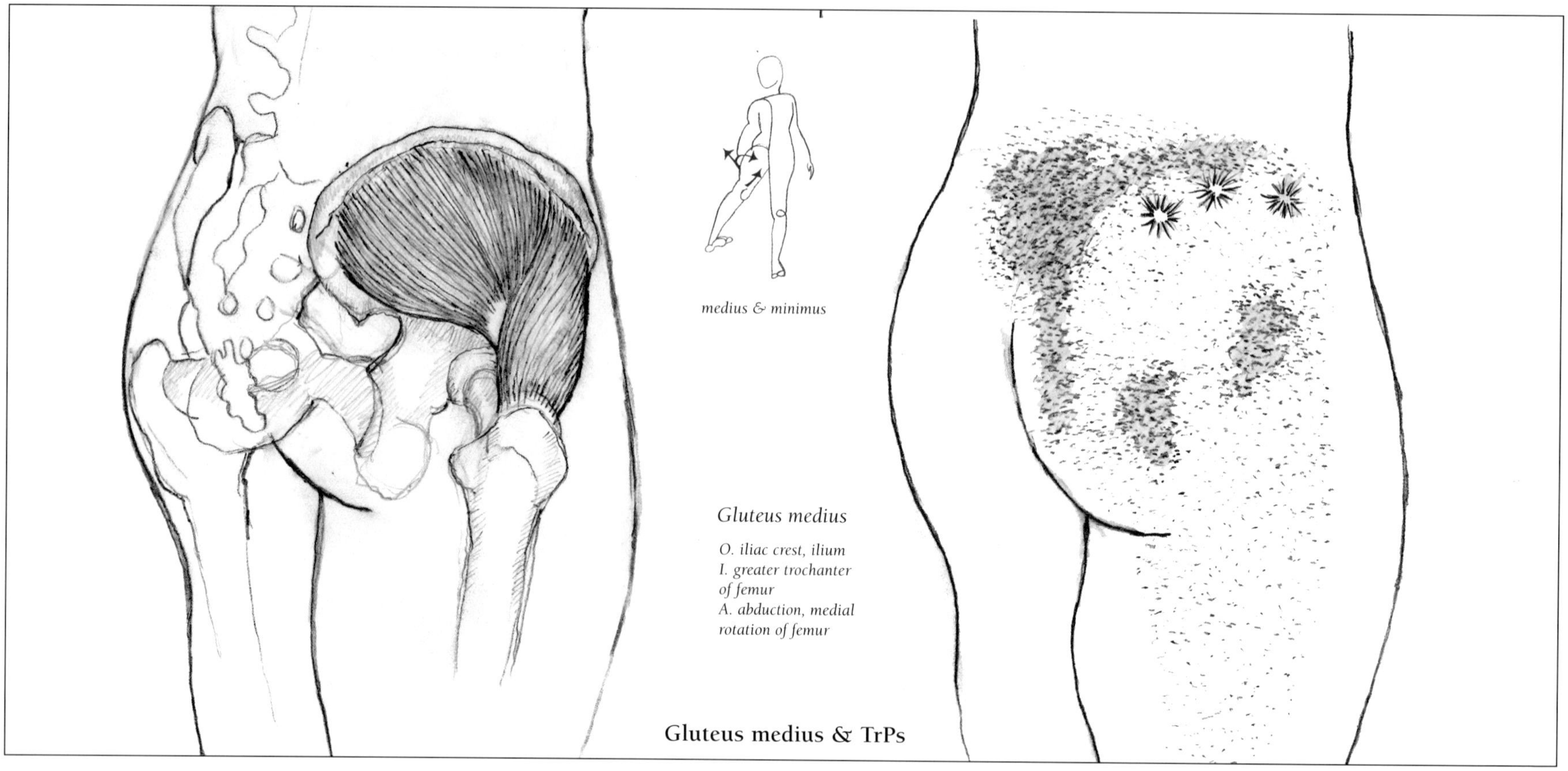

Gluteus medius & TrPs

GLUTEUS MEDIUS

AT LEAST 90% OF LOW BACK PAIN that we've seen is muscular. Of that, 90% involves the gluteus medius in conjunction with the quadratus lumborum and gluteus minimus. These ARE the major troublemakers.

At approximately twice the size of the gluteus minimus, the gluteus medius muscle is a major hip and torso stabilizer whether running, walking or standing on one foot. Athletes, particularly runners, often have over-use problems with this muscle. Muscular development alone won't necessarily protect one from developing trigger points even though well developed muscles are often resistant to trigger points.

You can quickly and effectively work trigger points in this muscle with our feet. While access by hand is initially easy, the large numbers of trigger points and sheer mass of this muscle makes it a real hand-trasher. Use your feet!

Trigger points themselves in the gluteus medius can be extremely painful when compressed – even more painful than their referral pattern. Warm the area thoroughly and enter gradually. Slowly compress trigger points to avoid the sharp pain that causes splinting and armoring. Just one or two applications of direct pressure can often completely clear this muscle of trigger points.

Most therapist-assisted stretches are difficult because of the sheer weight of the client's legs. A client's simple side-bending self-stretch is ideal to complete the treatment

No low back protocol should be utilized without consideration and thorough examination of the gluteus medius.

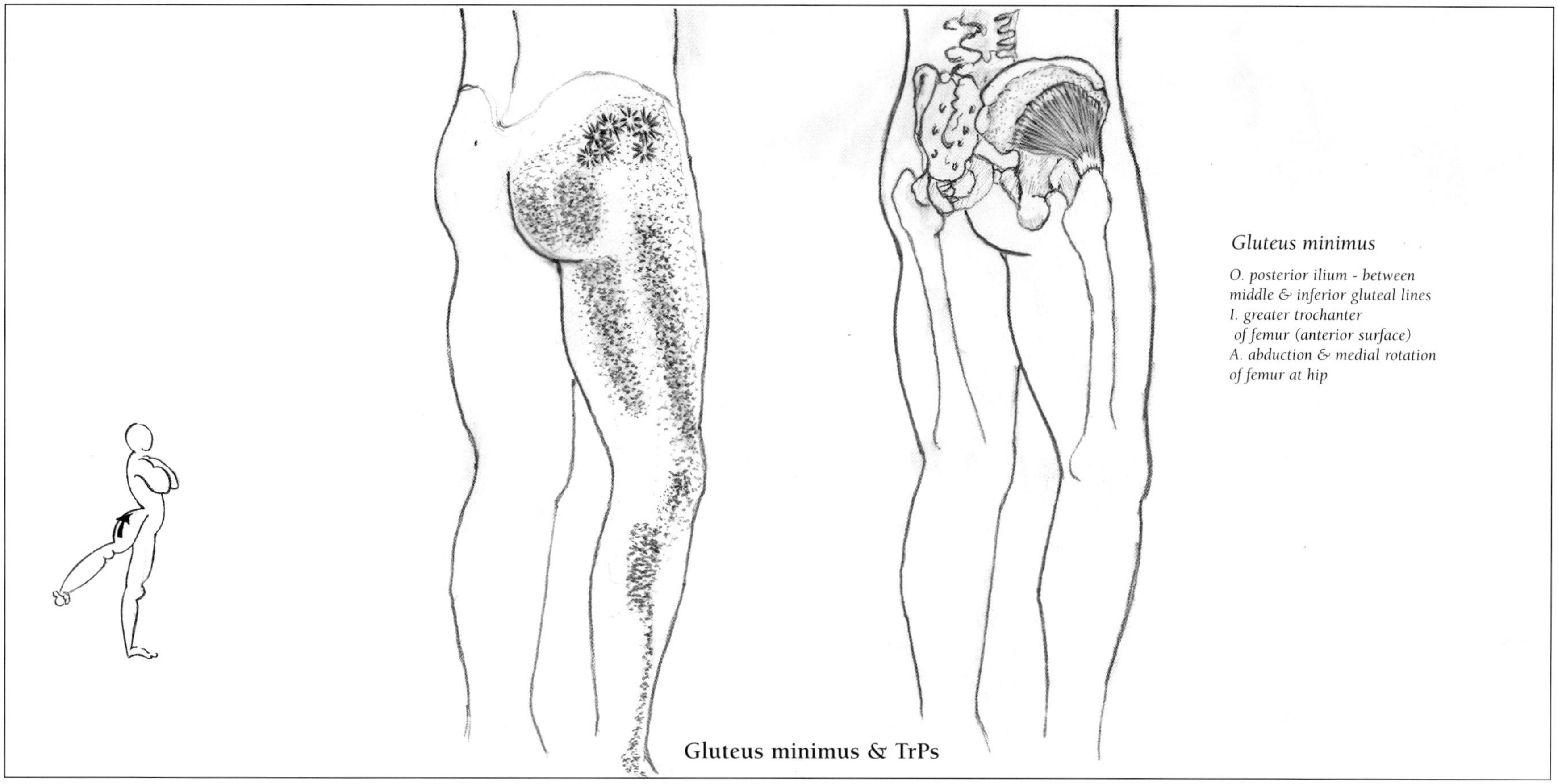

Gluteus minimus & TrPs

Gluteus minimus

The trigger point pain referral pattern of the gluteus minimus, covers a large portion of the vastus lateralis. It is often perceived of as a sciatic pain distribution. If a hands-on evaluation isn't utilized, it is easy to overlook gluteus minimus trigger points and think in terms of discogenic problems caused by nerve root pressure from a bulging disc.

The minimus, while difficult to differentiate from the other over-lying gluteus muscles, is as important to treat in chronic lumbar pain as is the gluteus medius.

Treating the minimus trigger points will often result in a major reduction of chronic pain after the first visit. Advise your clients to use moist heat to prevent post-treatment soreness and to help prevent recurrence of trigger points.

We've had clients who have undergone laminectomy operations (excision of the posterior arch of a vertebra) without success – they still hurt, generally in the region of the hamstrings. This fairly common result has its own label, "post-laminectomy pain syndrome." This pain syndrome can be caused by trigger points in the gluteus minimus, gluteus medius or the piriformis or from sciatic nerve compression by the piriformis.

Be aware of vastus lateralis trigger points or mid-region iliotibial band trigger points also mimicking a sciatic pain pattern.

If treating the gluts, piriformis, and tensor fasciae latae does not completely address the post-laminectomy pain syndrome, look to iliopsoas trigger points either unilaterally or bilaterally.

Greek Toe

If you encounter trigger points in any of the "gluts," the peroneus longus or vastus medialis, check for a 2nd metatarsal that is longer than the first (Morton's Foot or Greek Toe). When the extended 2nd metatarsalphalangeal joint is too prominent, a rocking, destabilized gait pattern results.

Instead of standing on a tripod (consisting of heel and the heads of the first and fifth metatarsals), these folks balance on only two points. Balance on two points is unstable. This instability can effect the ankle, knee, hip, and even the neck. Problems are most often accompanied by a callus on the outside of the big toe, on the bottom of the foot behind the second toe and a "hammer" toed second toe.

The simple cure for this situation is to provide added support in shoes (moleskin works) under the first and fifth toe's metatarsalphalangeal joint. Elevating these joints eliminates the second toes wobble-producing pivot and returns balance to the more stable tripod.

Remember that the gluteus medius overlies the entire gluteus minimus. Pain referrals will tell use which muscle is harboring the TrP. When we treat one, we treat both.

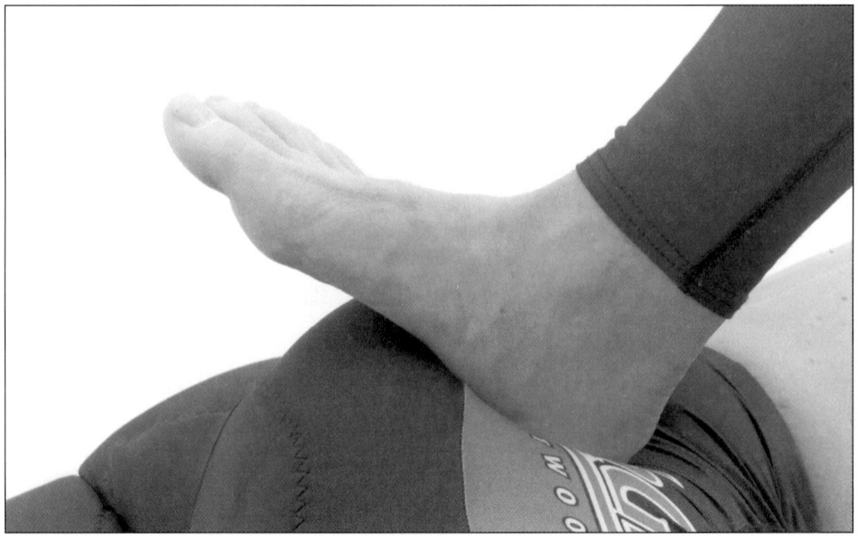

Direct heel pressure into major gluteus medius trigger point. Note therapist's relaxed toes.

Treatment

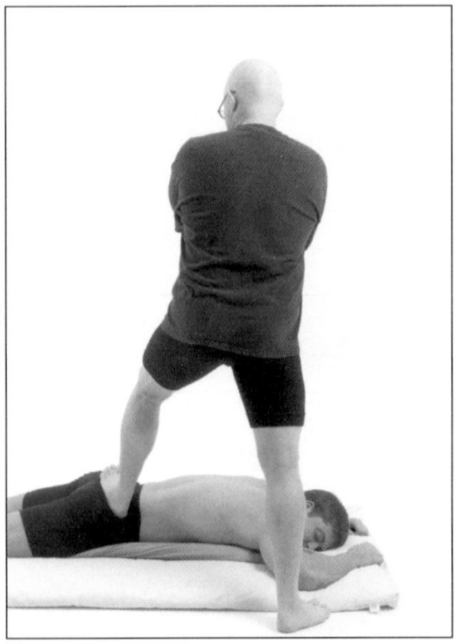

Gluteus medius, gluteus minimus warm-up. Hold for 20 to 30 seconds with a soft foot.

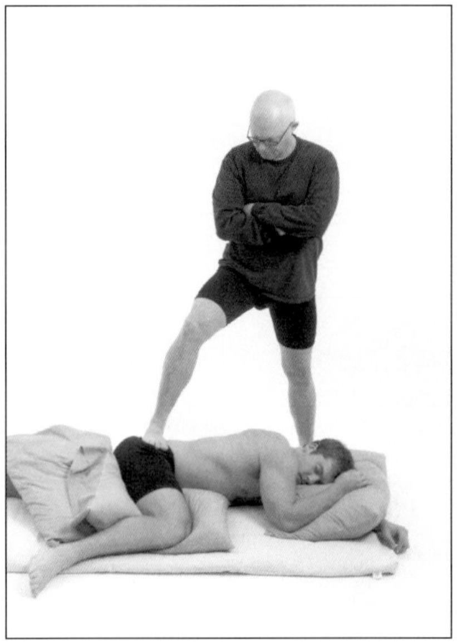

Note foot position for side lying warm-up of gluteus medius/gluteus minimus. Don't let the therapist's relaxed posture fool you – there is approximately 30 pounds of pressure on these muscles.

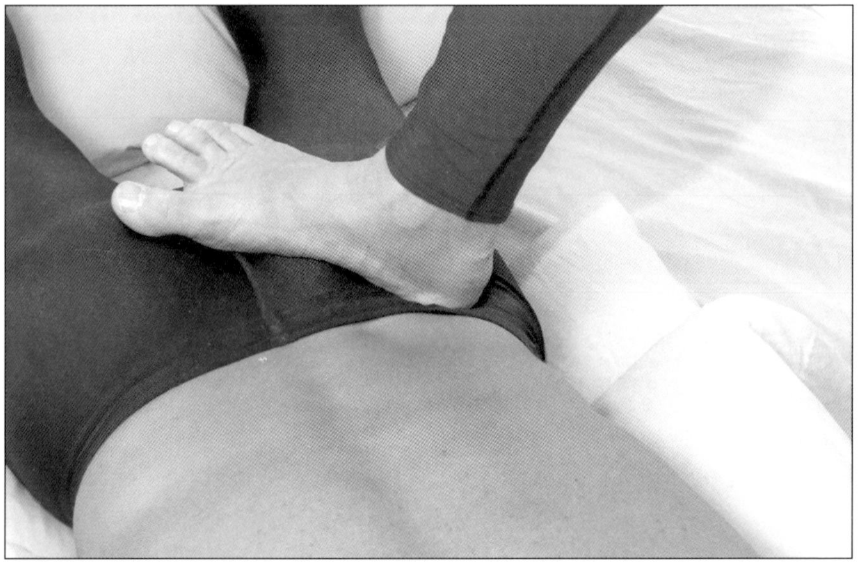

Direct heel pressure into gluteus medius trigger point. The heel is below the posterior pelvic crest.

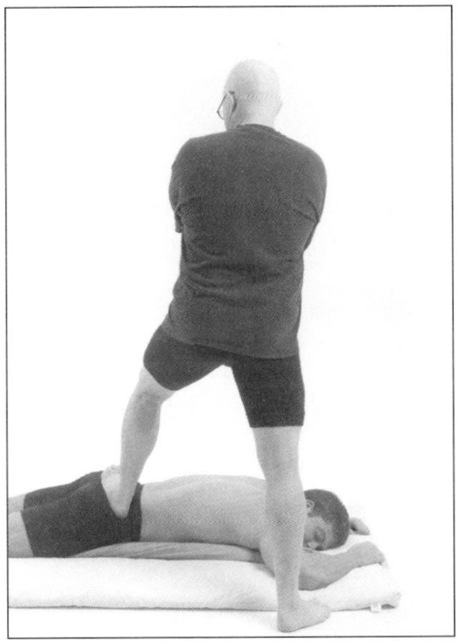

Direct heel pressure into gluteus medius/gluteus minimus trigger points. Even with a substantial portion of the therapist's weight on his support leg, there's now approximately 80 pounds of focused pressure.

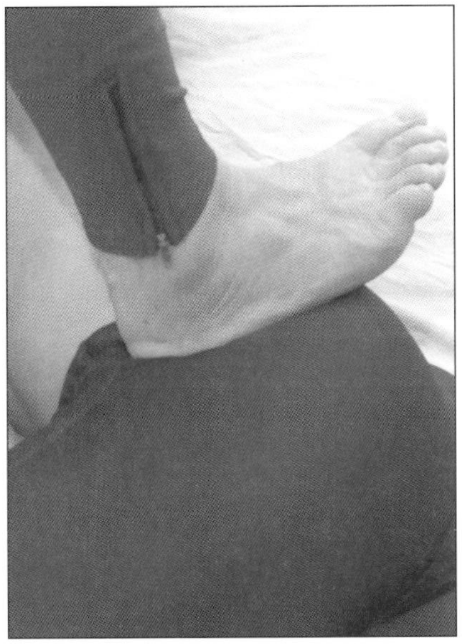

Close-up of direct heel pressure into gluteus medius/gluteus minimus trigger point from a superior position.

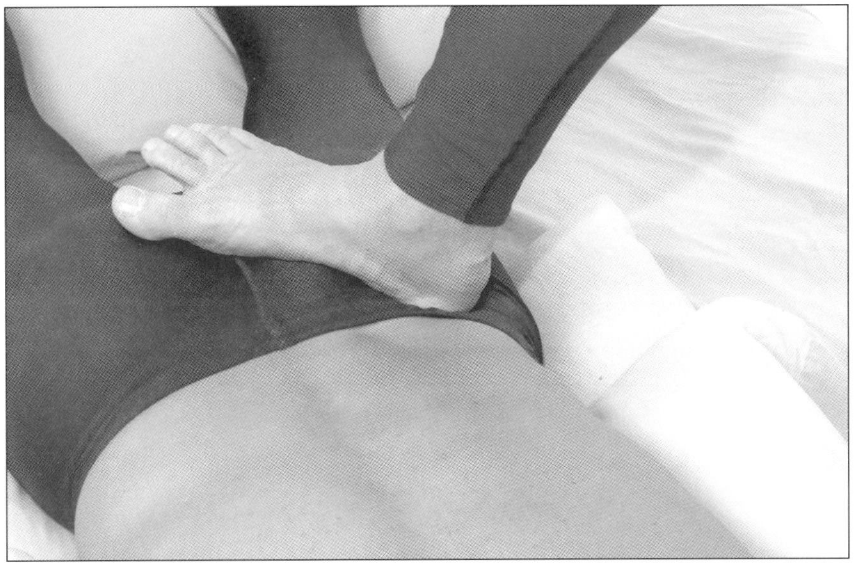

Therapist "gets it just right."

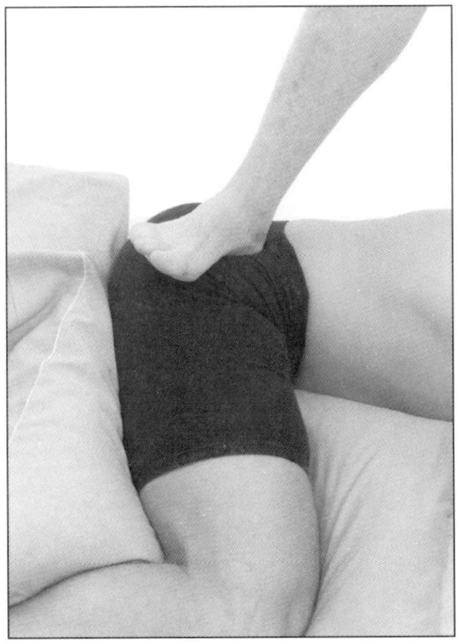

Posterior approach to the gluteus medius trigger point. Note angle of attack with the heel pressing at 45 degrees. Client is well bolstered and doesn't have to suport himself from rolling forward.

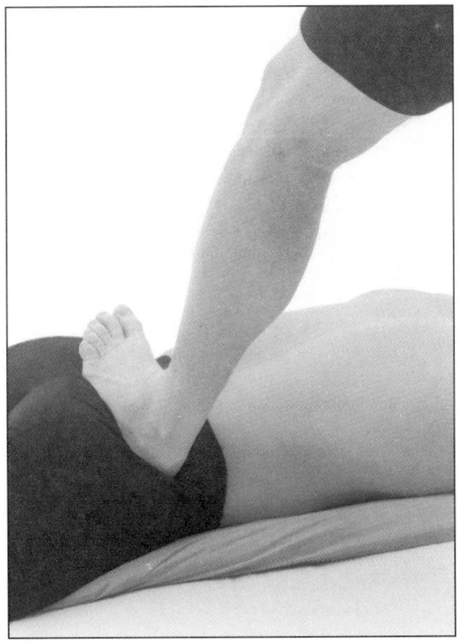

A downward drag prior to direct heel pressure into a medius TrP.

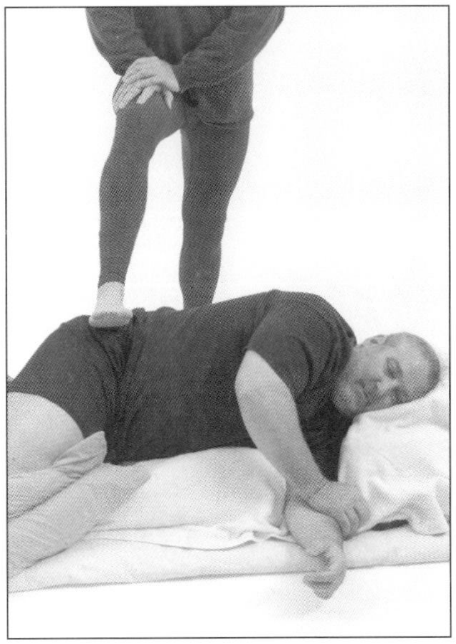

Larger clients require elegant therapist biomechanics…keep your hips level.

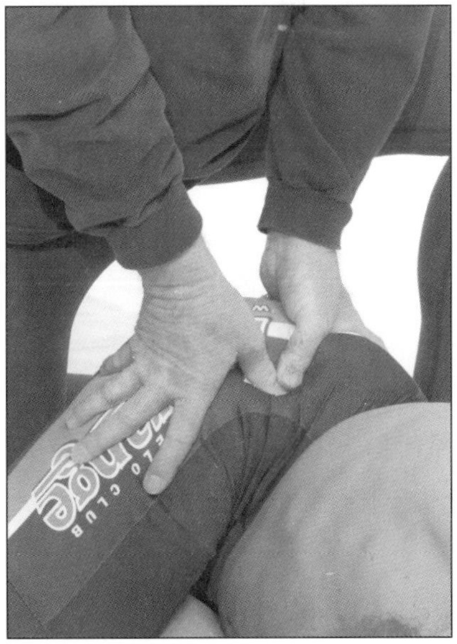

Treatment by Hand – direct thumb on thumb pressure. Elbows are straight but not locked. Sink slowly into the TrP. Don't muscle it – use your weight.

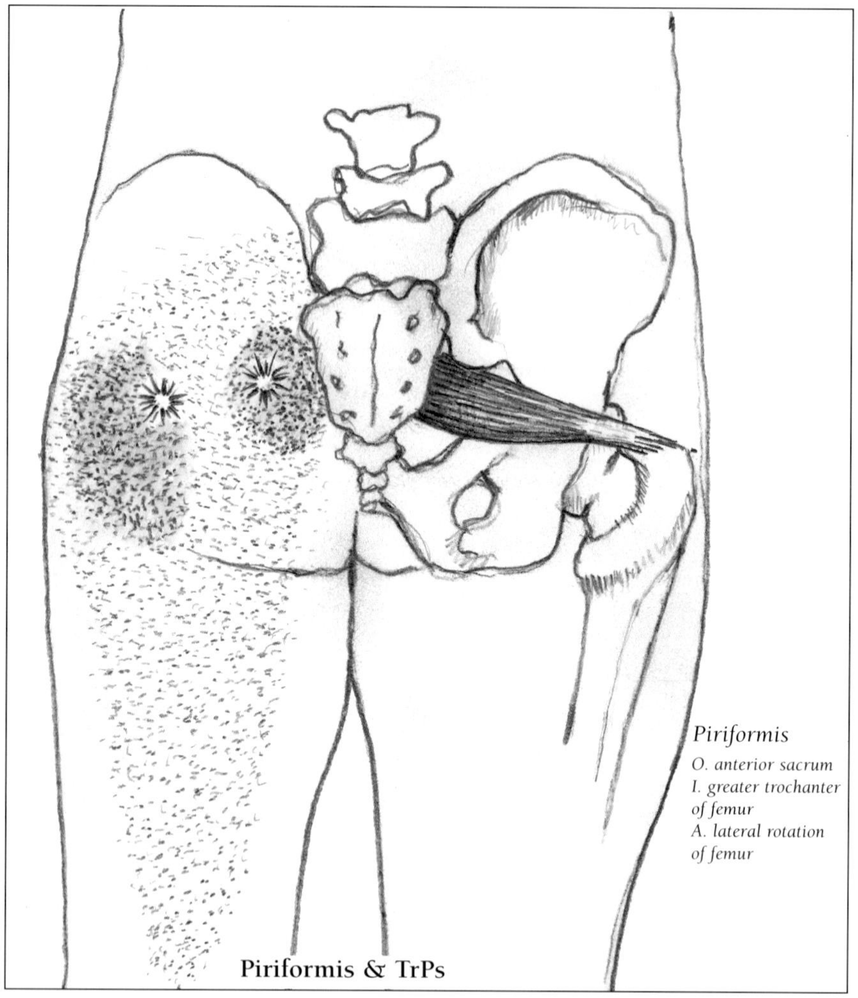

Piriformis & TrPs

MARY'S STORY

Mary, a fine massage therapist, also possessed a tactilely appealing gluteus maximus. Twice in her career, when receiving massages from glut-fixated therapists, she received compression injuries to her sciatic nerve. A high price to pay for overzealous therapy.

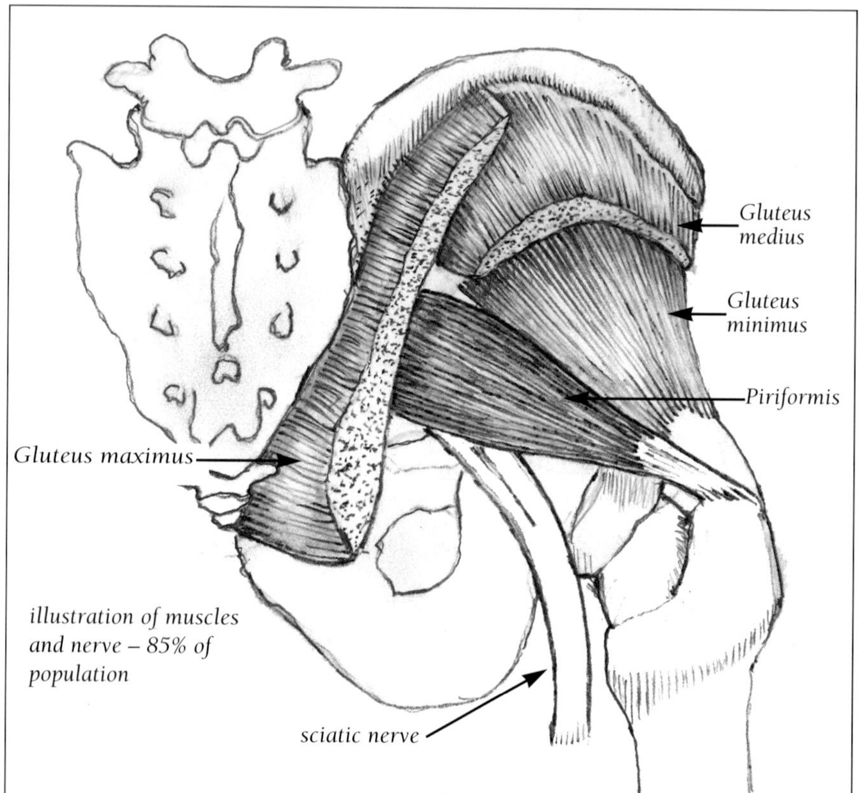

Sciatic Notch & Nerve

THE PIRIFORMIS muscle can entrap or compress the sciatic nerve and cause pain down the leg. The piriformis muscle can also have trigger points that cause (refer) similar pain patterns. No sciatic pain assessment is complete without trigger point palpation of this lateral rotator.

The piriformis should be palpated for trigger points if pain is experienced:

- in the hip
- posterior thigh
- down the back of the leg to the foot
- in the inguinal region of the groin
- while defecating.

Similar pain patterns can also be caused when nerves and blood vessels are pressed against the edge of the greater sciatic foramen.

On rare occasion, the nerve passes through the belly of the piriformis and can be entrapped. Releasing trigger points in the piriformis, followed by active or passive stretching, will take the tension out of the muscle. This allows it to relax and de-entrap, releasing pressure on the nerve.

Nerve compression can also occur when an enlarged piriformis muscle pushes the neurovascular bundle against the bony rim of the sciatic foramen. Because the piriformis nerve fibers, both motor and sensory, seem to be extremely sensitive to prolonged compression, this can be a very important source of pain.

When treating the piriformis it is critical to also treat the secondary trigger points found in the gluteus medius and gluteus minimus and the "go-gos." In our experience, many bodyworkers often mistake the "go-gos" (gemellus superior, obturator internus, gemellus inferior, obturator externus and quadratus femoris – all deep lateral rotators of the hip) for the piriformis.

The easiest way to make sure you are on the piriformis is to put your middle finger on top of the sacrum/coccyx intersection and thumb on top of the greater trochanter. Then find the midpoint and mark it with your index finger. Move just superior to this point, and you'll be on the belly of the piriformis.

Hooking the fingers on the posterior crest and rubbing the thumb transversely across the muscle is the easiest way to find the trigger point. A jump response and a sciatic pain pattern indicate trigger points are present. Treat the trigger point with direct pressure. If the piriformis is short and tight, but free of trigger points, treat by performing a CRAC stretch.

Caution

Don't compress the sciatic nerve for prolonged periods. The large sciatic nerve can be injured both by too long or too much pressure. Use special care while treating the trigger points near the greater sciatic foramen.

Special Note

Gluteals being held in chronic tension create male erectile problems and impotence. A tight, swollen piriformis can also impinge on pudendal nerves and blood vessels leading to inguinal (groin) pain. It can also cause frigidity in women and interfere with normal sexual function in both men and women.

Occasionally, trigger points are found at the origin of the piriformis on the anterior sacrum These can be palpated and treated either intrarectally of intravaginally. We refer these clients to osteopaths.

To locate the piriformis

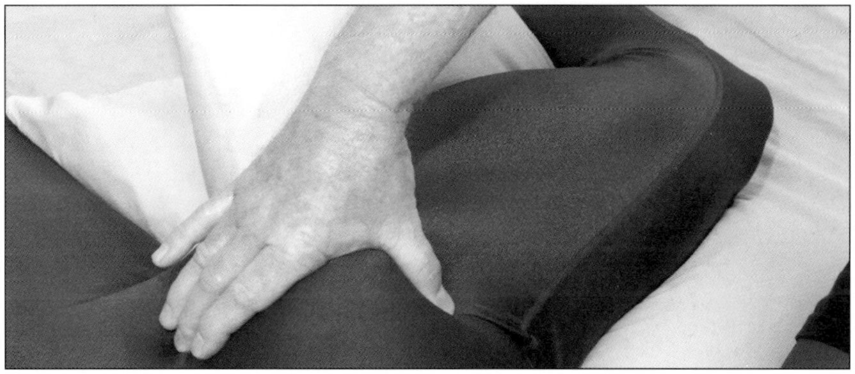

Place thumb on superior aspect of greater trochanter with middle finger resting on sacrum just above coccyx.

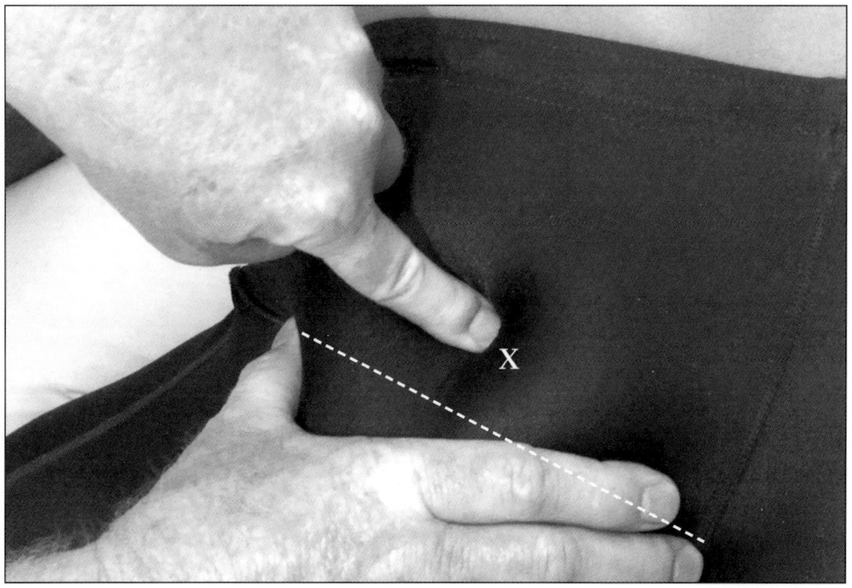

The piriformis is just superior to an imaginary line between your thumb and middle finger.

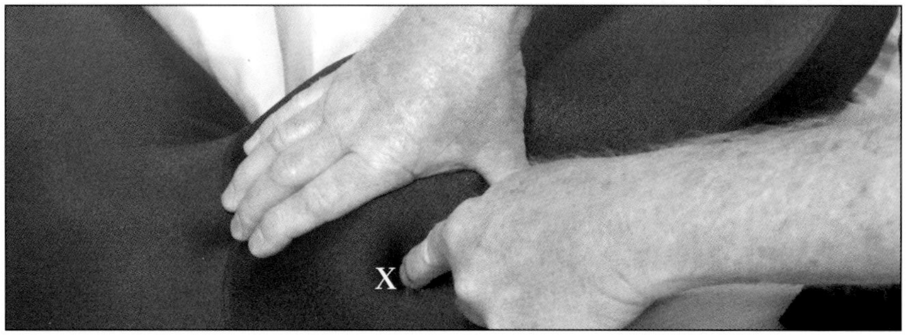

Major trigger points are found right here.

Treatment

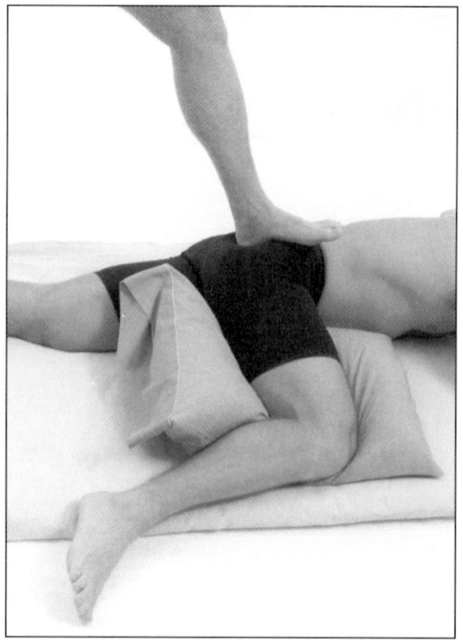

Direct pressure to the medial inferior portion of the piriformis. The client's hip is flexed and well bolstered.

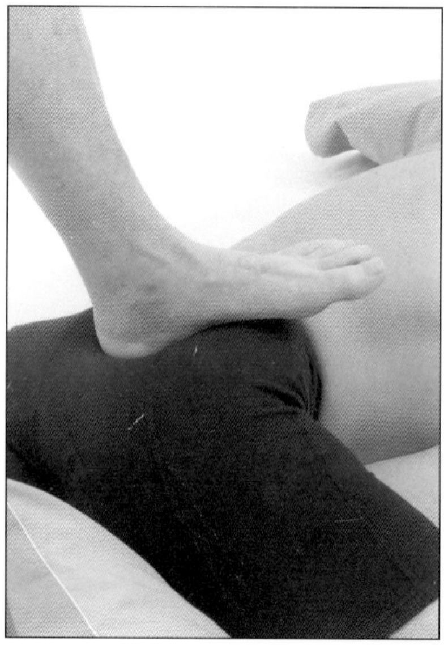

Exercise care to avoid direct pressure over the sciatic nerve.

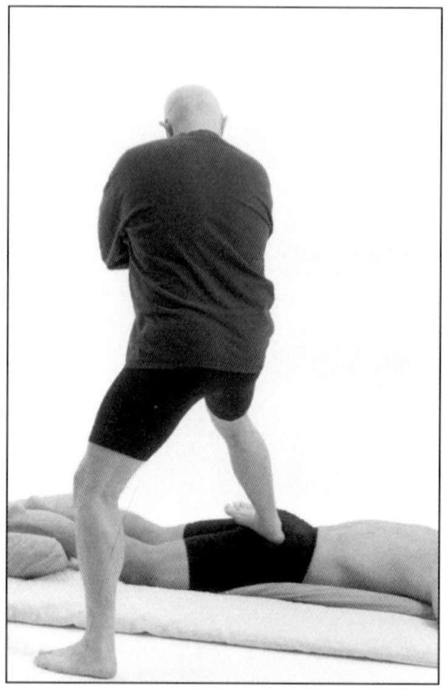

Another approach.

Serratus Posterior Inferior

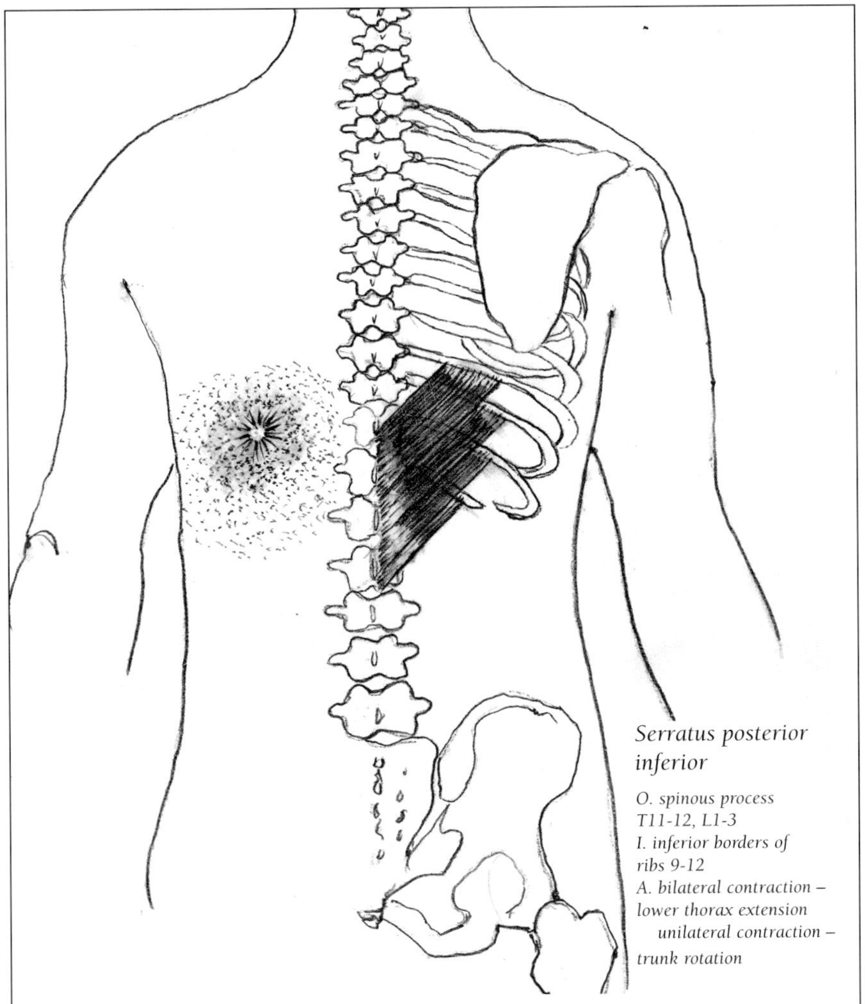

Serratus posterior inferior & TrPs

WHILE NOT REFERRING PAIN DIRECTLY into the lower back, these muscles seem to play a role in "locking-in" trigger points in the adjacent quadratus lumborum. This muscle may assist in forced exhalation pulling down and stabilizing the 9th through the 12th rib, although some myographic studies indicate otherwise.

It is unusual to find a case of muscular low back pain that doesn't have an extremely tender concomitant trigger point in the serratus posterior inferior.

Treatment

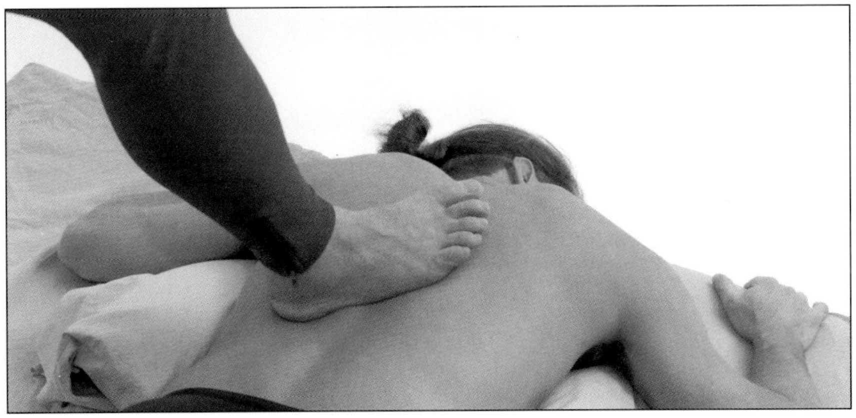

Direct heel pressure to the serratus posterior inferior trigger point. This TrP is generally found at the level of the 10th rib (just lateral to the bulk of the superficial paraspinal back muscles). Use your thumb (not your heel) on smaller clients.

Treatment by hand

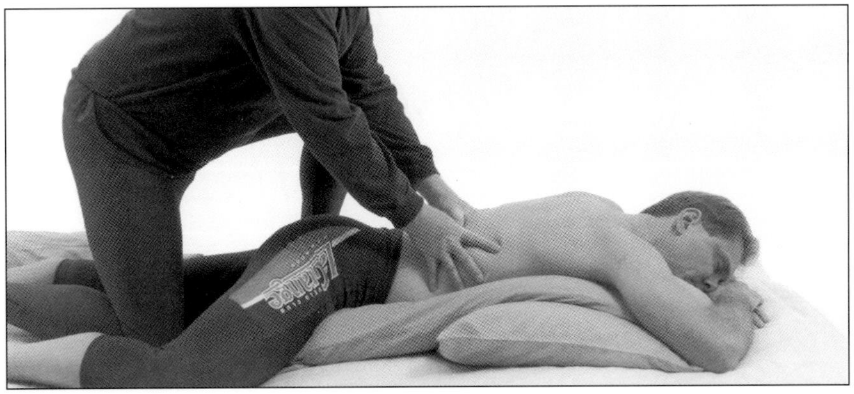

Note client bolstering and balanced therapist posture.

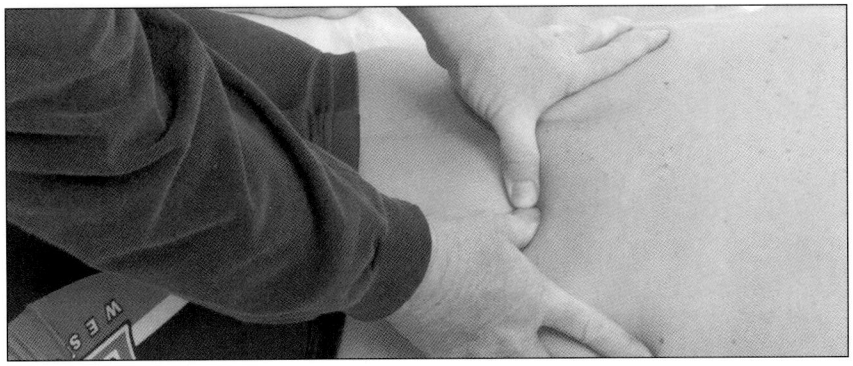

Thumb on thumb leaning into direct pressure.

Gluteus Maximus

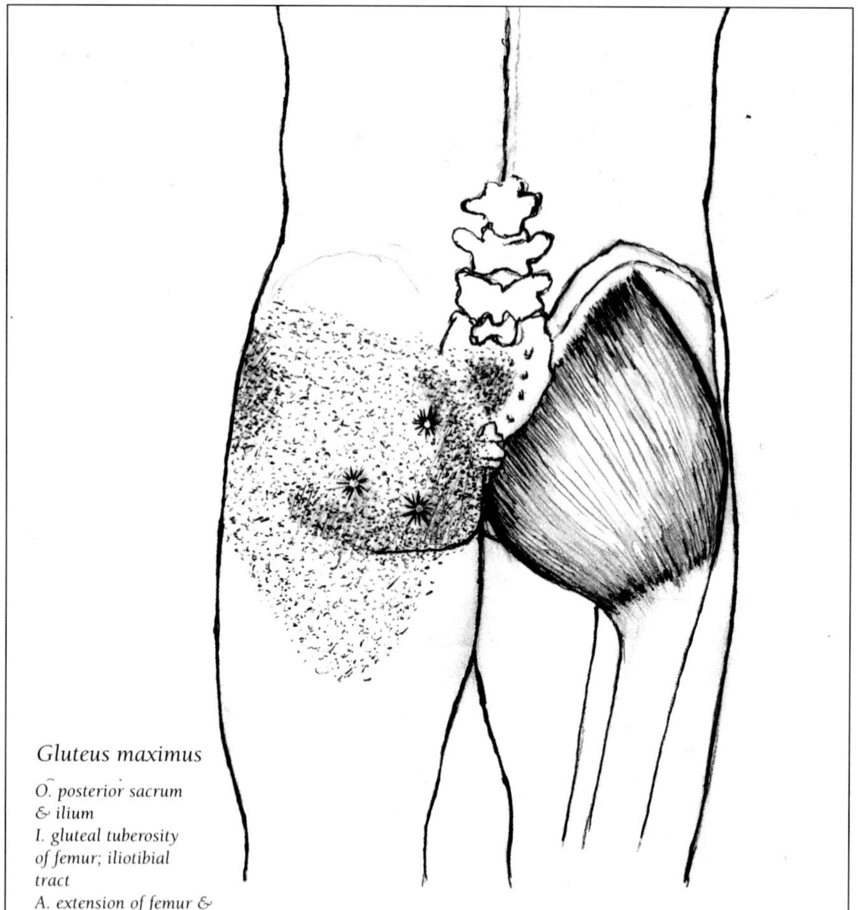

Gluteus maximus & TrPs

THE GLUTEUS MAXIMUS, while a secondary player in chronic low back pain, should still be treated in any lumbar pain protocol. This muscle can be severely stressed by prolonged sitting or by strenuous stair or hill climbing.

Pincer palpation can be the ideal method for treating trigger points in this muscle, but the sheer volume of the maximus makes it extremely difficult for many therapists to handle by hand. The heel works wonderfully.

Treat gluteus maximus trigger points so they won't rekindle trigger points in the other gluts – those that do play a more direct role in the generation of low back pain.

In some clients, the gluteus maximus is continuously contracted, often because of fear or habit. This results in formation of active and/or latent trigger points.

Some male clients will suffer reduced sexual desire and functioning because of the chronic tightening in the gluteal muscles. For women, this "holding" can result in frigidity. Treatment is enhanced client awareness. With awareness, clients can learn to relax their gluteals.

The Relax method

Ask your client to squeeze their glutes as tightly as possible while noting the sensation. Then ask them to relax and notice the difference. Repeat several times. These consecutive actions lead to greater awareness of holding patterns, and, over time, the ability to change the pattern to one of more relaxed gluteals. This protocol uses post-isometric relaxation to augment an awareness of relaxation.

Clients, with practice, will experience major changes in their holding patterns. Most afflicted folks will have to repeat this practice many times over an extended period (up to 6 months). Usually, within this time frame, they will feel the difference between tight and relaxed, and be able to maintain relaxation. Some clients use reminders such as Day-Glo dots placed on mirrors and in other commonly frequented locations to remind themselves to "let go."

Take care not to over-treat – don't become glut-fixated. Remember the sciatic notch and pencil-size sciatic nerve is covered by a major portion of the gluteus maximus. Injuries have occurred from overzealous gluteal kneading, stroking, and pressing. For best results whenever you work near major nerves, use the minimum effective amount of pressure and duration.

> The minimal therapy that will accomplish the job is the most effective therapy.

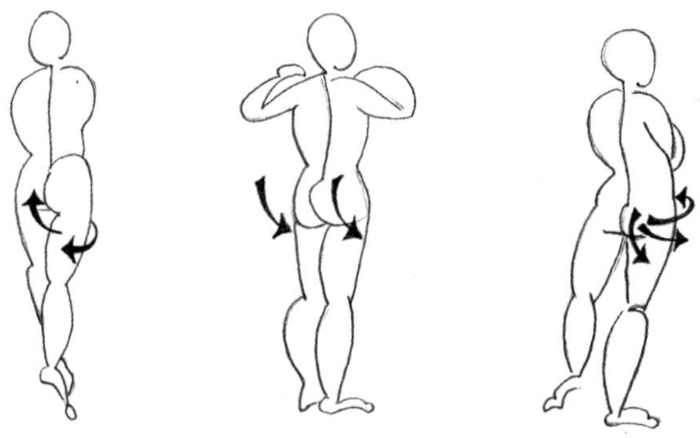

Treatment

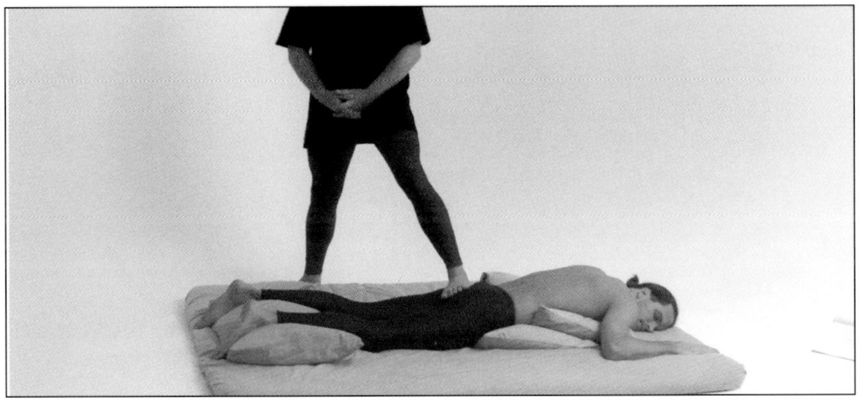

Gluteus maximus warm up. Note client bolstering and the therapist's relaxed posture and soft foot. Support leg is straight with knee unlocked.

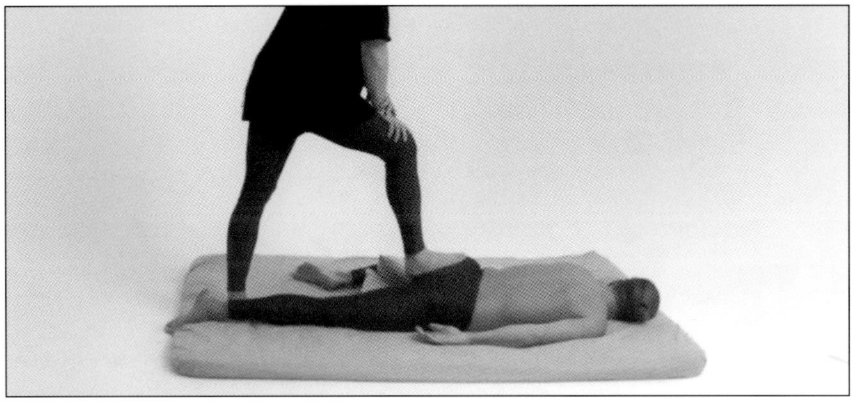

Alternative gluteus maximus warm-up. Hip bolstered with maximus on a moderate stretch.

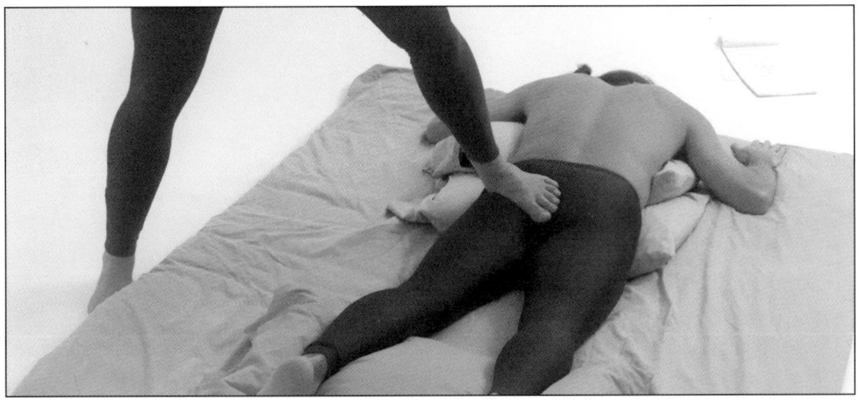

Gluteus maximus warm-up. Support leg is not on the futon. Moderate pressure is used. The success of the warm-up relies on the duration of the compression (approximately 20 seconds) to warm the tissue.

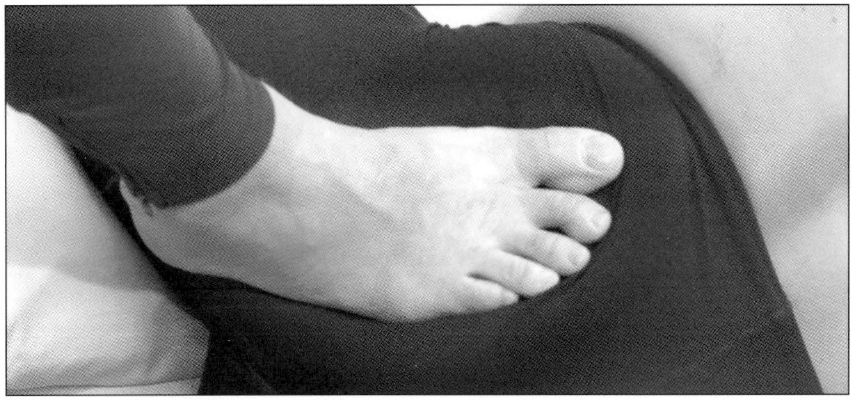

Warm-up close-up.

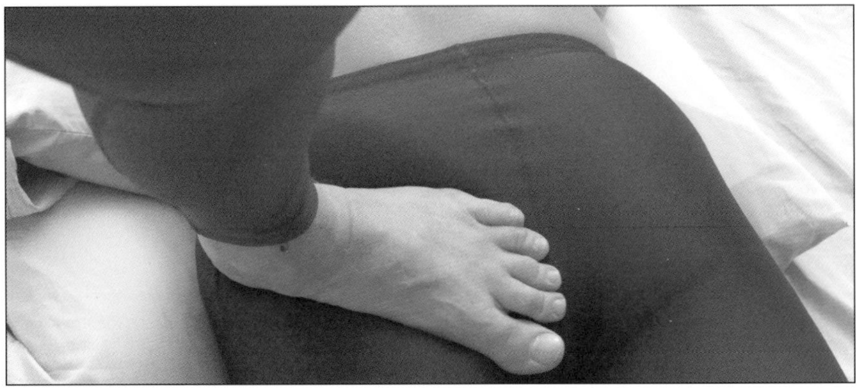

Knee over ankle equals less ankle stress.

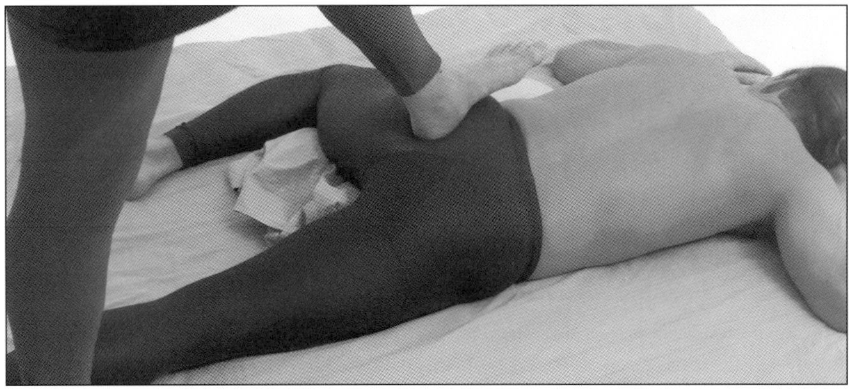

Direct pressure to a gluteus maximus TrP adjacent to the sciatic notch. Avoid direct pressure to the sciatic nerve.

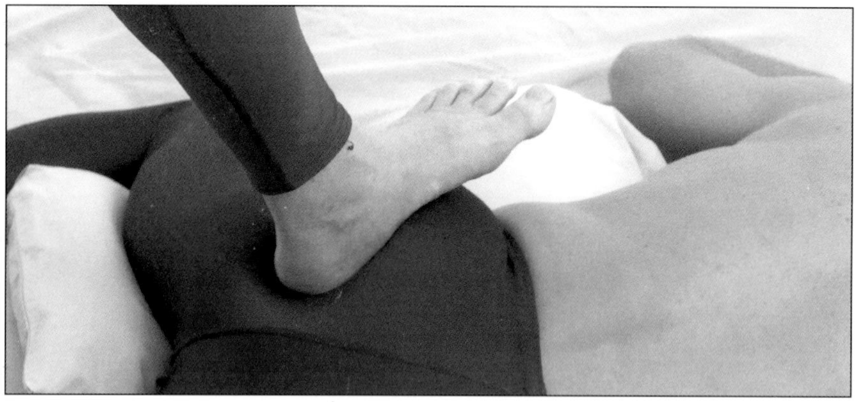

Direct pressure with a relaxed foot in moderate dorsiflexion.

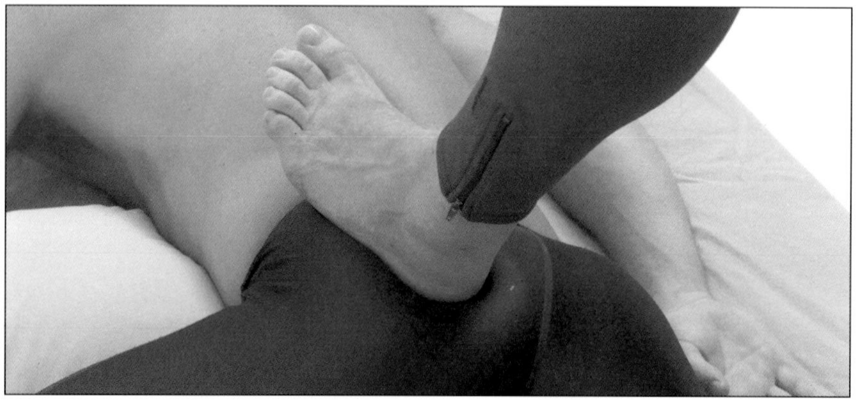

A broad heel is less painful than a thumb or elbow.

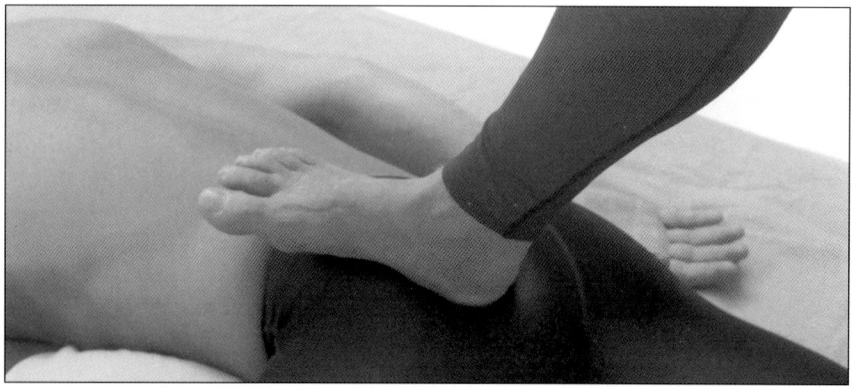

Protect support leg. Change feet frequently and take advantage of alternative angles of attack. Rotate your heel to stretch muscles.

Rectus abdominis

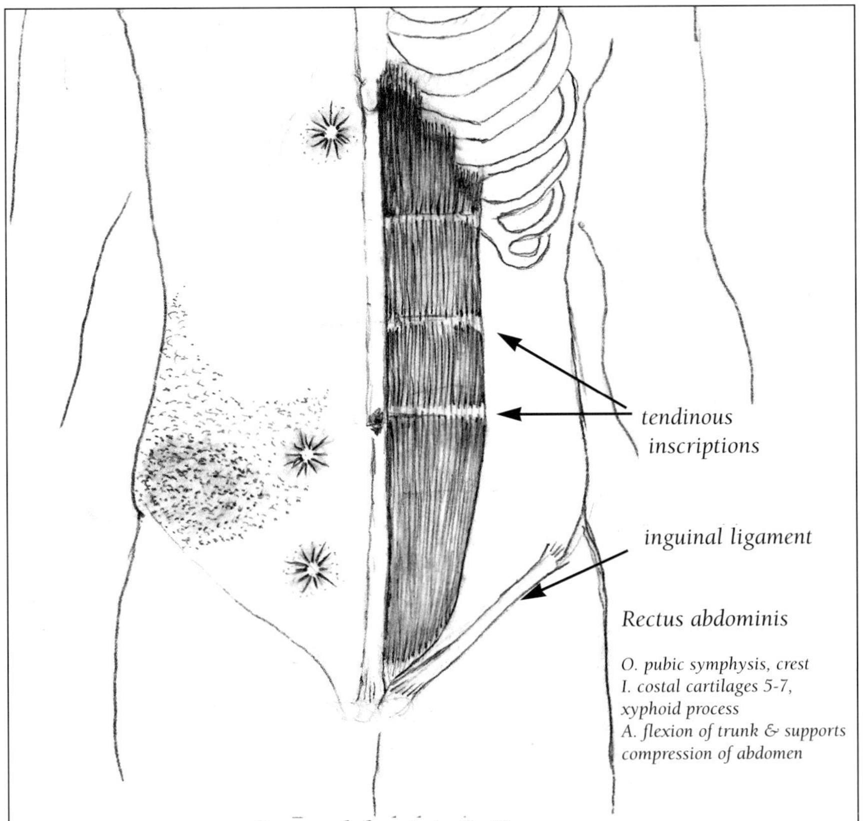

Recus abdominis & Trps

THE RECTUS ABDOMINIS attachments are frequently overlooked as a source of both mid and low-back chronic pain. Trigger points at the costal cartilage attachment of the ribs will refer in a wide band of pain across the mid-back. Trigger points in the pubic attachment are very common in people who do countless crunches or sit-ups. They refer a wide band of pain across the lumbo-sacral region just above the top of the ilium.

When the usual protocol of quadratus lumborum, gluteus medius, gluteus minimus, and piriformis doesn't yield results, go to the rectus abdominis. No need for feet here. Direct pressure with the thumb-braced-thumb will be efficient and effortless.

When some therapists push against trigger points on the rectus abdominis at the costal cartilage attachments, they use an incorrect vector to apply the direct pressure. Some practice may be required to get this application just right.

Trigger points in this muscle can mimic appendicitis and other visceral pains. We don't treat clients with the symptoms of appendicitis without first referring them for medical evaluation.

It is important for us to refer to a physician with knowledge of manual medicine. We recommend conservative treatments before more invasive ones. Sometimes who you see is what you get.

In many cases chronic pain is fairly straightforward and resolves with direct, soft tissue approaches. In other cases there seems to be such an interplay of emotion, nutrition, attitude, and stressful circumstances (past and present) that an intellectual understanding of the problem becomes difficult – possibly irrelevant.

We do what we can. If there isn't substantial improvement in 3 or 4 visits, we refer. This is our practice and, we think, a good policy.

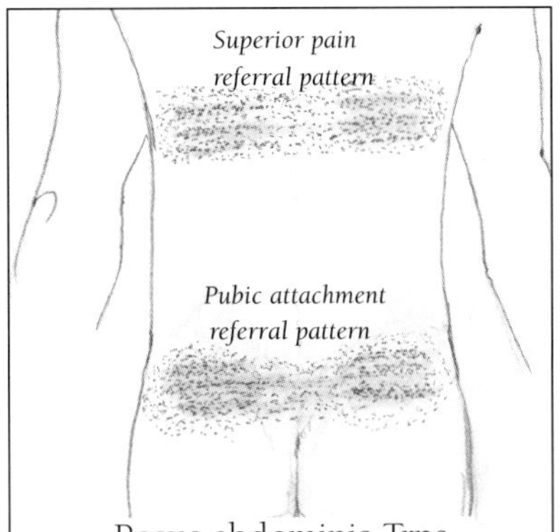

Recus abdominis Trps

Treating trigger points at both the origin and insertion of this muscle often aborts menstrual cramps. If done as a preventive treatment, cramps usually won't occur. As often observed in our workshops, cramps will diminish or cease 5 to 10 minutes after treatment.

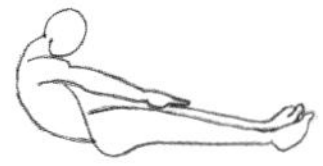

HER STORY

One young client had undergone two exploratory surgeries for bowel pain. Upon examination, we found trigger points that caused abdominal pain. Several treatments resolved her pain. We refrained from asserting TrPs as the cause. We don't diagnose.

The rectus abdominis is one of the few muscles that has referral patterns that cross the midline of the body. A trigger point in the right side can refer to the left. Trigger points here can also contribute to or be the cause of diarrhea.

Treatment

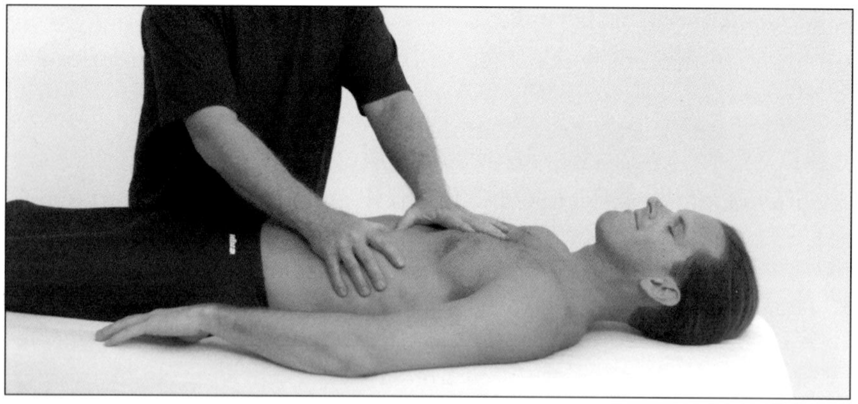

Address rectus abdominis trigger points from the opposite side of the body. Do not press on the xiphoid process. Trigger points are located from the xiphoid process all along the costal cartilage to the end of the rectus attachment.

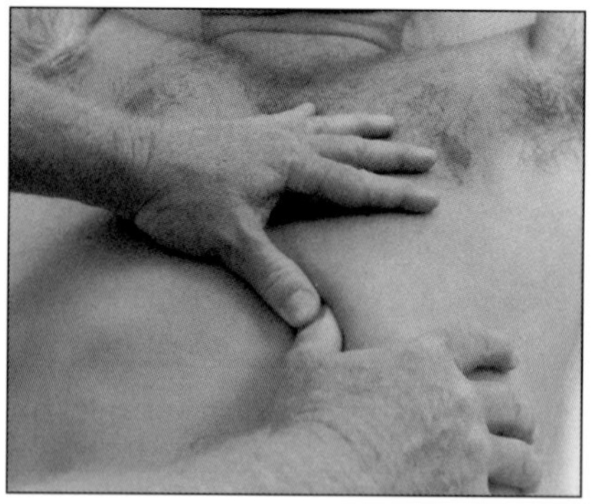

Direct pressure to the edge of the costal cartilage. The braced thumb pushes directly against the trigger point. The thumb is NOT under the rib pushing toward the diaphragm.

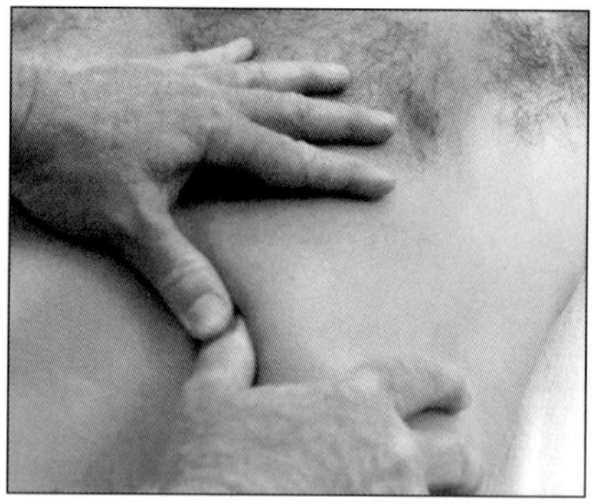

Use the broad aspect of the thumb and not the tip. This is less invasive and doesn't "jam" your thumb joints.

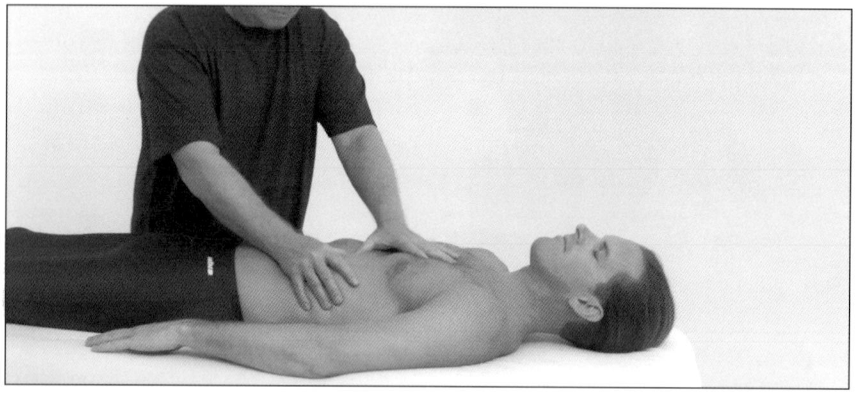

Palpate the lateral edge of the rectus abdominis (a client crunch helps delineate the muscle). This will be the outermost point for trigger points along the costal cartilage of the ribs.

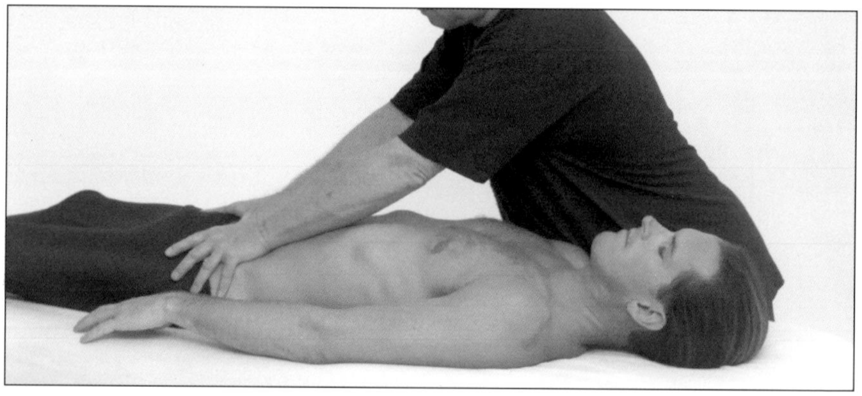

Direct pressure to the rectus abdominis attachment at the pubic crest. Gently sink into the muscle and push caudalward.

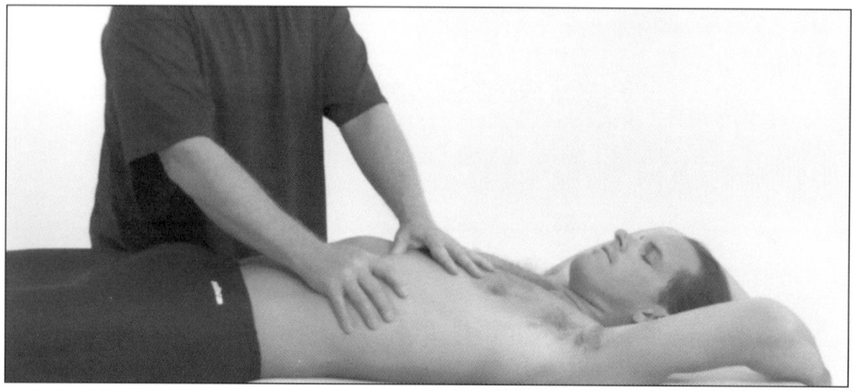

A slight stretch on the rectus abdominis potentiates the TrP treatment.

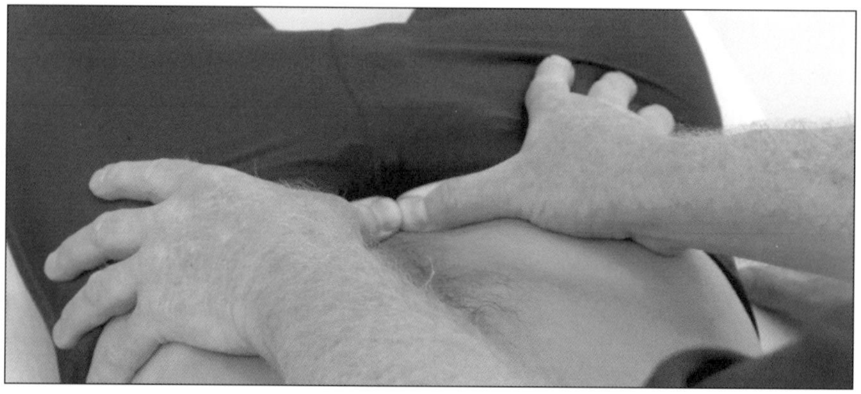

Hand position for ease of access to trigger points and client's emotional comfort.

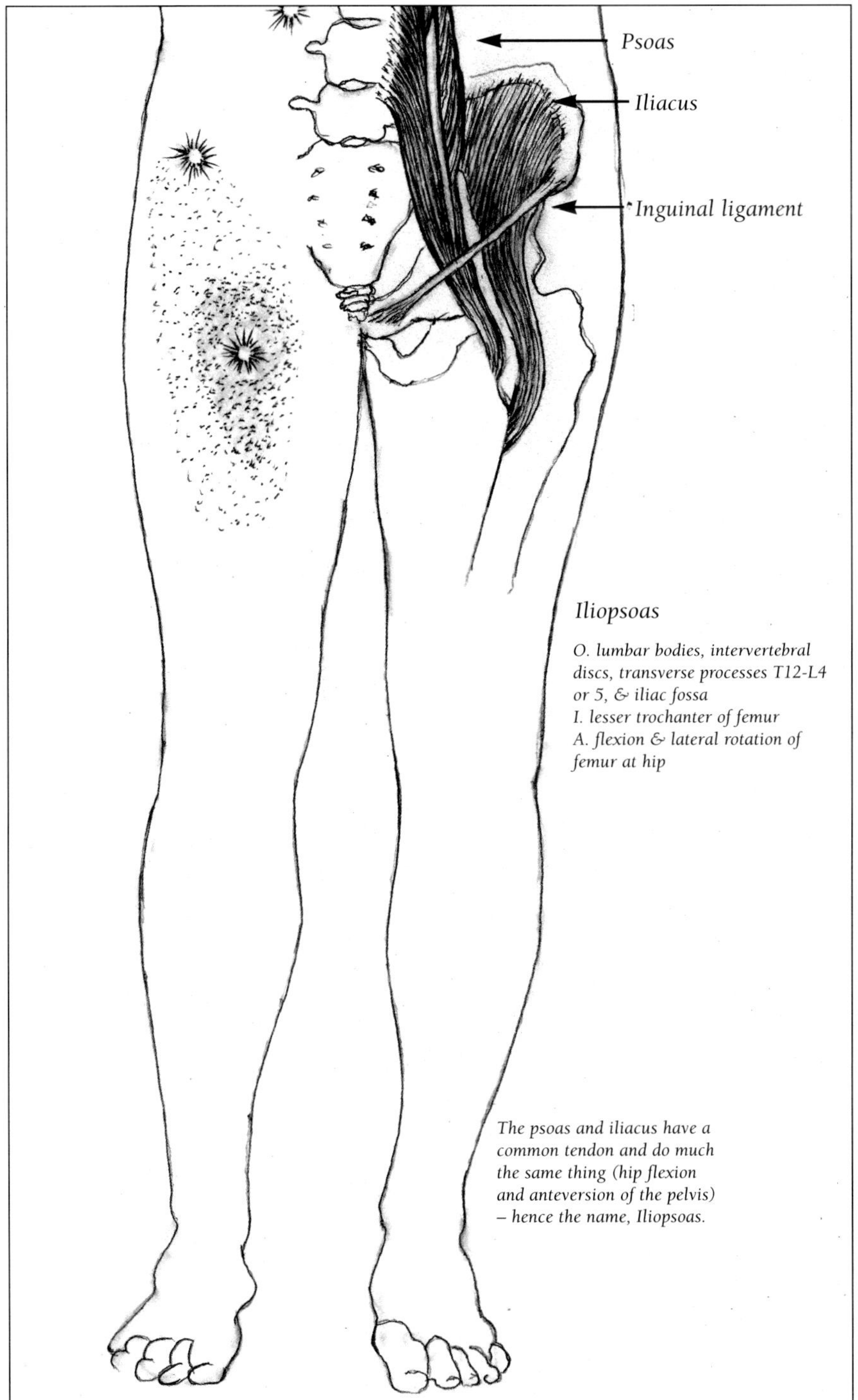

Psoas major / Iliacus & TrPs

THE PSOAS MAJOR and iliacus together comprise the iliopsoas. We've elected not to consider the psoas minor, since it purportedly exists in fewer than 1 in 5 people. Shortening and tightness of the iliopsoas are evident in those whose walk is stooped with an externally rotated leg.

A paradox exists with this muscle. Shortness can result in either a flattened lumbar curve, or paradoxically, in a hyperlordosis. Shortness will exaggerate the client's pre-existing lumbar tendencies. We find the majority of short psoas muscles (often unilateral) in men. In our experience, 10 to 15% of lumbar pain involves the psoas and/or iliacus. Test for shortness in the psoas.

Trigger points in the iliopsoas refer along the lower thoracic and lumbar paraspinals and/or down the front of the leg in the rectus femoris. Trigger point releases followed by stretching of this muscle have a strong salutary effect on walking, running and posture.

This is the muscle that coaches and trainers always warn neophytes about when doing straight leg sit-ups or leg-lifts. Because the muscle not only attaches to vertebral bodies, but also to the intervertebral discs, unilateral shortness may play a role in creating herniated discs in the lumbar region.

In our early days of teaching work on the psoas, our standing joke was that anyone who had their psoas lengthened by a stretch would feel like the "Keep-On-Truckin'" man in the Zap Comic strips… torsos just couldn't seem to keep up with their legs. We also found that unlocking the pelvis can lead to a flooding of sexual feeling. As ethical practitioners, we made a point of calling the client's home to warn their significant other.

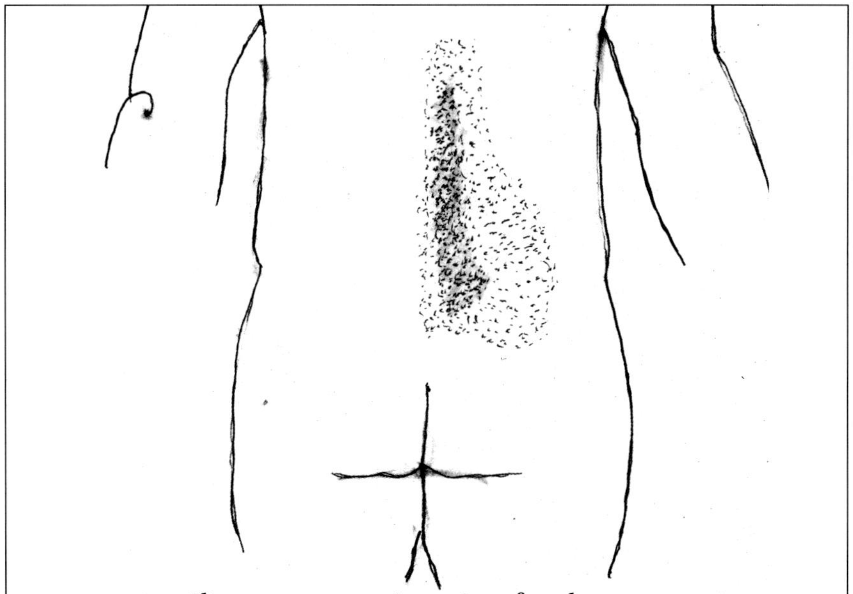

Iliopsoas – posterior pain referral pattern

Occasionally, tendonitis can occur in the musculotendinous juncture. This juncture is located in the inguinal triangle just medial to the sartorius. Cross-fiber friction works best for treating tendonitis in this region. Resisted hip flexion with pain is an indicator of iliopsoas tendonitis. Do not friction across the femoral artery, vein, and nerve. They are usually located just medial to the iliopsoas's musculotendinous juncture. With the hip passively flexed, find the femoral artery just below the inguinal ligament (you'll feel the pulse) and move slightly lateral. Between the femoral artery and the sartorius, you'll find the musculotendinous juncture of the iliopsoas – the likely spot for the tendonitis. It will be tender.

The psoas can shorten in response to prolonged sitting or squatting. Cab drivers, baseball catchers, tennis players and desk jockeys are all vulnerable.

Do not "strum" or otherwise aggressively work the psoas. By following our protocol for palpating the psoas, it can be worked in a fairly non-invasive manner.

An Internist M.D. friend recently told us of an emergency room case of a ruptured bowel purportedly caused by a massage therapist's work on a client's psoas. We do not and we recommend that you do not strum this muscle.

There are other ways to eliminate trigger points without direct pressure. If CRAC stretches are ineffective and we cannot safely access the psoas with direct pressure, we usually refer to a P.T. for spray and stretch. We prefer, however, to treat shortened iliopsoas muscles with CRAC stretches. If the CRAC stretch is insufficient to rid the client's pain and shortness, use direct pressure.

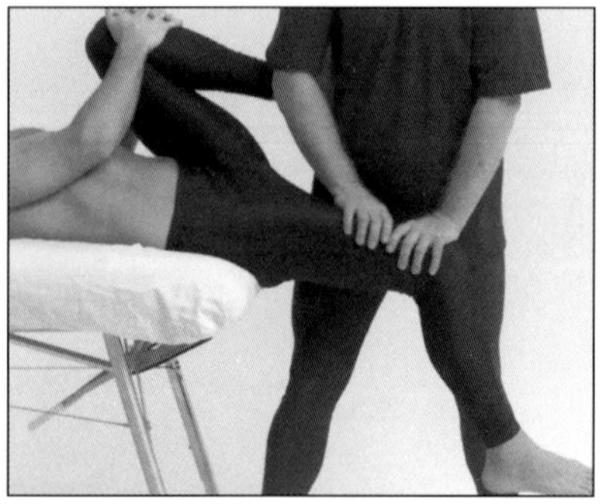

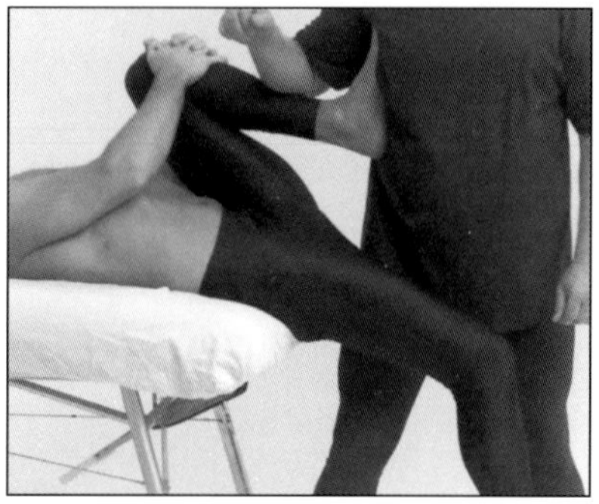

CRAC stretch to the iliopsoas:

- *The client lies with their greater trochanter at the end of the table.*
- *The client pulls one knee to their chest (prevents hyperlordosis and positions pelvis for stretch). This will also keep the client from kicking you.*
- *Offer resistance with both hands above the client's knee on the side to be stretched.*
- *Instruct client to flex their hip and pull their knee into the therapist's hands.*
- *The therapist always instructs clients to begin slowly and build to a 20% muscular contraction. This 20% prevents strain to the client and injury to the therapist.*
- *Instruct client to relax their hip, take a deep belly-breath and release while they push their heel toward the floor. The gluteal and hamstring contraction reciprocally inhibits the psoas, allowing a deep stretch.*
- *This stretch can be repeated several times. Re-test muscle length between stretches. We repeat stretch up to three times per session.*

Always avoid direct pressure on any inflamed tissue(s). Caveats for this muscle include:

- pregnancy
- irritable bowel syndrome
- colitis
- appendicitis
- pelvic inflammatory disease
- aortic aneurysm

Deconditioned clients will find themselves suffering post-exercise soreness if they don't initially do these stretches very moderately.

OTHER PSOAS PROBLEMS

Local pain, swelling, hard to walk: all could by indications of a psoas hematoma – often trauma induced.

Anticoagulation therapy: the iliopsoas is susceptible to hematoma. Don't work clients with psoas pain who are using blood thinners without medical check for hematoma.

Femoral nerve compression caused by hypertropy, atrophy, cancer, tumor, abscess and lymphoma: all possibilities in the psoas muscle.

Trigger points rarely occur alone in the psoas: it is also important to check for trigger points in the quadratus lumborum and rectus abdominis.

Tight hamstrings give the pelvis an unnatural tilt and overload the psoas causing or perpetuating trigger points.

HIS STORY

New clients should be treated moderately until you ascertain their response to friction massage, direct pressure and stretches. Use full contractions for CRAC stretches only with fully conditioned (very fit) individuals

A moderately-conditioned student considered himself very fit. He used full contractions for his back-extension CRAC stretches. He was less fit than he thought. Needless to say, he strained his quadratus lumborum muscle while performing the stretch.

To Locate Primary Trigger Points:

Direct pressure by hand to the two primary trigger points in the iliopsoas is highly effective. One is in the iliacus in the bowl of the ilium; the other is located in the inguinal triangle approximately at the level of the musculotendinous juncture of the iliopsoas.

Direct pressure to the third trigger point located in the psoas at the level of the umbilicus or just below must be approached gently and with a great deal of care both during palpation assessment and treatment.

With heavy-set clients, use a side-lying position to allow the gut to fall away from the area needing work. If there is too much fatty tissue for ease of palpation and treatment, use other approaches.

Treatment

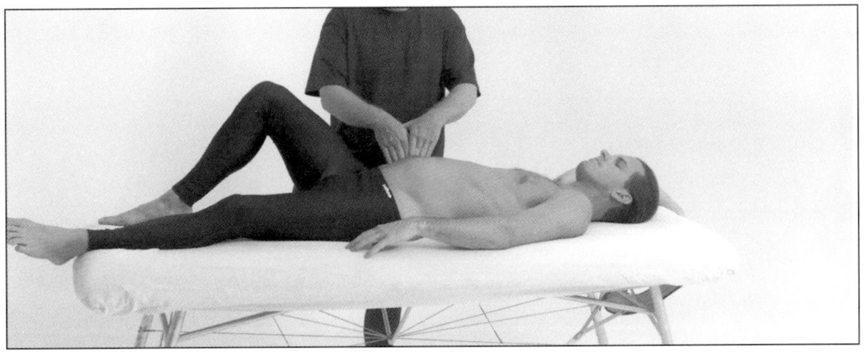

Client takes large belly-breath prior to your palpation of his psoas. Entry is made at a 45 degree angle at the edge of the rectus abdominis near the level of the umbilicus. Client exhales as you administer moderate pressure toward the spine. Hands are held in a spatulate position with fingers firmly (but not rigidly) extended.

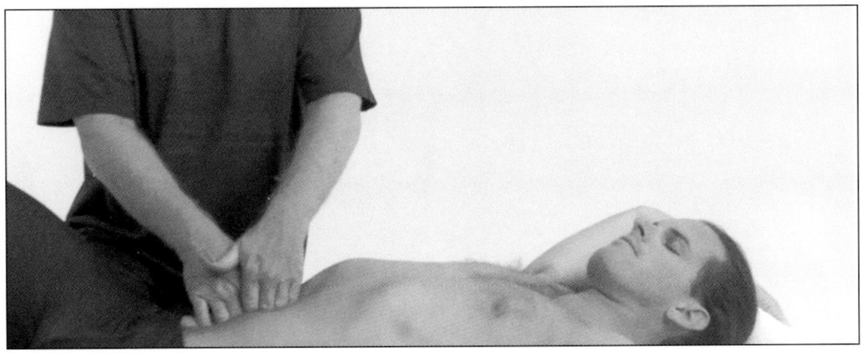

As client slowly releases "belly breath," you push gently toward the psoas. Initial entry should be made at about the level of the umbilicus.

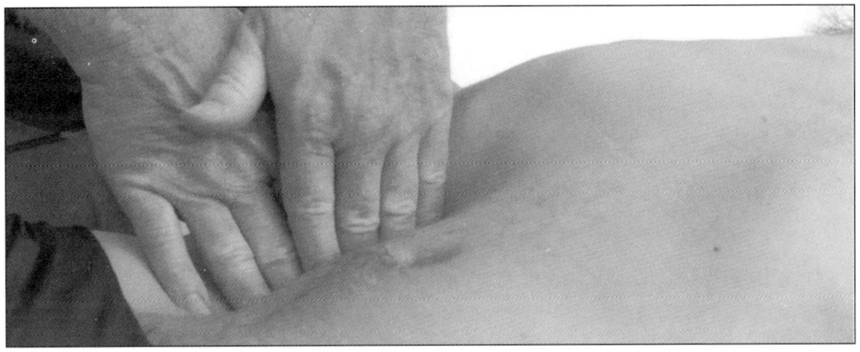

Close-up of direct pressure to the psoas. Palpate slightly above and below for TrPs. Carefully treat all TrPs with direct pressure.

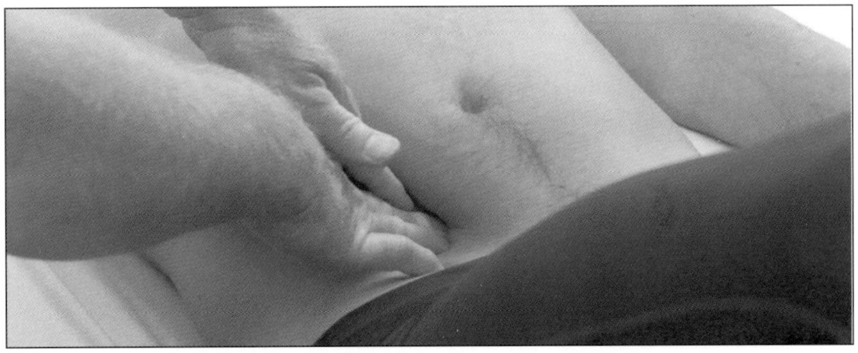

Note that the therapist's fingers are firmly but not rigidly extended.

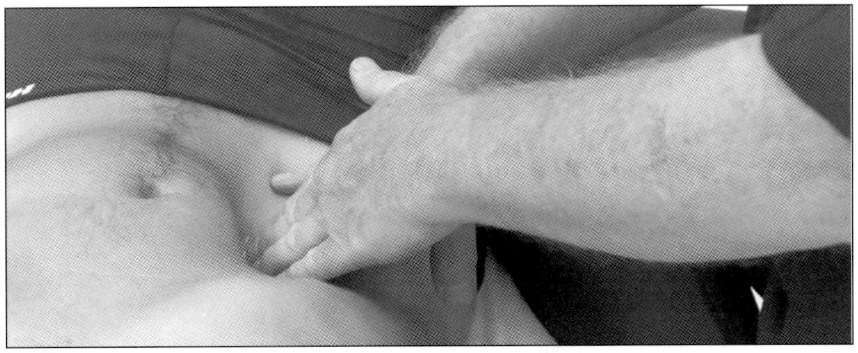

Many times the psoas is close to the surface and easily encountered. If not, have the client flex involved hip against resistance – this is easily accomplished by placing your hand closest to the hip against the client's thigh. The psoas contracts, broadens and comes closer to the surface for easier access.

If there is pain, sink your hand a little further into the belly as the client releases the hip contraction. Hold this direct pressure for 15 to 20 seconds.

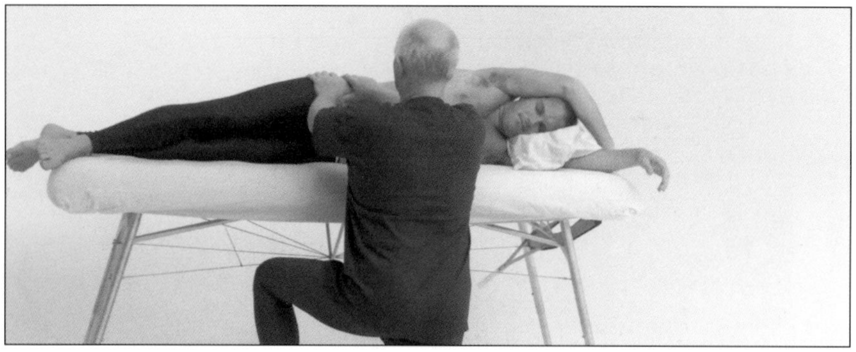

Address the iliacus with the client side-lying. Bolster the neck well.

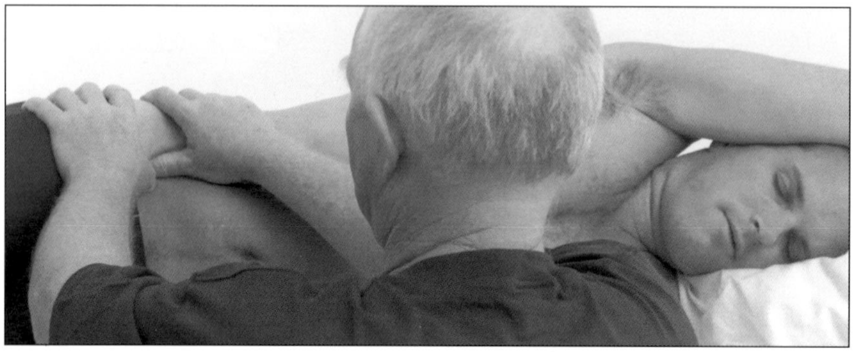

The gut drops toward the floor giving us good thumb access to the belly of the iliacus.

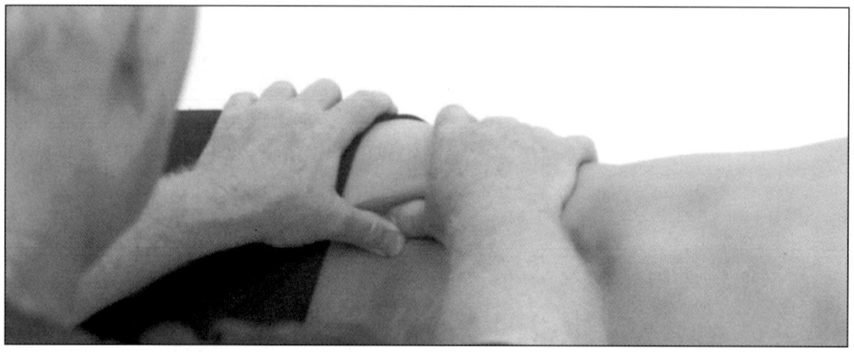

Don't over-stretch your client's skin when accessing the iliacus. Lift skin (bunch) toward ASIS before sliding into the iliacus.

Stretch Test for the RIGHT Iliopsoas.

Client pulls left leg to chest. If the right knee comes up from the table, the right iliopsoas is short. Clients with knee problems should pull against their hamstrings to avoid knee damage. Persons with an inflamed rectus femoris origin may feel a pinch or pain in the left hip as the knee is pulled toward the chest. Change the angle of pull slightly and/or decrease the intensity of the pull.

If the involved (lower) leg straightens (extends) with or without the thigh coming up from the table, the sartorius, the rectus femoris, or the tensor fascia latae, (or any combination of these 3 muscles) is short.

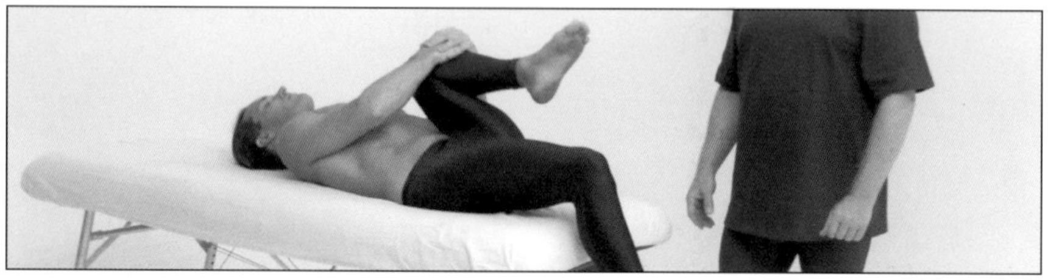

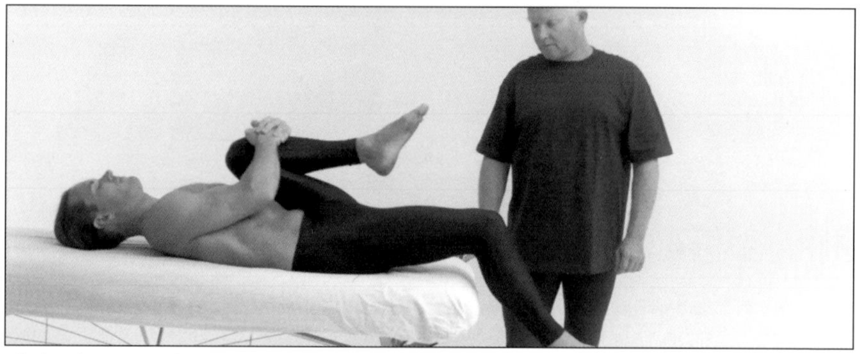

Slight elevation of the right knee (above the table) indicates a moderate shortening of the right iliopsoas.

CHAPTER 11

Leg and Foot Pain

THE CONTOUR OF THE MUSCLES of this region and the human foot must have been made for each other. This is the easiest, most comfortable region of the body for compressions and direct pressure. It just feels right.

We find numerous tendon injuries in this region, all quite easy to find and address with cross-fiber friction. Compressions and direct pressure from the heel are quick to clean up trigger points, adhesions, or just plain old fatigued muscles.

Extensive caveats are offered for the occasional serious problems that require medical attention. Compartment syndromes, blood clots and inflamed veins are a few of those covered.

From hamstring pulls, iliotibial band syndrome, groin pulls of the adductors, tennis leg in the gastrocnemius, to Achilles tendonitis and the inversion sprain ligaments of the ankle – they are all covered here in sufficient detail to give you the tools you need to make a salutary impact in a short period of time.

Before You Begin

Safe, effective leg and foot treatments are enhanced by first reading the *Indications, Client Intake, Contraindications, Deep Compressive Massage, Endangerment Sites, Trigger Points, Cross-fiber, Fascial Release, Stretching* and *Hydrotherapy* sections.

Note the specific procedural notes and cautions. They will help you effectively treat your client without harm. Protocols and guidelines are included to help you know when to treat and when to refer.

Hamstrings

Biceps femoris
Semitendinosus
Semimembranosus

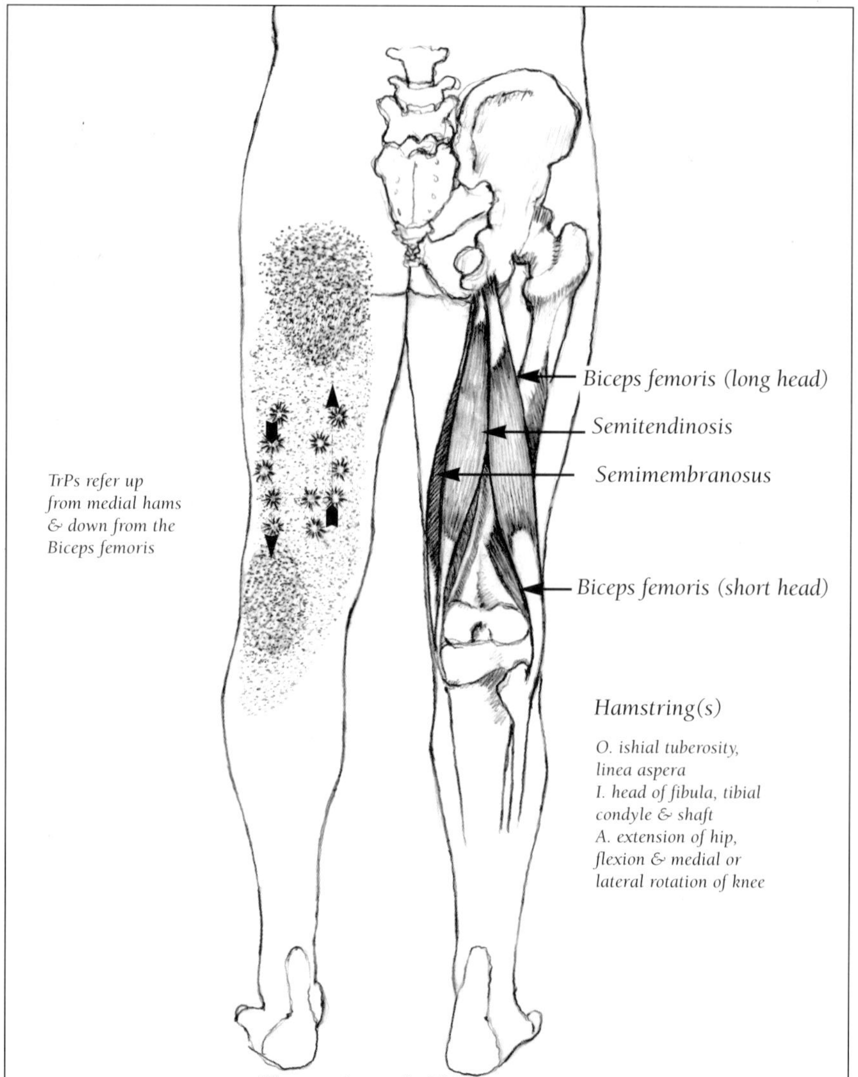

Hamstrings & TrPs

HAMSTRINGS RESPOND WELL TO COMPRESSIONS and direct heel pressure. The muscles are bulky enough to tolerate firm, diffuse pressure. The painfully scarred hamstrings found in athletes respond positively to direct pressure with a twist. Prolonged, firm pressure has a strong psychotropic effect on clients. A few minutes of sustained compressions will generally drop clients into very deep parasympathetic states. We often begin our massage work at the hamstrings to evoke this healing state.

The upper portion of the hamstrings can become weak and fatigued with long distance running. Over time, the hamstrings loose their capacity to relax and lengthen during hip flexion while running. The resultant strain on the slow-to-release hamstring results in microtrauma at the ischial tuberosity. Prolonged microtrauma ultimately will develop into a clinical level, painful tendonitis. Compressions and deep transverse friction can abort this process. The therapy should be combined with upper hamstring strengthening and on going stretching. To strengthen the superior aspect of the hamstrings, use the glut-ham machine or similar exercises.

Painful strains in the hamstring body will also respond well to prolonged transverse stretching with prolonged compressions. Work slowly back and forth transversely to tease open the adhesions in the scar. Remember, in the early healing process, non-weight bearing, non-resisted movement helps to create strong, pain-free, flexible, and pliable scars. The scar should then heal without the painful adhesions.

Prolonged sitting in one position, as driving without stretch breaks, can cause jelling pain and activate latent trigger points. When working with trigger points, first warm the muscle with moderate, rhythmic compressions. Palpate the muscle looking for jump signs and other trigger point indications. Then take the muscle through its range of motion, noting any restrictions. Use direct heel pressure on the trigger points. Follow with a gentle, prolonged stretch, more compressions, and a final range of motion assessment. Also check for trigger points in the antagonist quadriceps and psoas muscles.

Generally, trigger points in both the semimembranosus and semitendinosus refer up to the gluteals while the biceps femoris trigger points refer down to the knee.

The hamstring muscles are often involved in low back pain even though their trigger points don't refer pain directly into the lumbar region. Significant shortness of these muscles causes a posterior tilt to the pelvis. This flattens the back, decreases the normal shock-absorption of the lumbar curve, and predisposes the lumbar musculature to tightness. Fatigue and weakness in the hamstrings predispose them to pulls, especially in minimally stretched, long distance runners. Premature stretching of a pulled muscle can result in a painful adherent scar at the site of the tendonitis. Don't stretch recently torn hams.

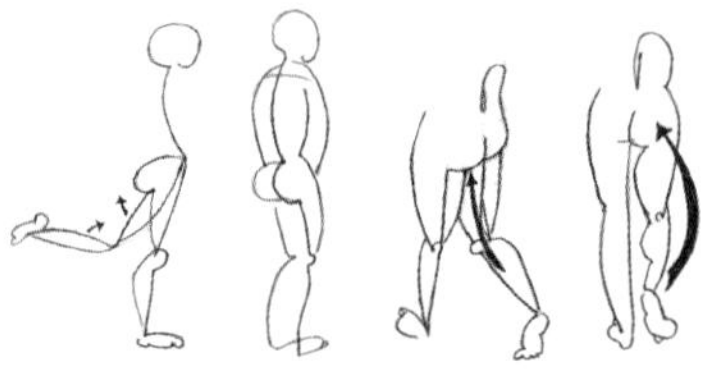

Cautions

Seek specific medical advice before working with anyone you suspect is a candidate for or who has had, recent knee surgery. Downward pressure to the hamstrings can stress the knee joint.

Avoid fresh scars, bruises, varicose veins, adductor hiatus area (Hunter's Canal) and the back of knee (popliteal space).

Treatment

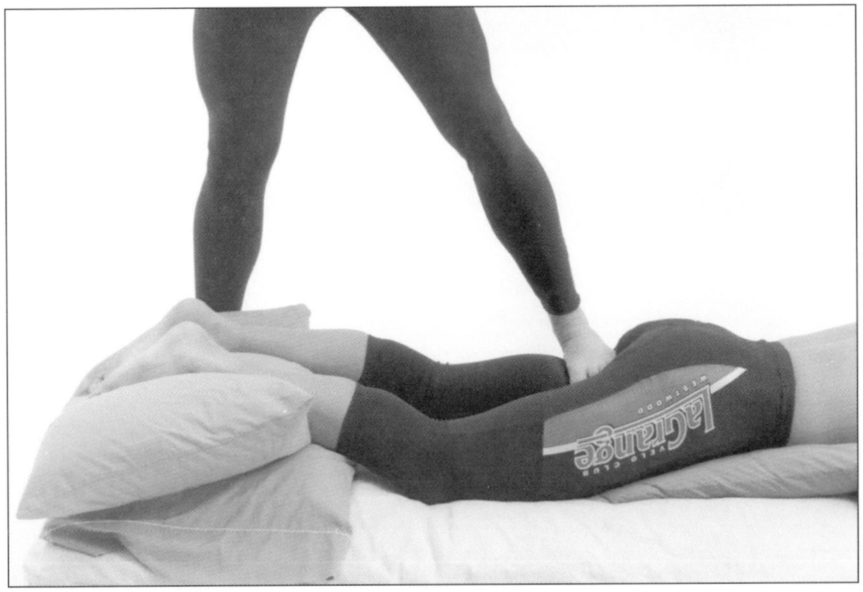

With a full, soft-foot, gently compress hamstrings. Each compression takes about 10 seconds. Use 5 to 10 compressions to thoroughly warm the muscles.

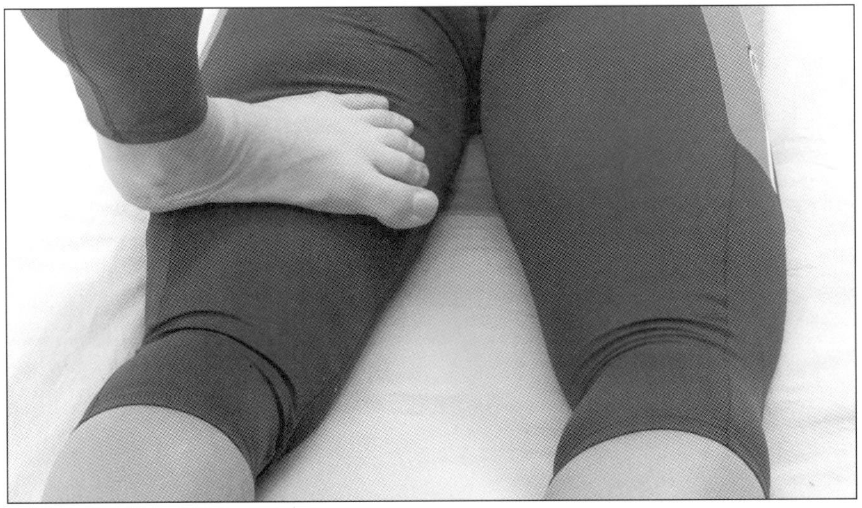

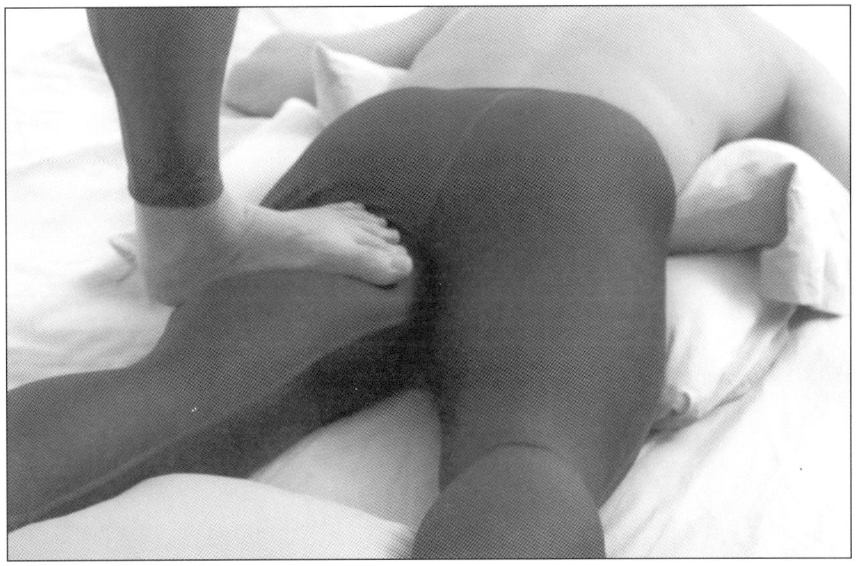

Prior to compressing a medially rotated hamstring, pull laterally with your foot to insure proper placement of the muscle over the femur. Stepping onto the femur in the superior portion of the thigh with this medially rotated hamstring may place the sciatic nerve in jeopardy.

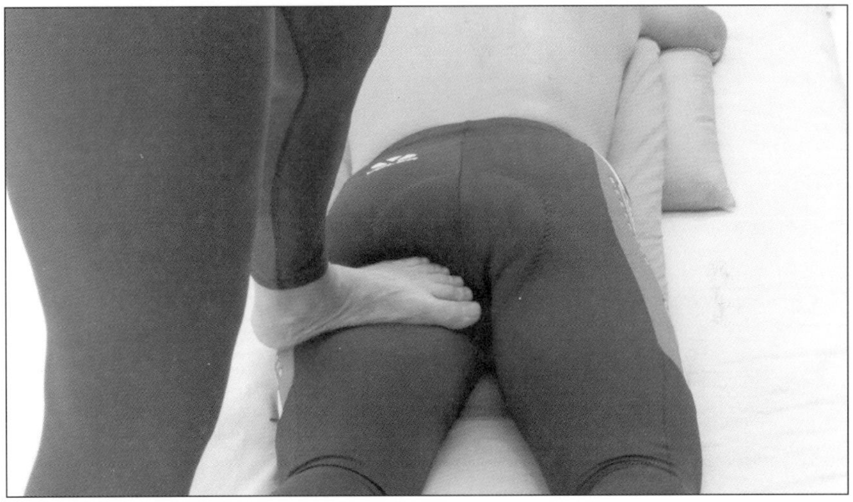

The sciatic nerve lies adjacent to the femur at the level of the ischial tuberosity. The biceps femoris muscle does not overlie and protect the sciatic nerve. Stepping directly onto the femur at this level may compromise sciatic nerve function.

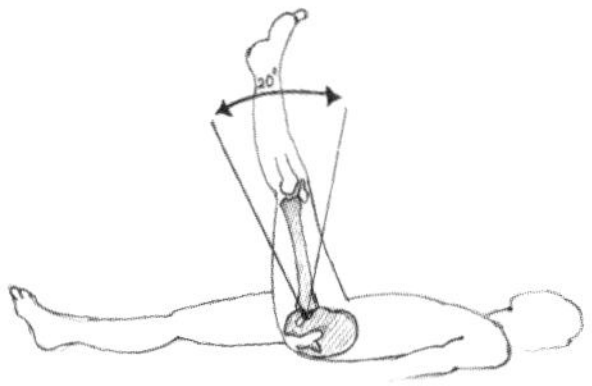

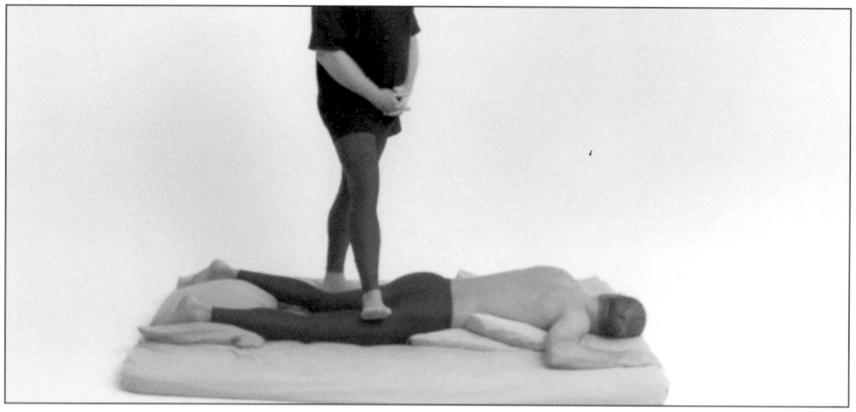

Direct heel pressure into client's medial hamstrings. Stepping across the body provides a good angle of attack for hamstring TrPs.

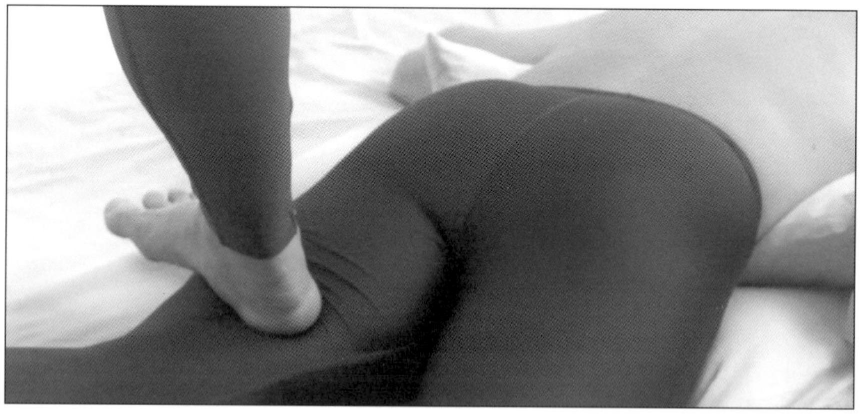

Direct heel pressure to the edge of the semimembranosus. Roll the medial hamstrings laterally.

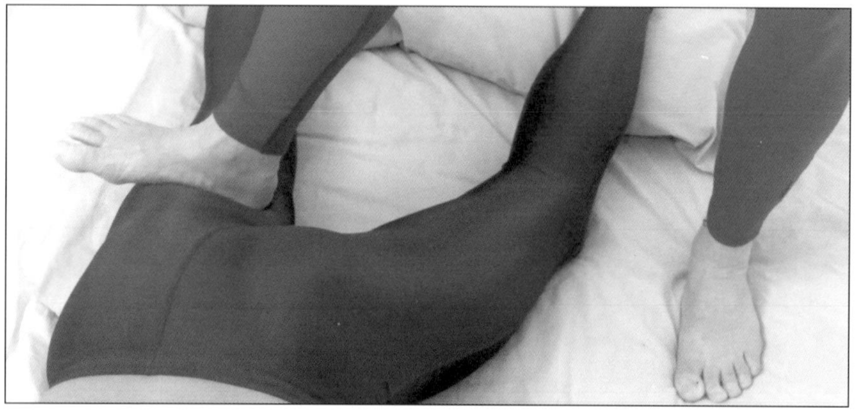

Direct pressure to the medial hamstring. Trigger points are generally more distal; this region often contains adherent scars.

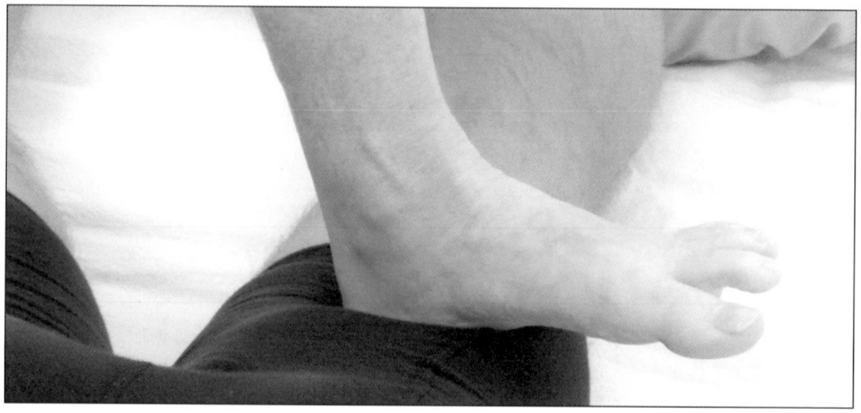

Precise positioning. Prolonged pressure.

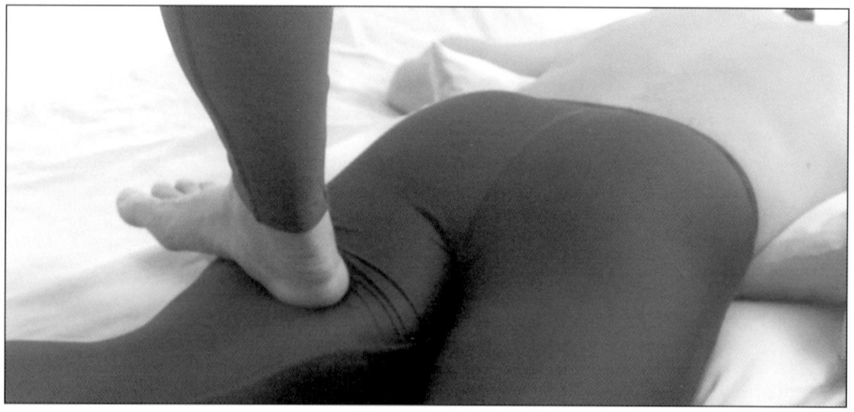

Work from this point distally for medial hamstring trigger points.

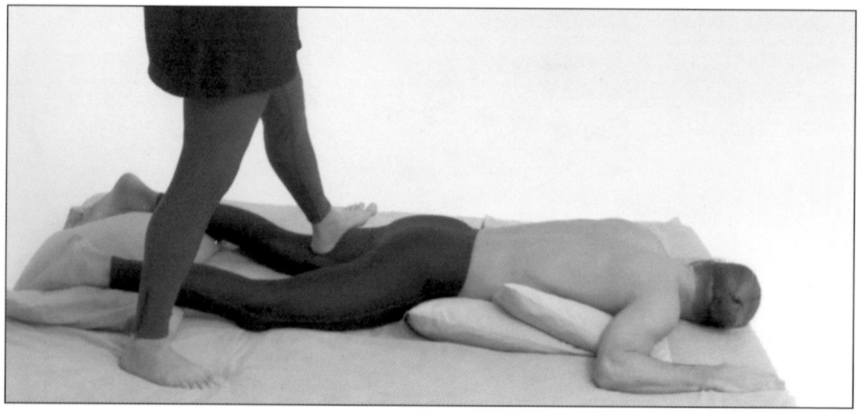

Switch support legs to change the angle of attack and enhance efficiency. This also helps you avoid fatigue.

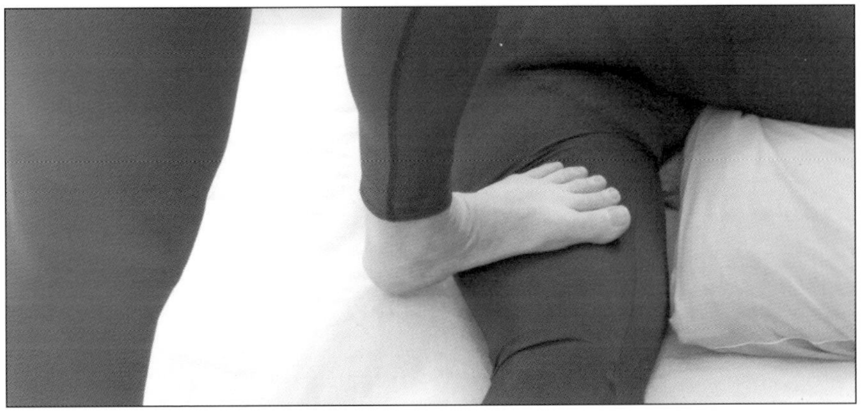

Side-lying approach to distal medial hamstring.

Table Work

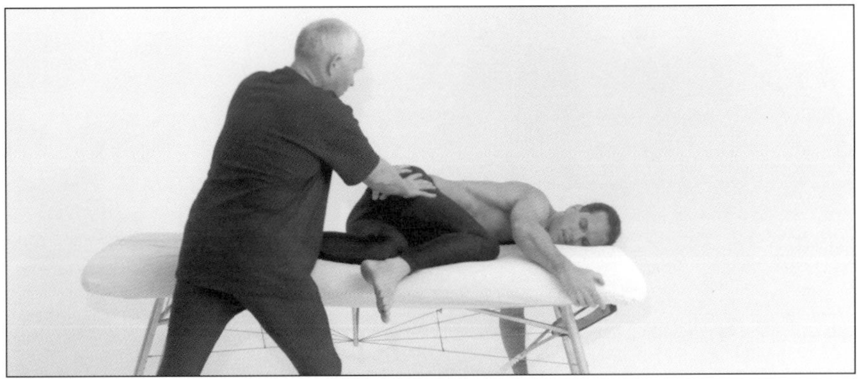

To treat a hamstring tendonitis at the ischial tuberosity use cross-fiber friction. Good biomechanics make this demanding treatment manageable.

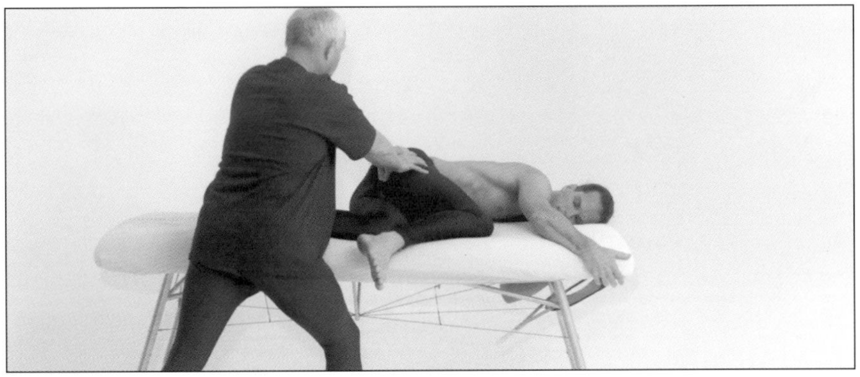

Lean into your thumbs. The "lean" gives sufficient pressure to provide the mechanical effect required to treat these thick, deep tendons.

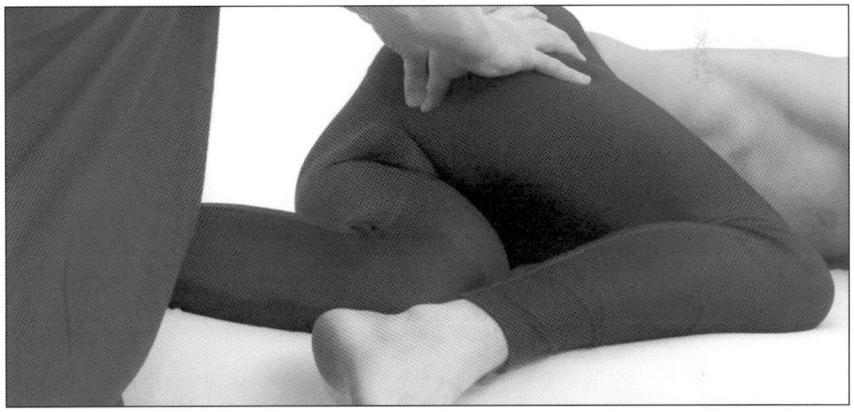

Begin cross-fiber friction on the medial aspect of the tendon at the ischial tuberosity. The client's flexed hip brings the hamstring tendons closer to the surface.

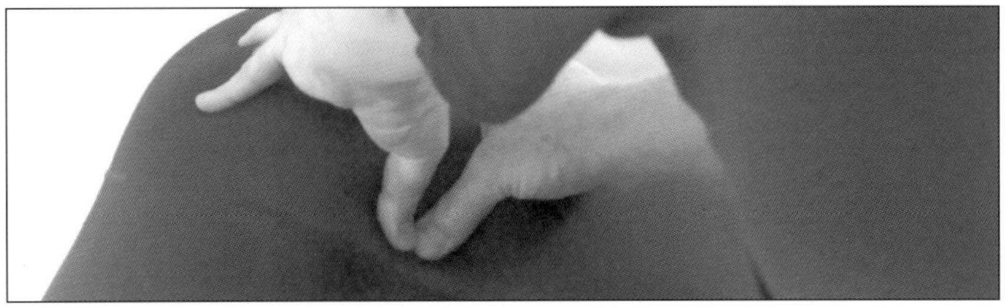

Use two thumbs. Following a successful first treatment, subsequent sessions will usually last 4 or 5 minutes. A successful treatment includes tolerable post-treatment discomfort for the client and unharmed thumbs for the therapist. If well tolerated, treatments on this tendon can be given daily. Take several brief breaks during the session and "flutter stretch" to relax your hands.

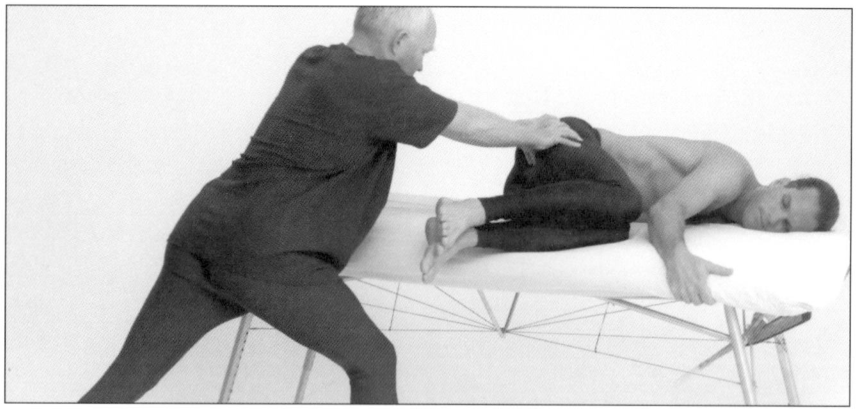

Don't "muscle" this treatment…pressure created by leaning into the tendon is sufficient.

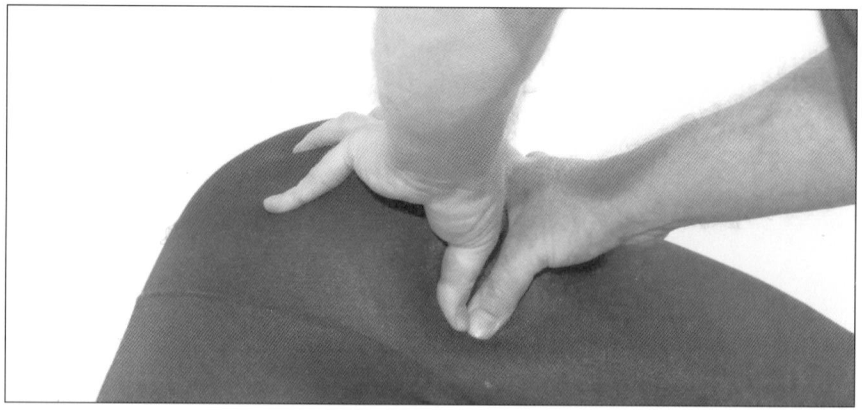

The exact site of the lesion can be medial, lateral, or across the entire tendon. Pain will be your guide.

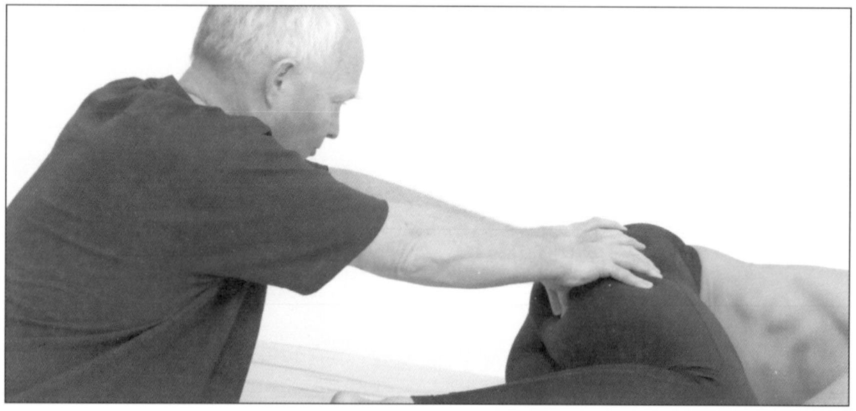

Arms are straight, but the elbows are not locked. The treatment is dynamic and comes from the floor.

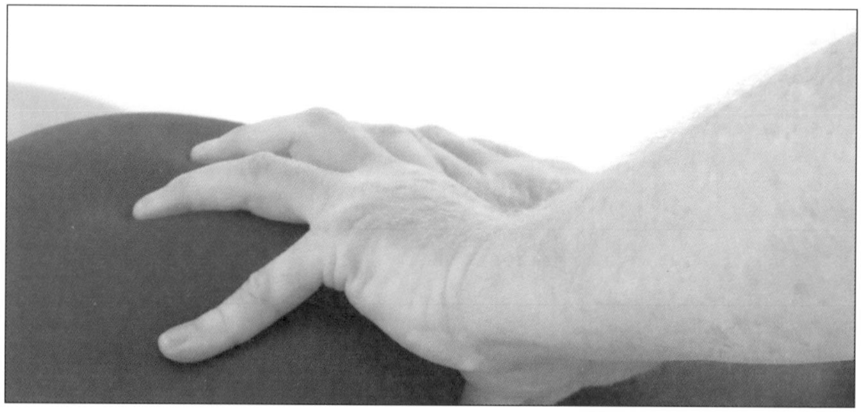

The frictioning movement comes primarily from your shoulders; slightly from the wrists, and not at all from thumb flexion. Thumbs sink in deeply on the medial aspect of the hamstring.

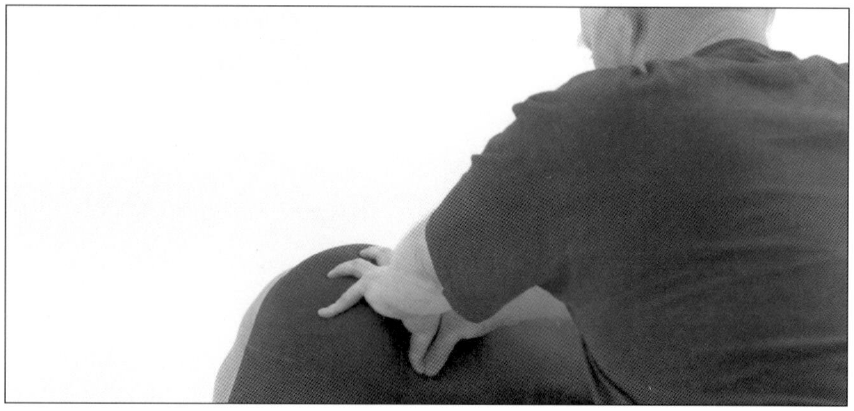

Works at a 90 degree angle to the client's hamstring. Any other angle diminishes effectiveness.

Tensor fascia latae and Iliotibial Tract

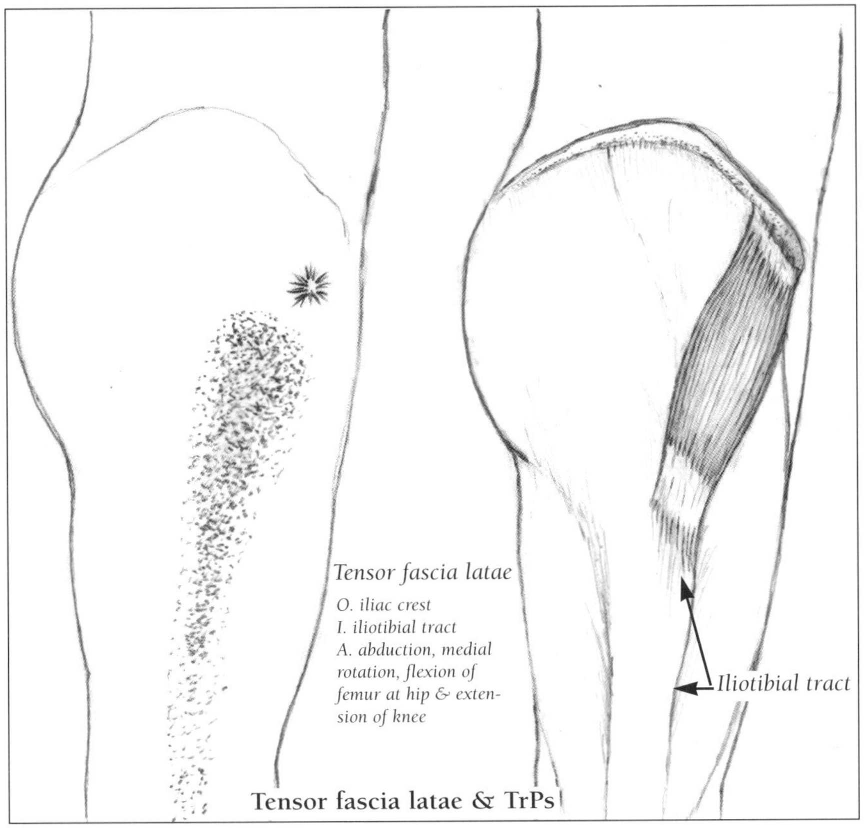

Tensor fascia latae & TrPs

The tensor fascia latae (TFL) can be troublesome to just about everyone, with athletes particularly vulnerable. The anterior and posterior parts of this muscle play differing roles in the stance and swing phase of walking, jogging and running. Cyclists and backpackers can overload this muscle from prolonged overuse and weight-bearing activity.

Runners and cyclists who have iliotibial band syndrome (a painful tendonitis of the iliotibial tract at its insertion to the tibia and fibula) will have concomitant painful trigger points in the TFL muscle and down the iliotibial tract. These TFL trigger points refer pain into the region of the greater trochanter and occasionally down the lateral thigh to the knee.

The trigger points in the iliotibial band tend to refer pain locally, with sporadic sciatic pain distribution in the hamstring. When TFL trigger points are active, clients will find it almost impossible to lie on the effected side.

The TFL is a synergist in hip flexion, medial rotation, and abduction. When the synergistic muscles of the hip become fatigued from overuse, trigger points form in the TFL. A compensatory pattern can result in which the TFL is used as a prime mover with resultant fatigue and "associated" (satellite and secondary) trigger points.

Several major trigger points located in the vastus lateralis or midrange region of the iliotibial band produce a broad referral pain pattern that mimics sciatic pain. Look for this one on older cyclists who don't stretch regularly.

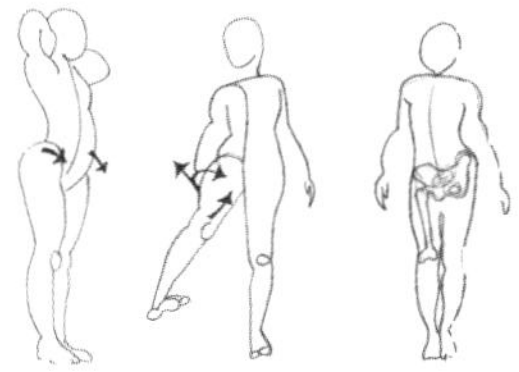

Treatment

To treat iliotibial tract tendonitis, use cross-fiber friction to the lesion – usually located in a 4 to 5 inch area just above the tibial tubercle. Then use a side-lying CRAC stretch to lengthen and relax the tensor fascia latae muscle. The stretch here rarely exacerbates the trigger points, and makes entry into the soft tissue less painful. Then use direct pressure to the trigger points in the band and muscle belly. Include prolonged direct pressure to the vastus lateralis for secondary trigger points.

You can apply a gentle fascial stretch with your whole foot for 2 to 3 minutes – sometimes it takes longer. Hold the stretch until you experience a release – your client will "feel" it. Because of the time involved and the attention required, some practitioners prefer to be comfortably seated during this procedure. Our experience suggests that trigger points in skin and superficial fascia can usually be released through this gentle, prolonged stretching.

NOTE

Trigger points in the TFL create general soreness and a referred pain pattern that can mimic trochanteric bursitis – a condition often caused by a or direct pressure on the bursa. In some cases when climbing stairs or steep hills, a tight iliotibial band mechanically exacerbates trochanteric bursitis as it snaps back and forth over the bursa. If your client is extremely sore in this area, refer for treatment. Direct pressure could aggravate the problem.

While a relationship exists between trigger points, joint pain, and bursitis, it is not yet fully understood. For clients with trochanteric bursitis, working trigger points in the surrounding musculature usually brings relief.

The tensor fascia latae muscle carries strong emotional responses in some people. With ischemic pressure, tears or deep sobbing often spring forth – often without apparent reason. This is not at all unusual. We recommend you begin your work here slowly and gently.

Caution

When treating trigger points in the illiotibial band, use moderate pressure. Too much force can cause armoring and extreme pain in the underlying vastus lateralis.

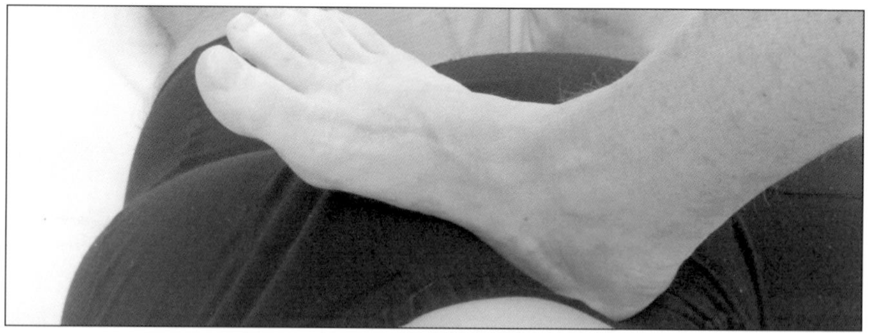

Heel pressure into a tensor fascia latae TrP.

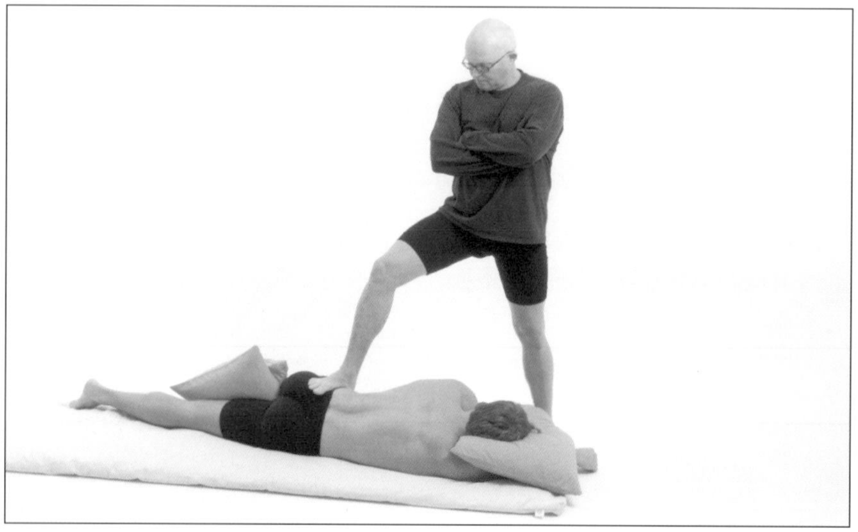

Good warm up position for the tensor fascia latae. Use 2 or 3 pillows to help support the client's hip.

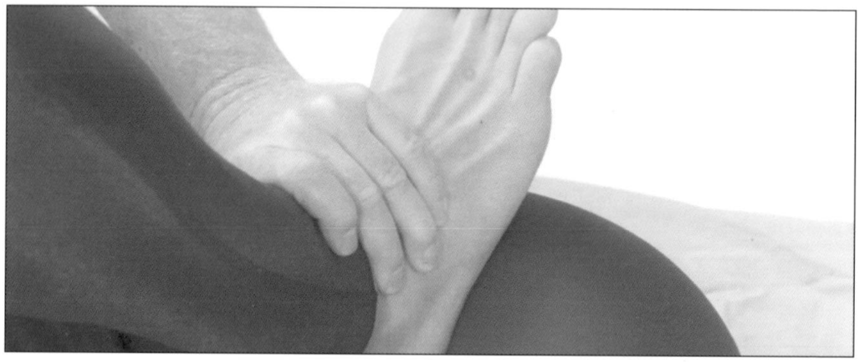

Client helps position therapist's foot to get it "just right." Client involvement equals efficacious treatment.

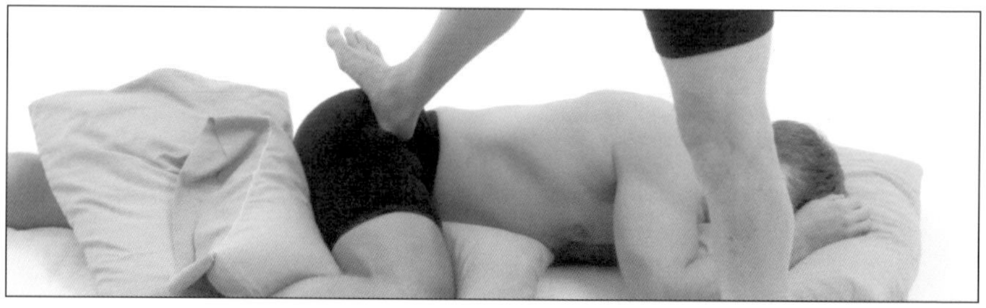

Enter slowly. Tensor fascia latae TrPs can be extremely painful.

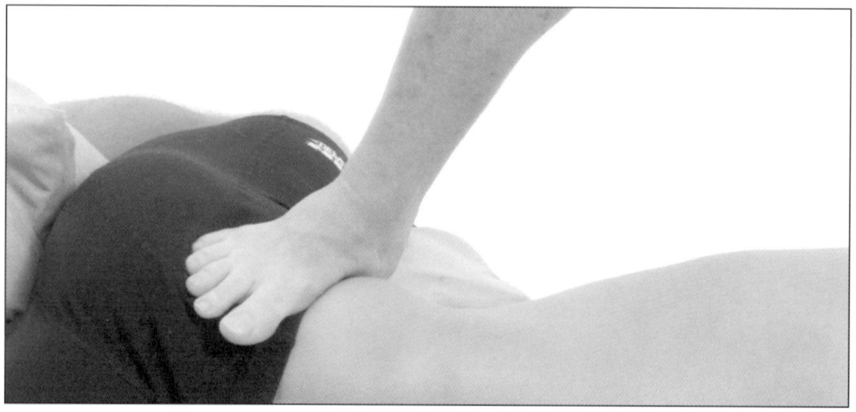

Soft-footed warm-up.

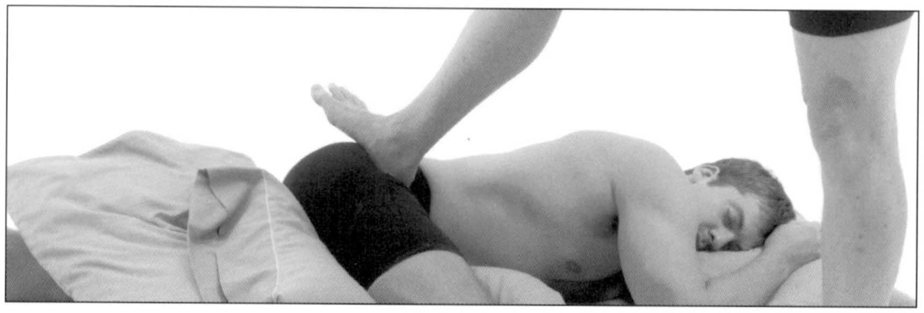

Direct pressure from the heel two or three times, each for 15 to 20 seconds, should eradicate the TrP and ensure maximum reactive hyperemia and microcirculation.

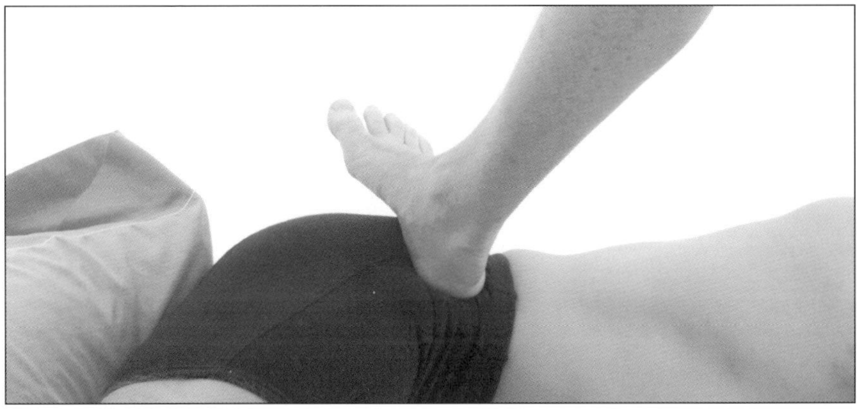

Direct pressure to tensor fascia latae TrP.

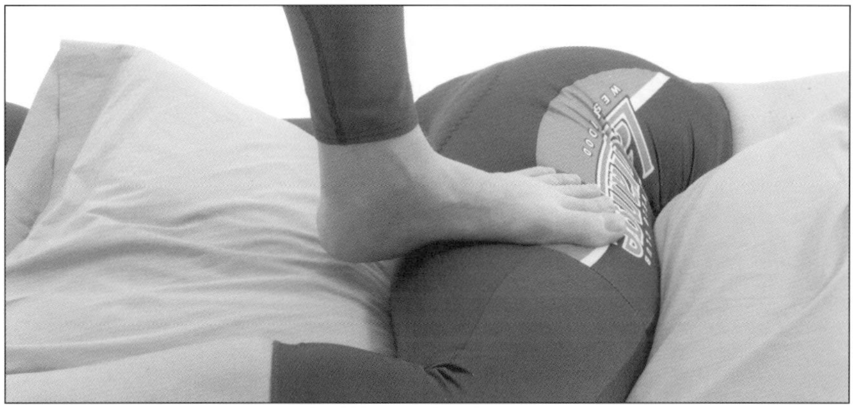

The ball of the foot is used to apply direct pressure to ITB TrPs.

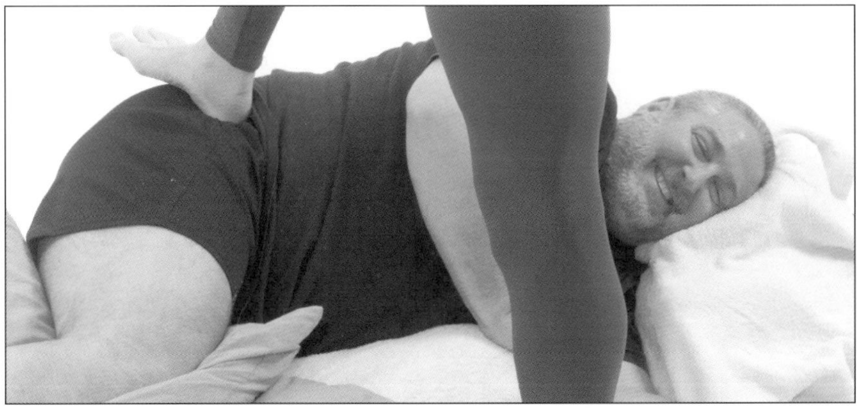

Imagine treating this champion power-lifter by hand.

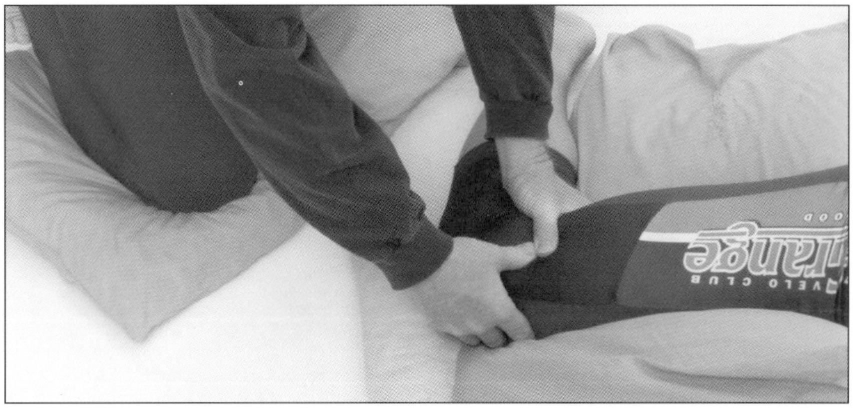

Cross-fiber friction over the last 5 inches of the distal portion of the iliotibial band.

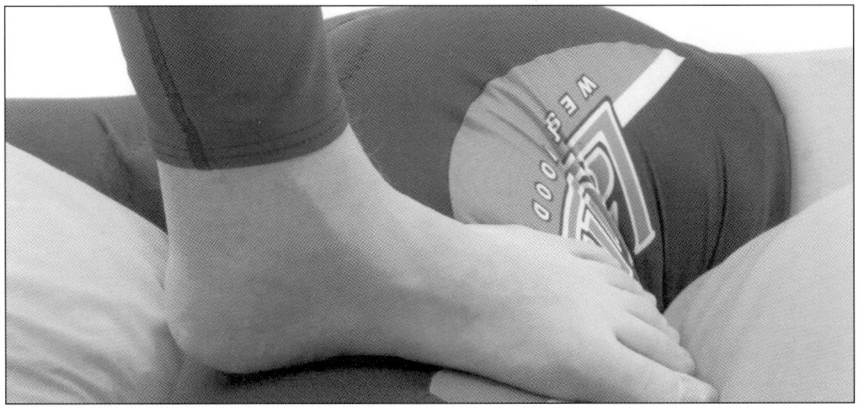

Soft-footed compression and prolonged duration prepare the iliotibial band (ITB) for a less painful TrP treatment.

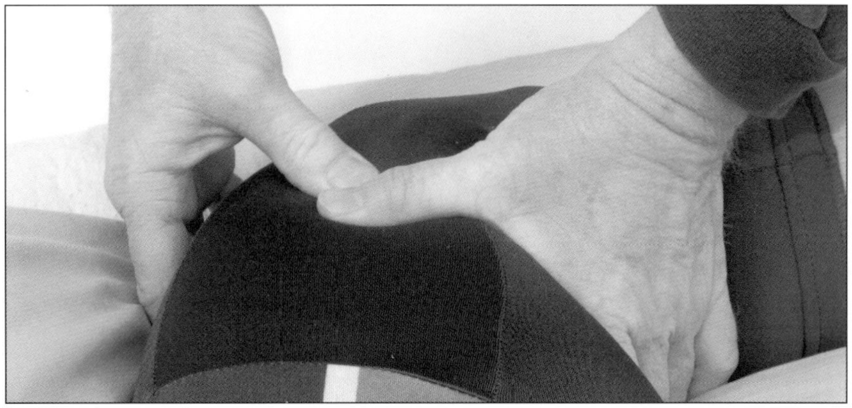

Friction is administered through your shoulders and down into your thumbs, e.g., a rotational movement.

Rectus Femoris
Vastus lateralis
Vastus medialis
Vastus intermedius

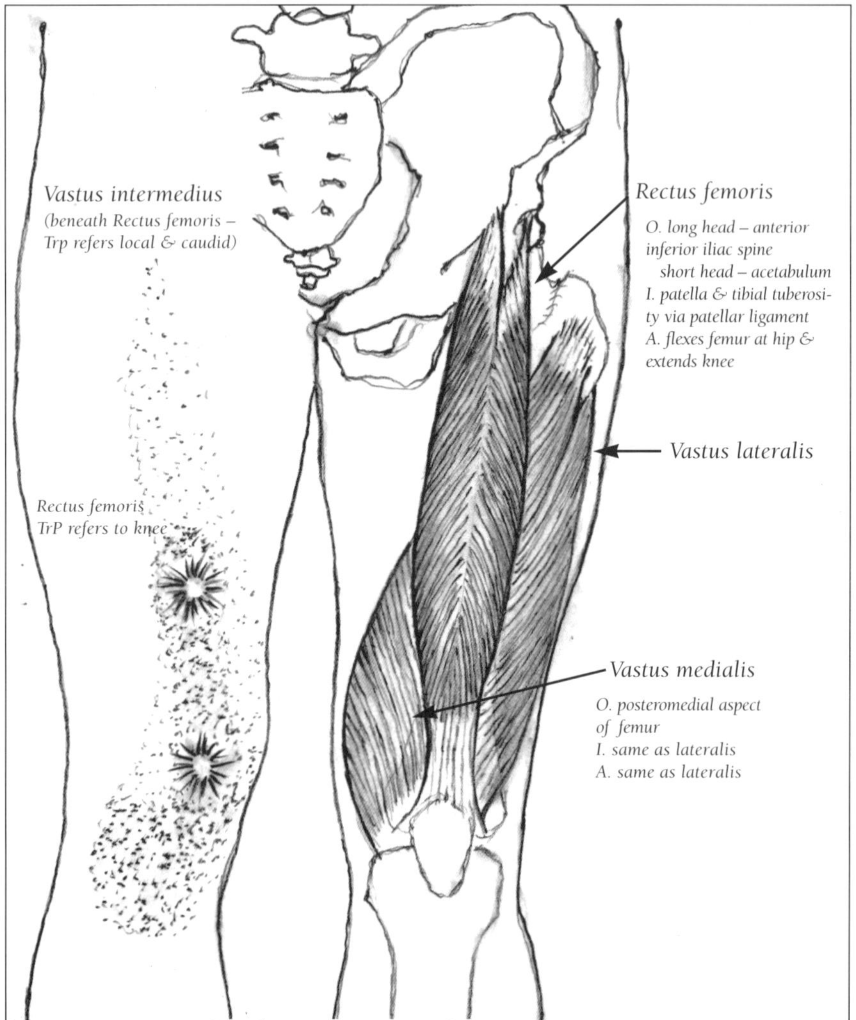

Quadriceps Femoris & TrPs

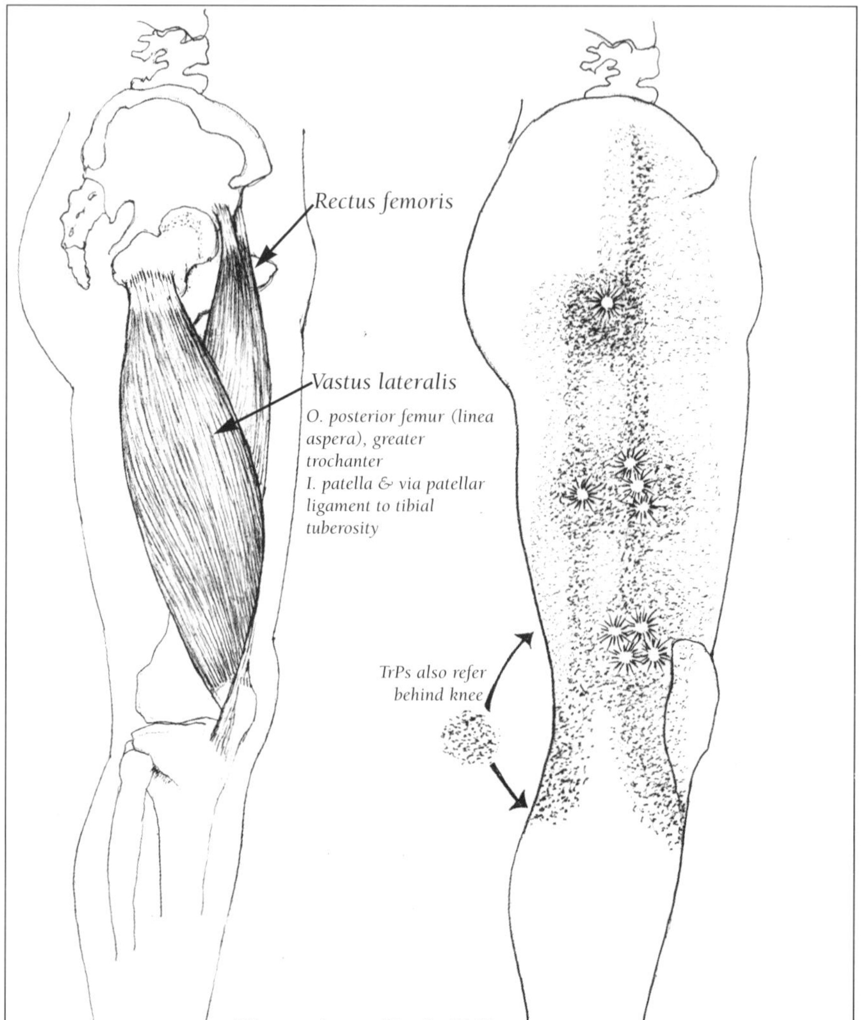

Vastus lateralis & TrPs

TRIGGER POINTS are generally found midpoint in the rectus femoris and the vastus lateralis, and in the distal portion of the vastus medialis. These muscles cause intense and debilitating pain when harboring trigger points. Sleeping side-lying with vastus lateralis trigger points compressed against the bed, commonly creates pain and interferes with sleep.

Sleep deprivation increases pain dramatically. Adequate sleep makes people more stress-resilient, with fewer secondary negative effects from pain.

Mid-muscle vastus lateralis pain, near the iliotibial band, can have a pain pattern broad enough to be mistaken for sciatica. More than a few laminectomies have been performed because of misreading this pain source.

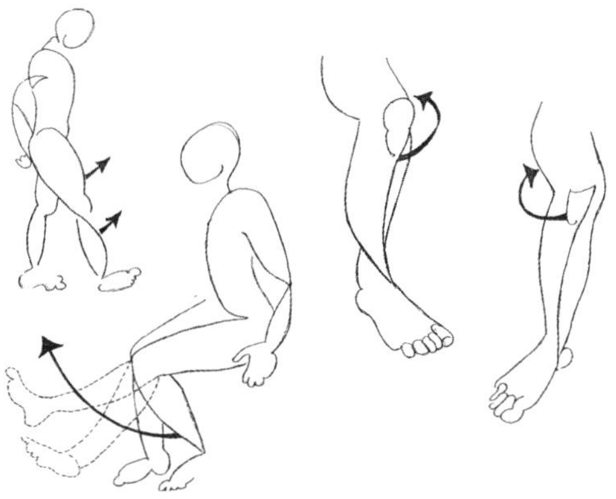

> **GEORGE'S STORY**
>
> George came in stooped, grimacing and massively sleep-deprived following two full years of what he described as "unrelenting sciatic pain." Initially we thought he was suffering post-laminectomy pain originating from the quadratus lumborum or psoas. Treating both these muscles provided only minor relief.
>
> Our next choice was to treat the piriformis – the most common source of sciatic pain – along with the gluteal group and the hamstrings. This treatment brought some relief and better sleep, but still we hadn't found the crux.
>
> George was a big, strong man in his 70s who had been an avid long-distance cyclist. Thinking deeper about his problem, we noted greatly reduced flexibility during knee flexion. Suddenly it dawned on us the likely culprit could be vastus lateralis trigger points. Sure enough, we found three major vastus trigger points.
>
> After eliminating these trigger points, we initiated a quad stretching program for George. He began to sleep well, stand straight, and he got back on his bike. George now uses self-care with a tennis ball for trigger points and he continues with his stretch program.

The next most common problem involves trigger points in the distal vastus medialis. Travel and Simons note that trigger points here can cause the knees to "buckle" and do so without any discernible pain! It is very distressing to walk or run while uncertain of when your knee will give out.

Athletes with chondromalacia (knee-cap pain) need to be regularly checked for this trigger point. Eradicate these trigger points to facilitate building of medial quad strength through weight training. This will insure better patella tracking. The medial quad cannot be adequately strengthened while harboring this trigger point.

The vastus intermedius trigger point pain distribution is broad and wide down the front of the leg. Care must be taken when searching for this trigger point. If there is a deep hematoma (Charley-horse or Cork) our direct pressure may slough off osteoblasts and create myositis ossificans (a bony growth within the muscle). A surgical incision can remove this growth, but it tends to reoccur. Hematomas must not be subjected to cross-fiber friction or other massage techniques.

> A good rule of thumb: do not to treat a blow to the anterior thigh if there is a possibility of deep bruising. "Cold" hydrotherapy is indicated. Review our hydrotherapy recommendations (pg. 172).

The primary rectus femoris trigger point is usually found close to its origins. It refers directly into the patella. This problem must be differentiated from the occasional rectus femoris tendonitis located above the usual trigger point location.

The sartorius has its origin just superior to the rectus femoris. Sartorius trigger point pain refers down the anterior medial aspect of the leg. A sartorius tendonitis at the pes anserinus attachment (combined insertion of the tendinous expansions of the sartorius, gracilis and semitendinosis muscles) is also common.

The adjacent insertions of the tendons of the sartorius, gracilis, and semitendinosus muscles are found on the superior medial aspect of the tibia. A tendonitis located here usually requires a few sessions of deep transverse friction to abort. However, take care not to friction a pes-anserinus bursitis. Functional assessment (resisted contraction) is used to differentiate a tendonitis from a bursitis. The pain of tendonitis will increase when the muscle is stressed with an isometric contraction.

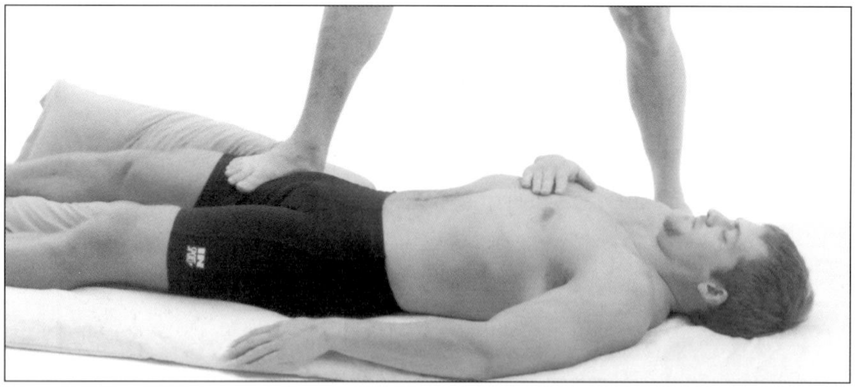

Rectus femoris & vastus intermedius warm-up.

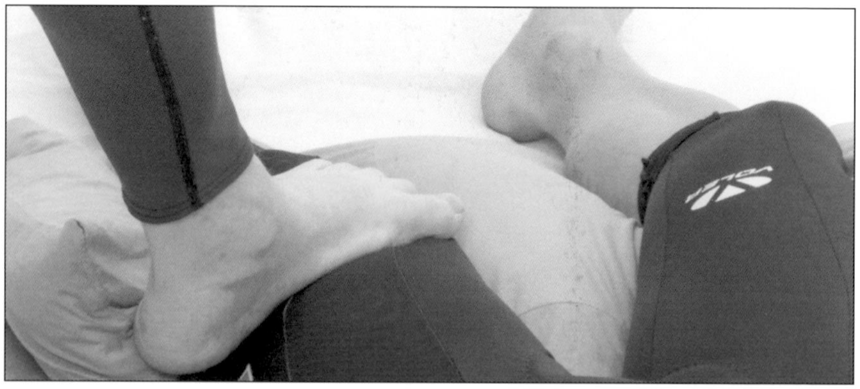

Warm-up of distal quads.

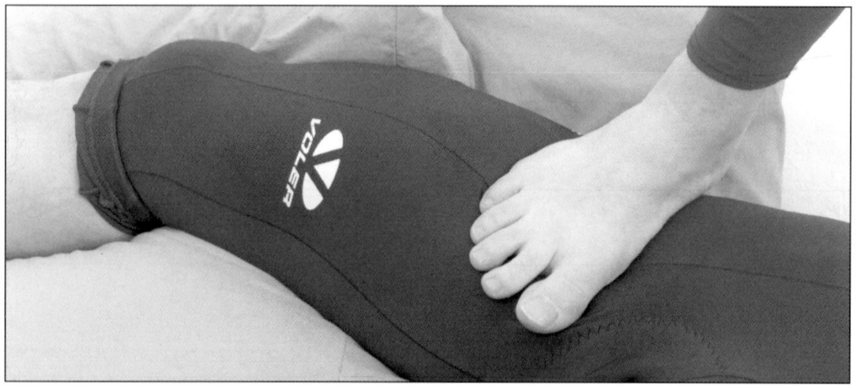

45 degrees gives direct pressure and a stretch.

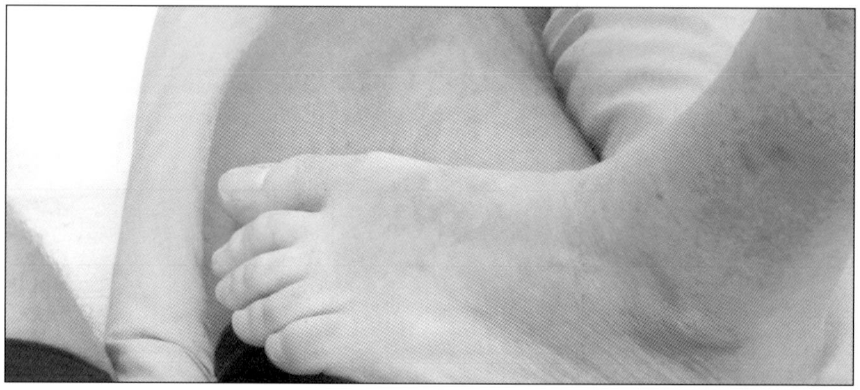

Roll the vastus lateralis medially before direct pressure. Positioning the muscle either medially or laterally with your foot for the best angle-of-attack is an important barefoot skill.

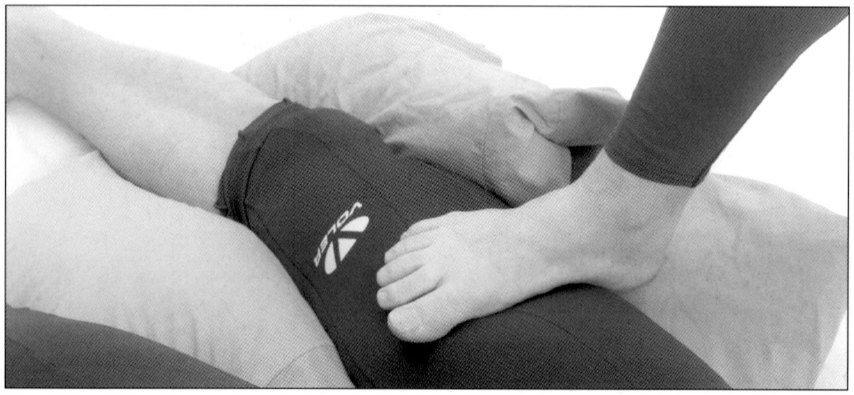

Roll the vastus lateralis medially and compress it for warm-up.

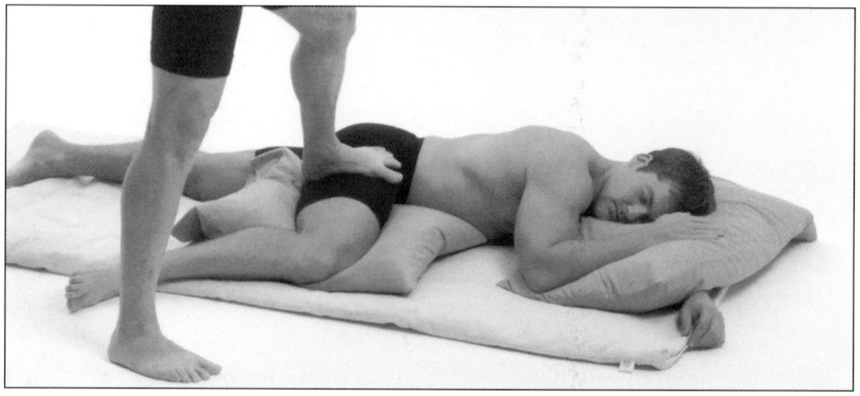

Good bolstering for addressing the vastus lateralis. Sink gradually into the muscle to avoid disturbing your client's hypnogogic state. Protective armoring is always avoided.

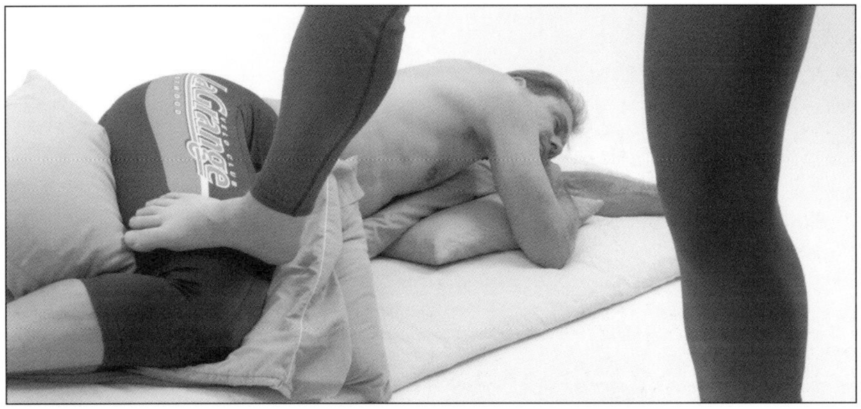

Distal vastus lateralis warm-up.

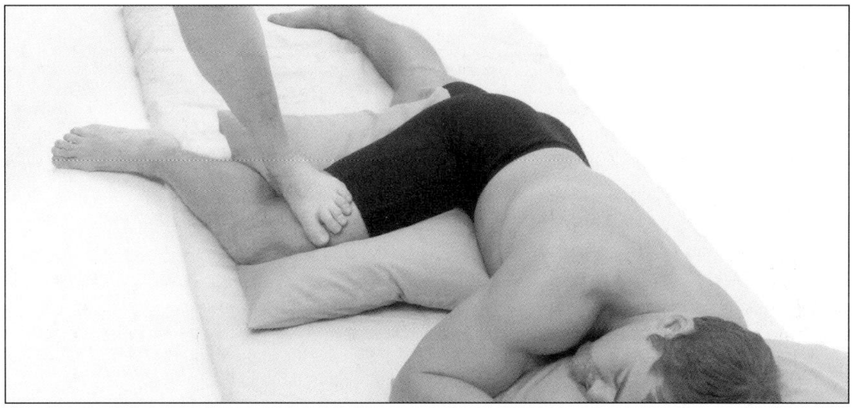

Another approach to the vastus lateralis.

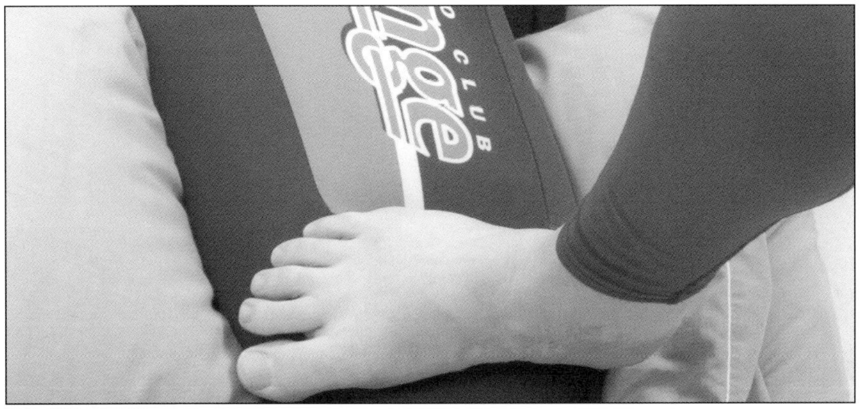

Distal vastus lateralis can be very tender – use moderate pressure.

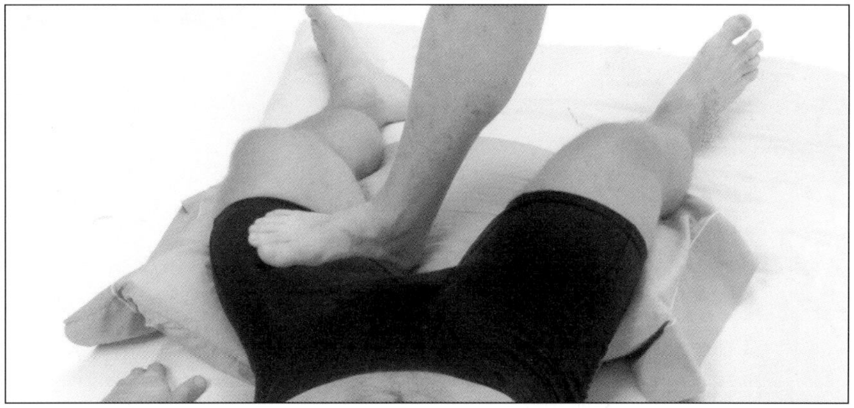

Simultaneous warm-up for the vastus medialis & long adductors.

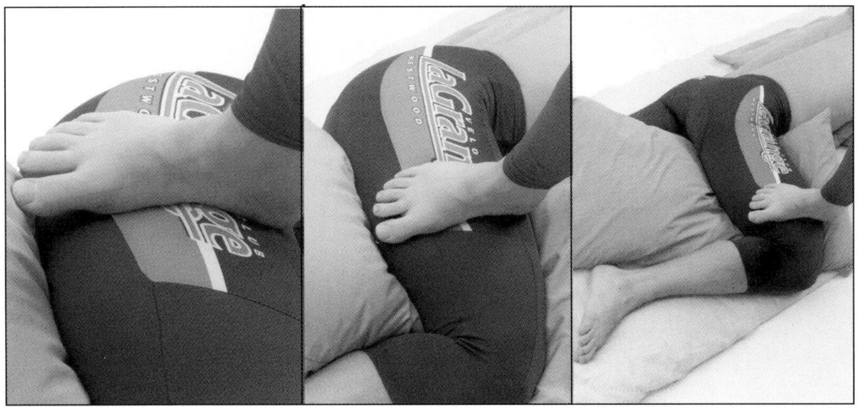

Warming up the vastus laterals.

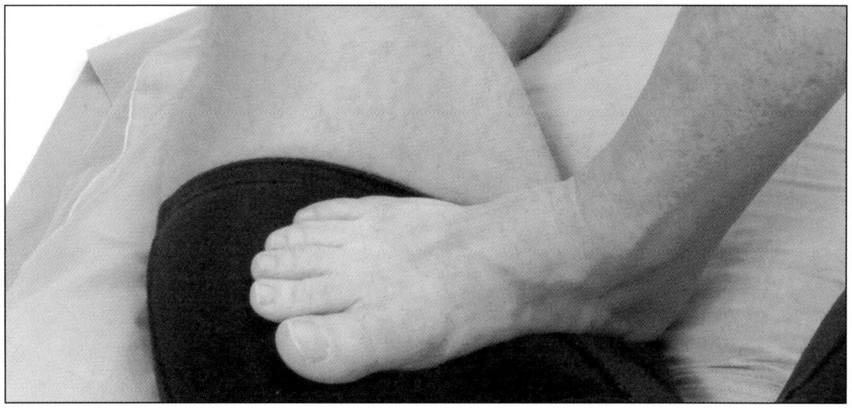

Moderate pressure is used on the medial thigh to avoid compression injury to vulnerable veins, arteries or nerves.

Treatment: Rectus femoris tendonitis.

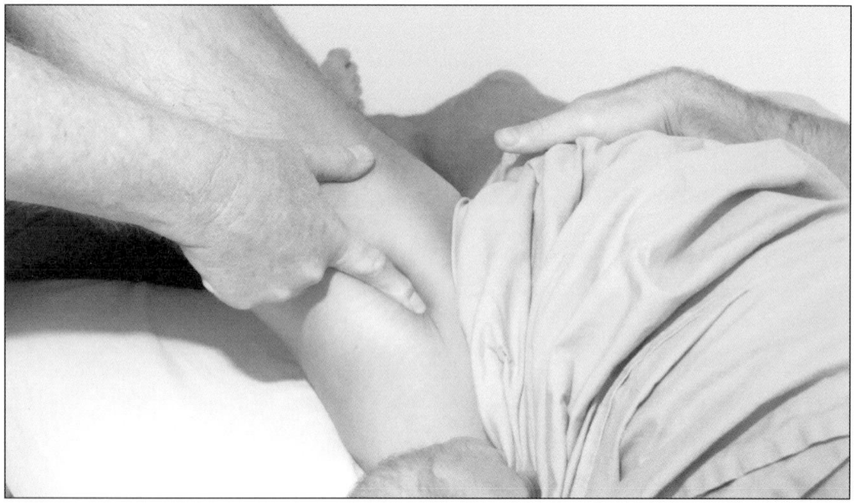

Tendonitis of the rectus femoris origin. This common "runners' problem" requires friction massage at the exact site of the lesion. Prior to treatment, differentiate between the adjacent origins of the rectus femoris and sartorius. The origin of the sartorius is at the anterior superior iliac spine. The primary origin of the rectus femoris is at the anterior inferior iliac spine. In our photo, the rectus femoris lies lateral to the therapist's index finger. To differentiate the rectus femoris, have your client simultaneously flex their slightly abducted and laterally rotated hip while one of your hands offers resistance against their knee and the other at the medial malleolus. This simultaneous flexion and medial rotation will contract both the sartorius and rectus femoris. Then simply press in the space between the two muscles near their origins. If these instructions seem complex, simply read and visualize several times. While both origins may be somewhat tender, the rectus femoris origin is the usual site of pain in the proximal (upper) anterior thigh. Another possible source of pain in this region is the musculotendinous juncture of the iliopsoas muscle.

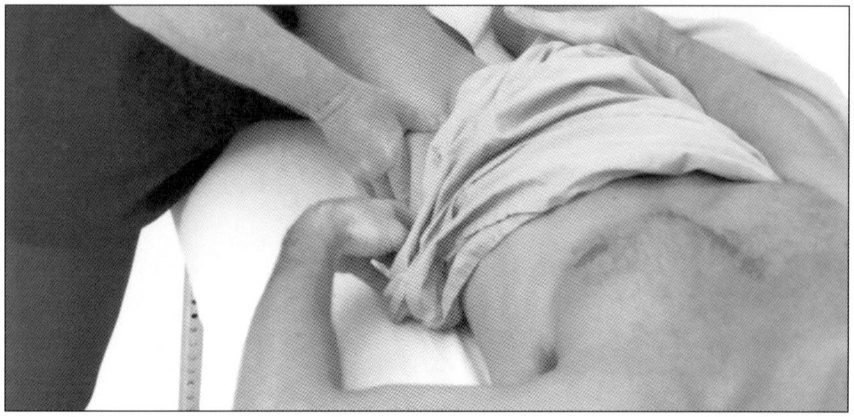

Cross-fiber friction across the rectus femoris just below the anterior inferior iliac spine.

Jumper's Knee

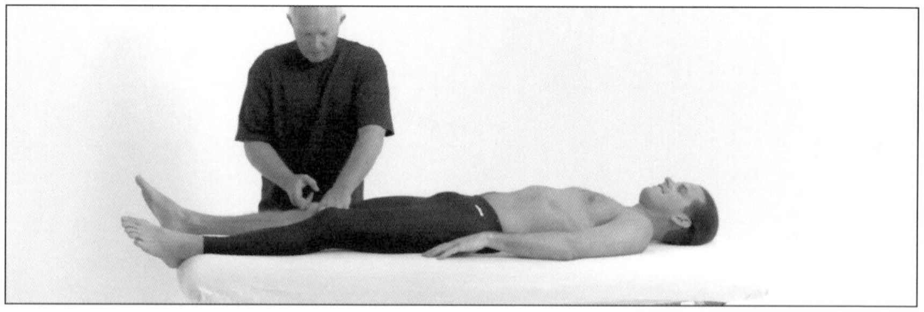

Cross-fiber friction to infrapatellar tendonitis (Jumpers Knee).

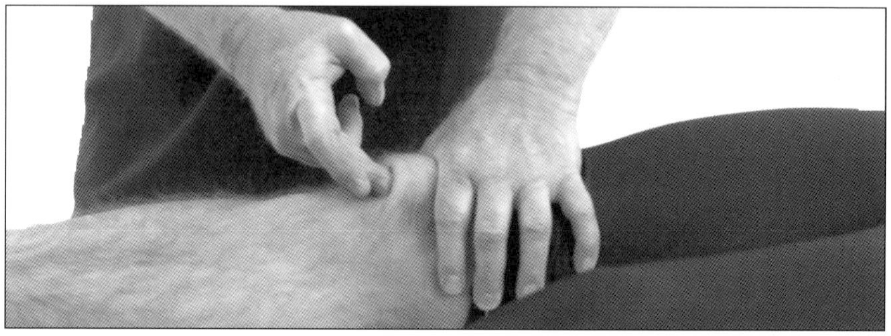

Some therapists friction down into the infrapatellar tendon and completely miss the exact site of the lesion. To insure cross-fiber friction to the exact site of the lesion, rock the inferior pole of the patella upward by pushing down (with the webbing between your thumb and index finger) on the superior pole of the patella (toward the floor). With the inferior pole of the patella rocked upwards, press into the edge of the patella medially, laterally, and in the middle. The most painful spot will be the lesion. Examining the photo carefully will help you understand this work.

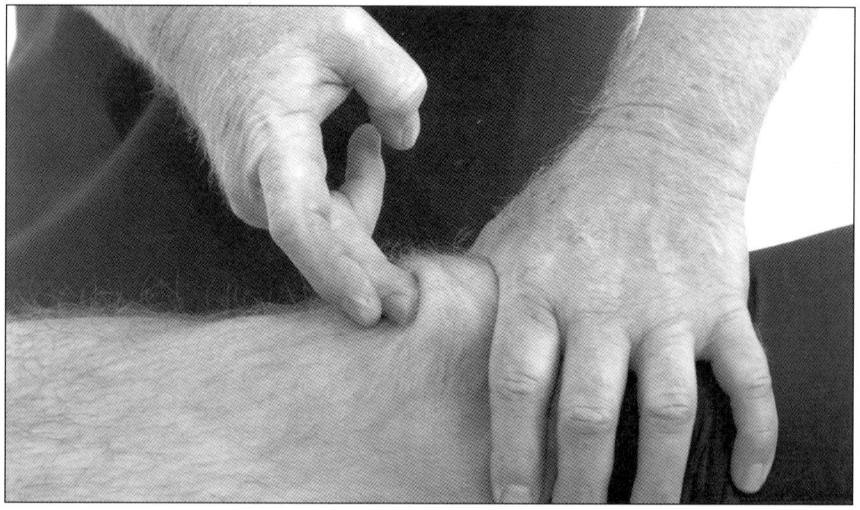

Cross-fiber friction is administered in a "sawing" motion, back and forth for 1 minute on the initial treatment.

ADDUCTORS

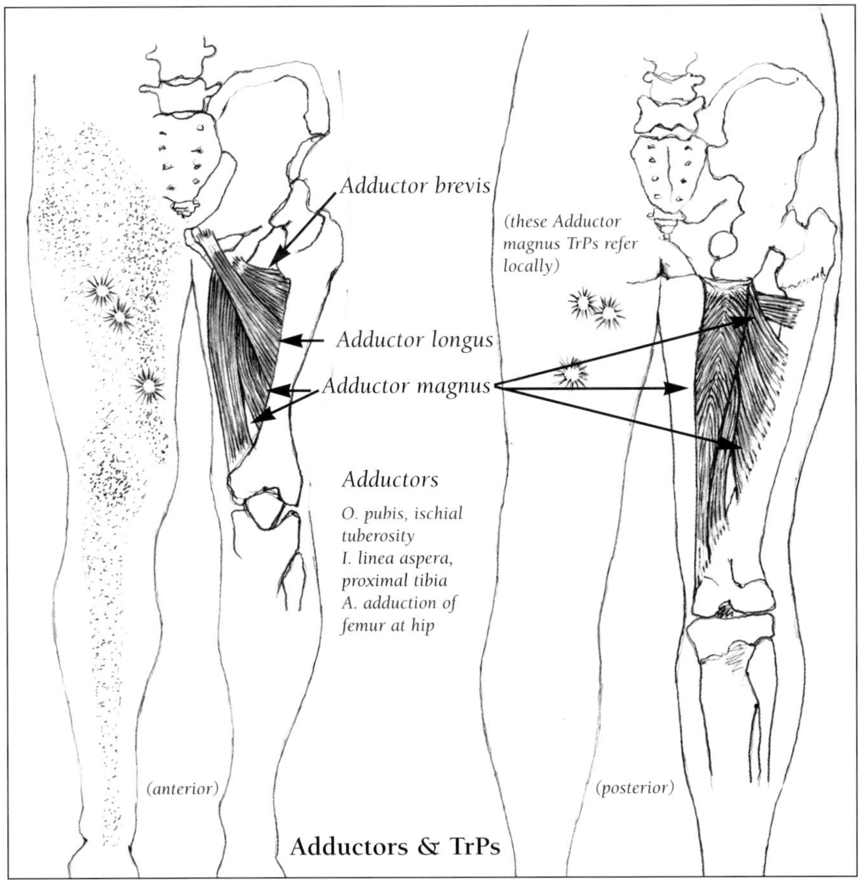

Adductors & TrPs

THE ADDUCTORS OF THE HIP play a role in standing, walking and running. Primarily hip adductors, they also assist in hip flexion, hip extension and gait stabilization.

Adductor strains are typically caused by quick or extreme abduction. Chronic adductor longus groin strains customarily occur in athletes, with direct pressure and cross-fiber friction often resolving the problem.

Treatment is usually administered to the adductor longus belly approximately two inches from its pubic attachment. Breaking down old adherent scar tissue with cross-fiber friction is frequently necessary to prevent recurrence.

Tendonitis also occurs in the pes anserinus attachment of the gracilis. It presents with a sharp, burning sensation. Brief, moderate friction massage often aborts this process if done as soon as the client senses the problem. Gracilis groin pulls occur at the pubic bone attachment. While less common than adductor longus pulls, they occur frequently enough to be a part of any bodywork assessment for groin pain. Typically, friction massage will be administered right at the attachment to the pubic bone. Because of the proximity to genitalia, use discretion.

> Proper warm-up, plus pre- and post-exercise stretching, will prevent many groin pulls.

Adductor trigger points can refer up into the groin, into the pelvis and down into the knee. These trigger point referrals mimic both knee pain and groin pulls. Adductor magnus trigger points commonly cause pain within the pelvis. This pain is often difficult for clients to pinpoint. Fairly deep, medial posterior palpation close to the origin with the client side-lying is necessary to locate these adductor magnus trigger points.

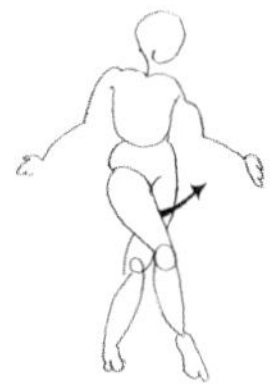

Foot Treatment

• As a warm-up for treating the adductors, have your client side-lying. Warm the adductors from pubic ramus to knee with gentle to moderate compressions. Assess for tightness, local and referred pain.

• When trigger points are found, use prolonged heel (or lateral edge of foot) direct pressure. Follow with work to the adductor magnus from the pubic ramus to the knee with your client prone. Avoid strong pressure over the adductor hiatus (Hunters Canal).

• With the client supine, work the adductor longus and brevis muscles. First warm and assess and then treat with moderate, prolonged direct pressure on trigger points and fascial restrictions.

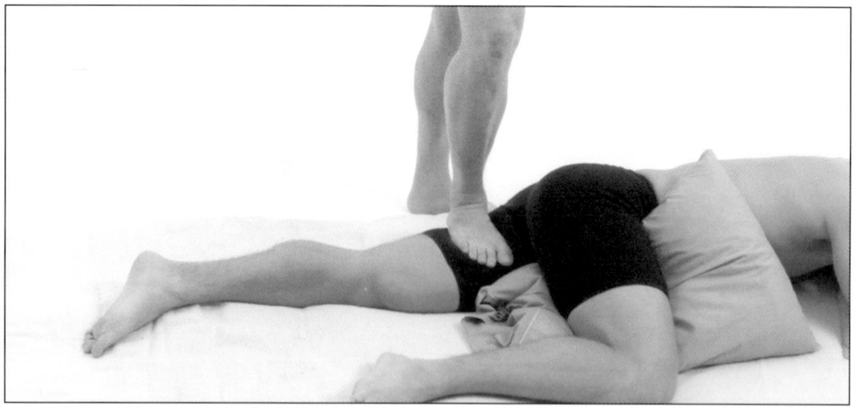

Side-lying approach to warm up the adductor magnus and medial hamstring.

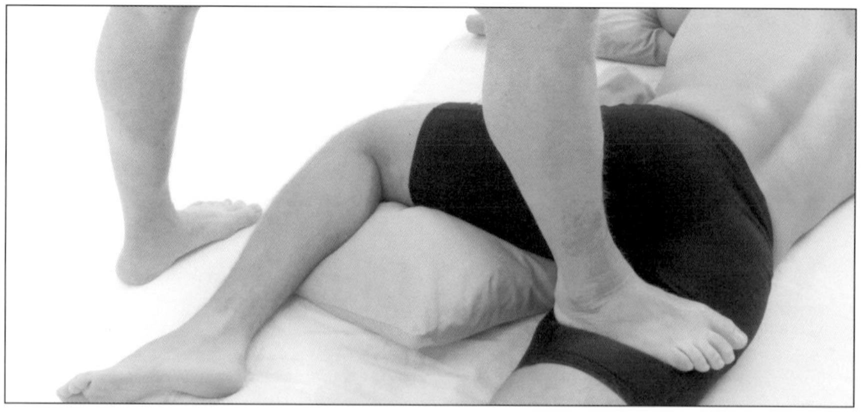

Anterior approach to the long and short adductors.

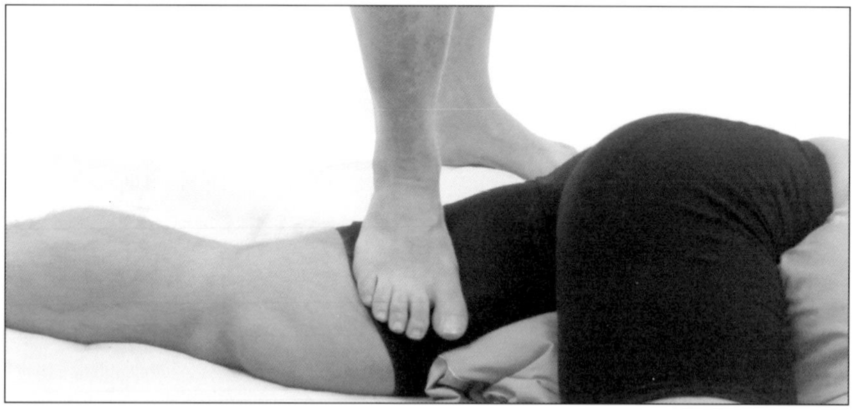

Adductor warm-up lateral and superior to Hunter's Canal.

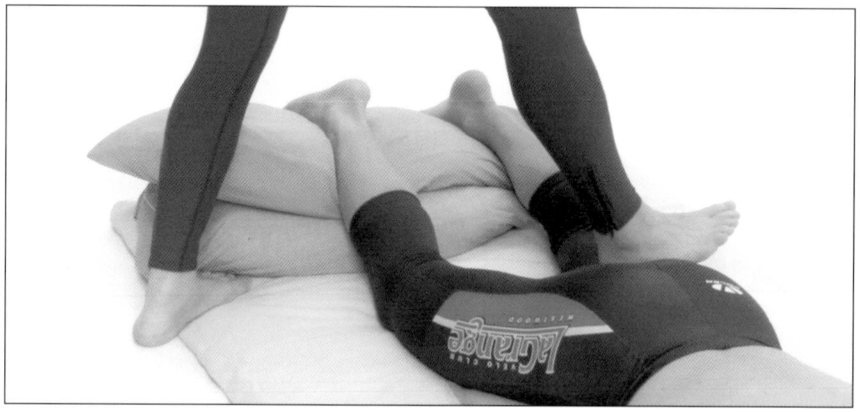

Direct pressure into the adductor magnus.

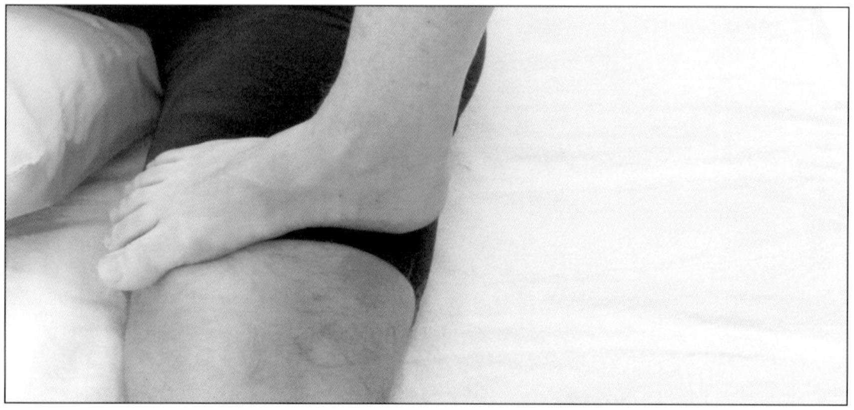

A proper fit…

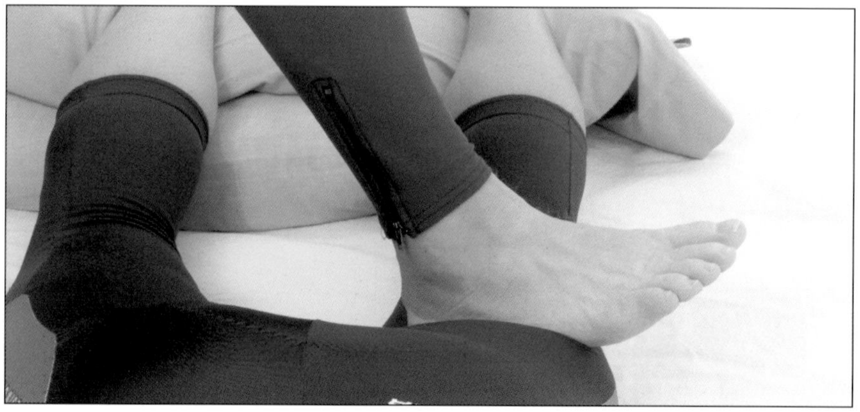

Deeper pressure to aductor magnus.

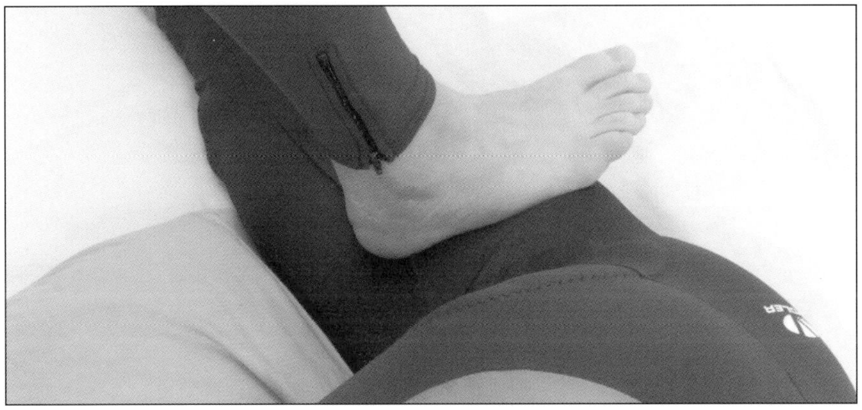

Direct pressure to the adductor longus.

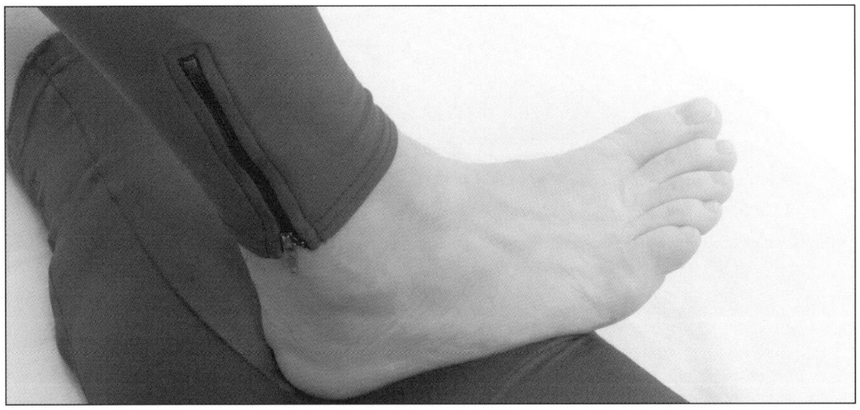

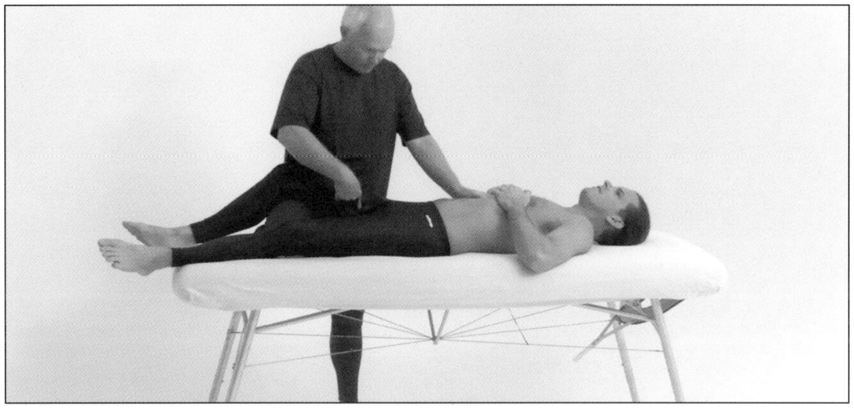

Cross-fiber friction for typical groin pulls. Most often the problem is in the adductor longus or the origin of the gracilis. Therapist's right leg bolsters client's slightly medially rotated and flexed hip.

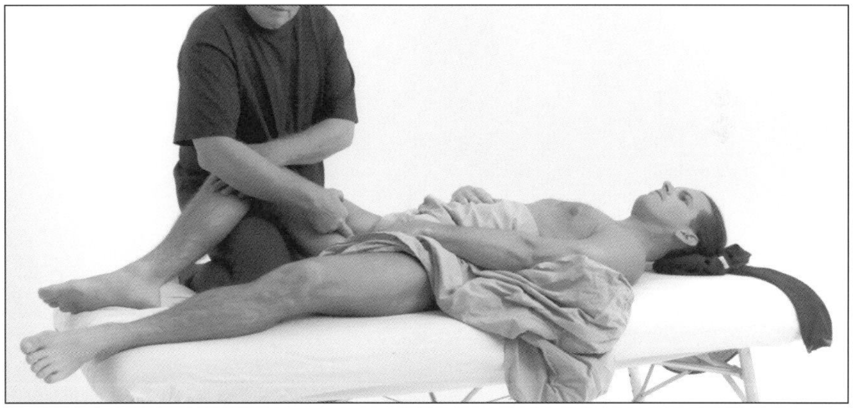

To differentiate adductor longus from gracilis prior to treatment, client gently adducts knee against therapist's hand. The adductor longus is found above the therapist's finger and the gracilis below.

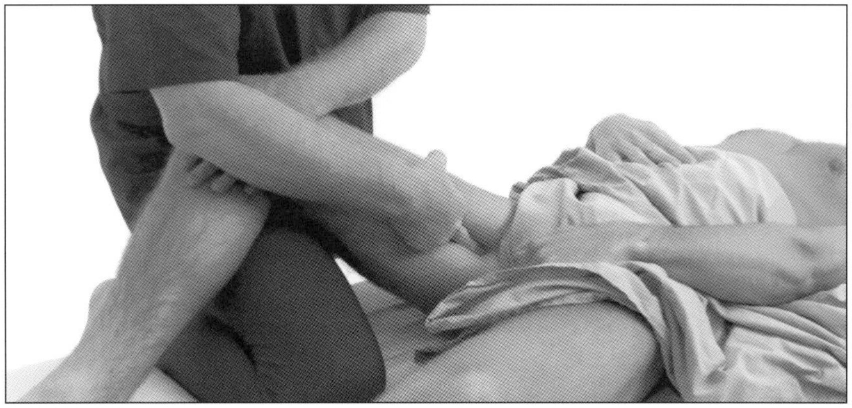

When treating the adductor longus, the pincer grip will wrap around the gracilis right here to reach deeper into the adductor magnus.

Hand Treatment

Locate (palpate) the femoral artery, nerve and vein before compressing the pectineus or adductor magnus muscle with the client side-lying or prone.

Cautions

- Do not over-treat.
- Don't friction a pes anserinus bursitis.
- Avoid deep pressure into the adductor hiatus.
- Avoid direct pressure or friction massage across the femoral artery, vein and nerve.

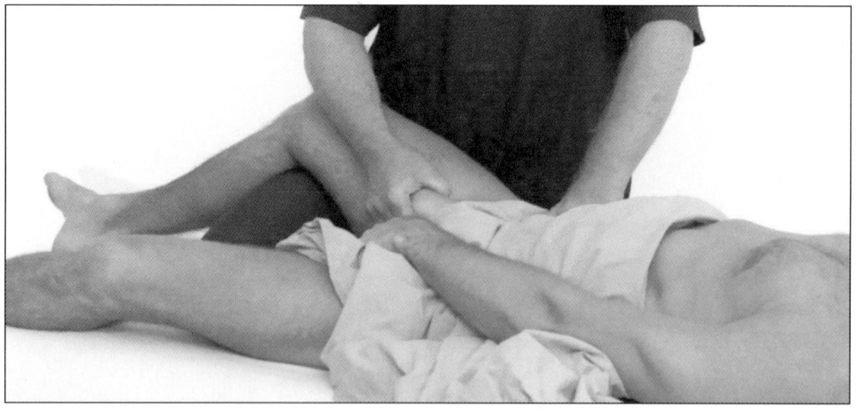

A strained adductor longus will be seen more often than a gracilis pull. To treat, grasp the belly of the adductor longus , approximately 2 inches below its pubic attachment in a pincer grip with the lesion between the thumb and index and middle finger. Friction transversely to the fibers of the muscle.

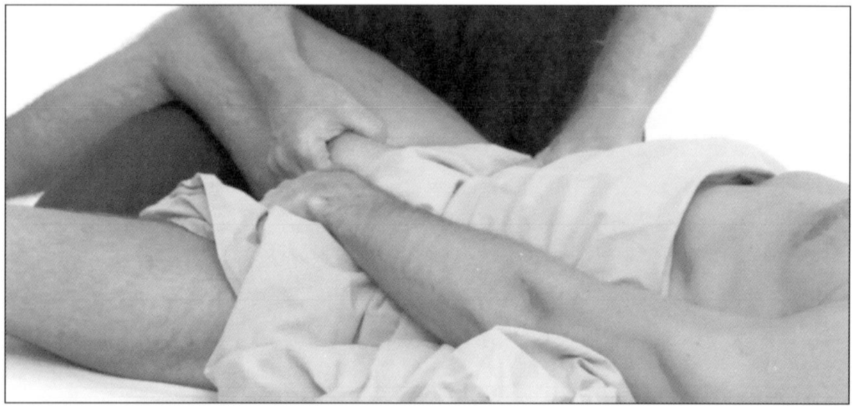

Friction is moderate with only a small degree of abduction at the hip. Any greater abduction at the hip (or stretching) will exacerbate the lesion.

Floor Treatment

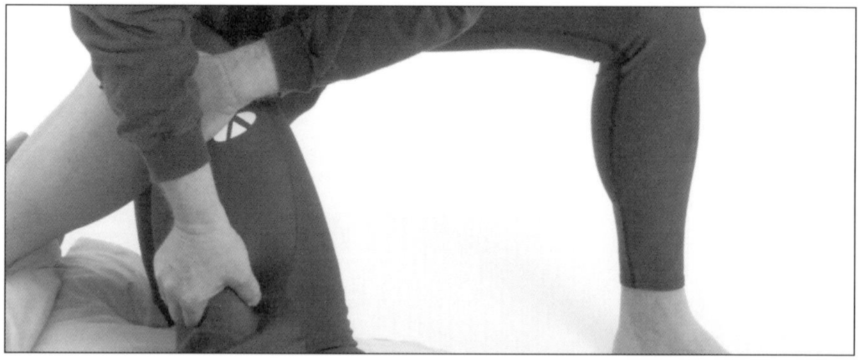

Floor treatment of adductor longus groin pull.

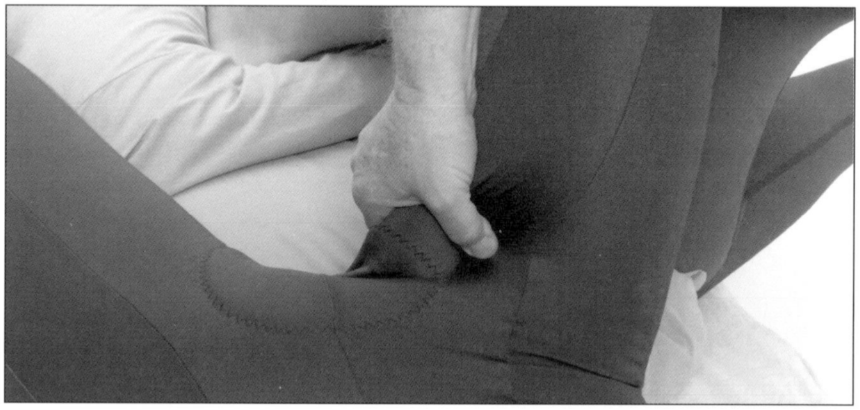

Hand forms a "claw" that neither opens nor closes during treatment once the lesion has been located.

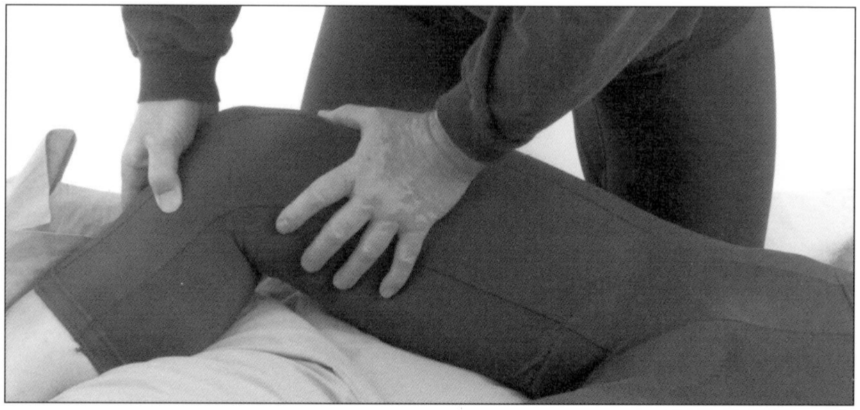

Cross-fiber friction pes anserinus attachment of the gracilis. This tendonitis often has a burning sensation as opposed to the more common TrP deep ache.

Gastrocnemius

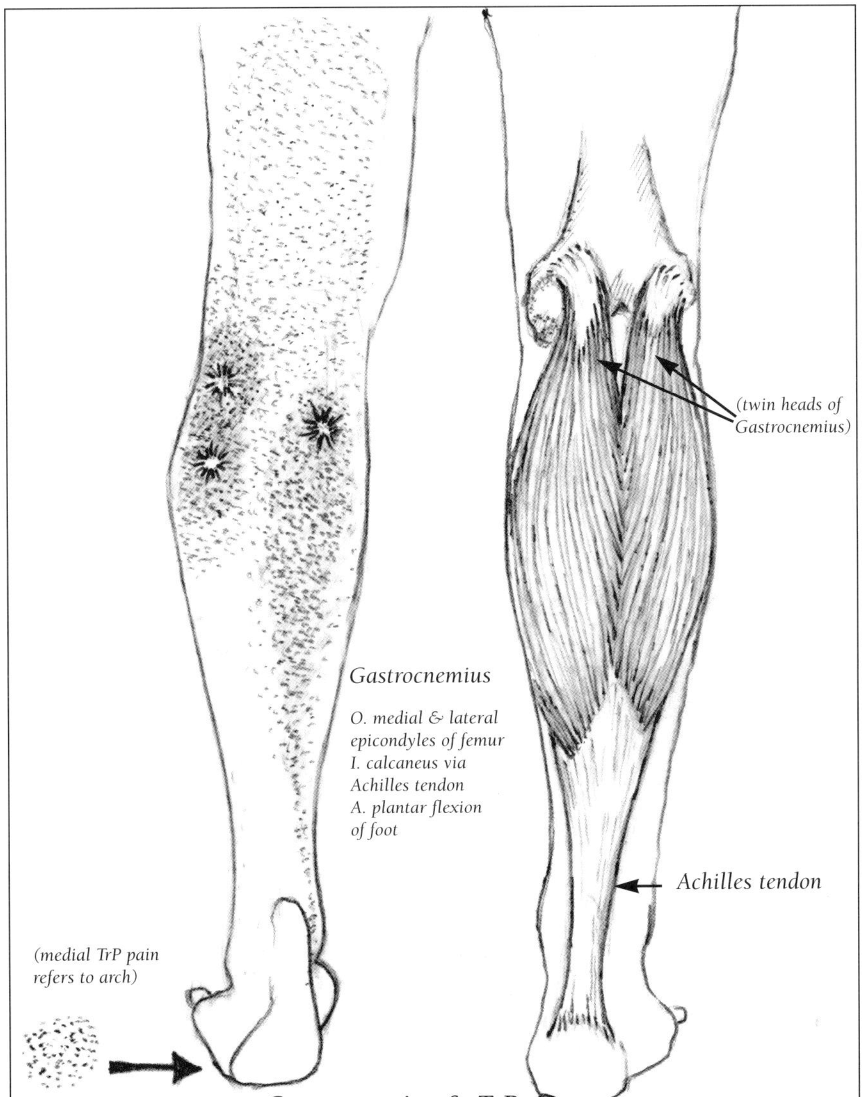

Gastrocnemius & TrPs

THIS TWO OR OCCASIONALLY THREE-HEADED MUSCLE forms a functional unit (triceps surae) with the underlying soleus muscle. The gastrocnemius provides for ankle plantar flexion or knee flexion. Both muscles play a role in ankle and knee stabilization. Vigorous plantar flexion involves the gastrocnemius as well as the soleus and deep to flexors. As knee flexion approaches 90 degrees, the polyarticular gastrocnemius becomes inoperative.

Trigger points in the medial head of the gastrocnemius can cause nocturnal calf cramps. Eliminating these trigger points can result in better sleep and happier clients. Pincer palpation is often the easiest way to treat trigger points in this muscle. If our client is large, use direct pressure from either the heel or ball of the foot. We usually work with a side-lying client or from the contra-lateral side of the body with a prone client.

Vigorous walking, jogging, or running up a steep incline, or a sudden over-stretch, can activate trigger points in this muscle and/or cause Achilles tendonitis – particularly if it has been shortened by overuse or improper footwear. Cowboy boots or high heels inevitably shorten this muscle. Instruct your client to stretch regularly as preventive care.

A gastrocnemius trigger point referral into the distal hamstring can mimic a medial hamstring pull. A gastrocnemius trigger points referral into the plantar surface of the foot can mimic a plantar fascia tear. Carefully palpating the tendon and the muscle belly for pain will give us clues as to whether a tear or a trigger point is operative.

Occasionally a trigger point will be found in the Achilles tendon proper. Be careful when applying direct pressure in this area to avoid the tibial nerve and the posterior tibial vein and artery.

Don't work on tears. Tennis leg is a tear in the distal portion of the medial head of the gastrocnemius. Direct pressure or compressions here in early healing stages can exacerbate the problem by tearing the newly forming scar. Avoid pressure to the popliteal space.

We query female clients complaining of deep calf pain as to whether they are using birth control pills. These pills can increase the likelihood of clotting. Chronic exertional compartment syndrome (often bilateral and commonly reversible with rest) needs to be differentiated from an acute compartment syndrome – a medical diagnosis.

Cautions

Refer immediately with any of the following warning signs as they can indicate a calf clot or phlebitis. Also true with soleus.

- Temperature difference between the feet or a lack of pedal pulse.
- Deep pain in the calf region accompanied by swelling and pain on walking (sometimes even at rest).
- Calf tenderness, redness, diffuse warmth and foot pain.

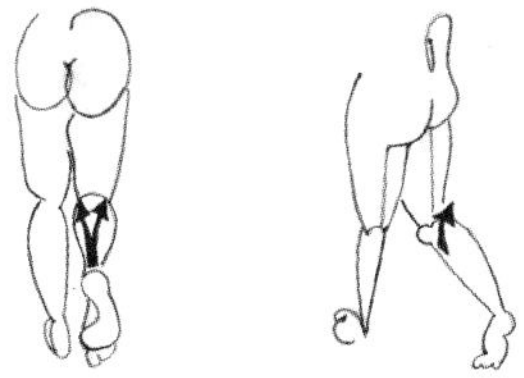

Treatment

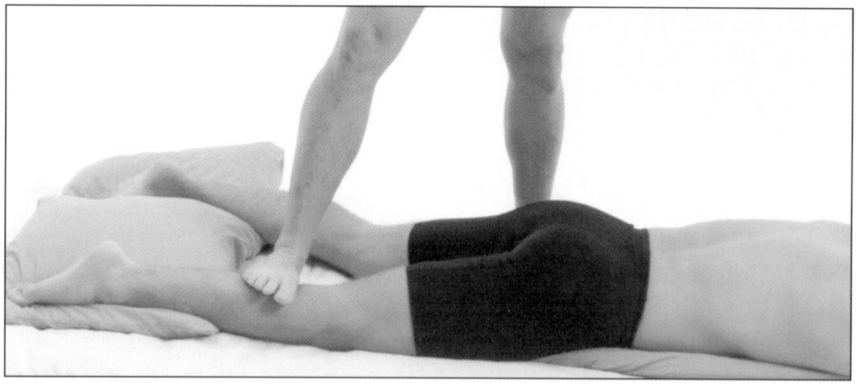

Cross-body treatment. Therapist is at his ease with weight evenly distributed between his support leg and his client's muscle. By extending his torso and standing upright, pressure can be lifted from the client's gastroc without "pushing off" the muscle, possibly causing excessive pressure on the gastrocnemius.

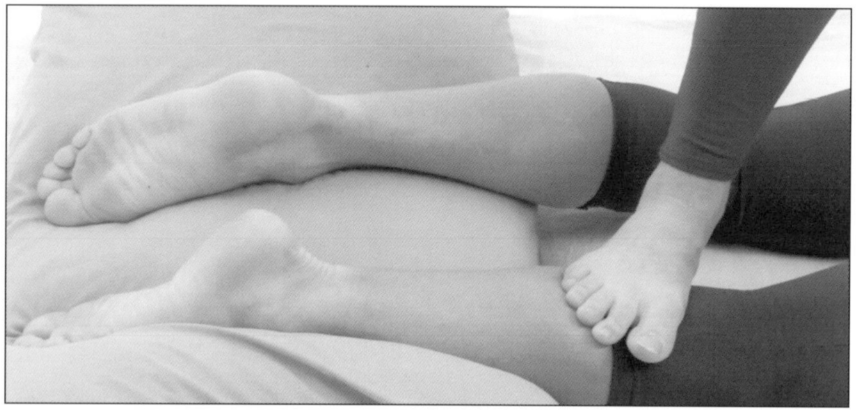

Pressure is focused through 5th metatarsal head.

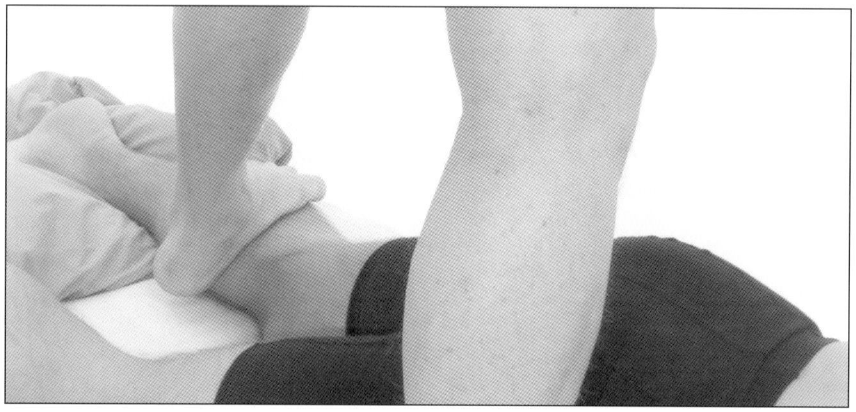

Therapist rotates medial gastrocnemius laterally for focused pressure.

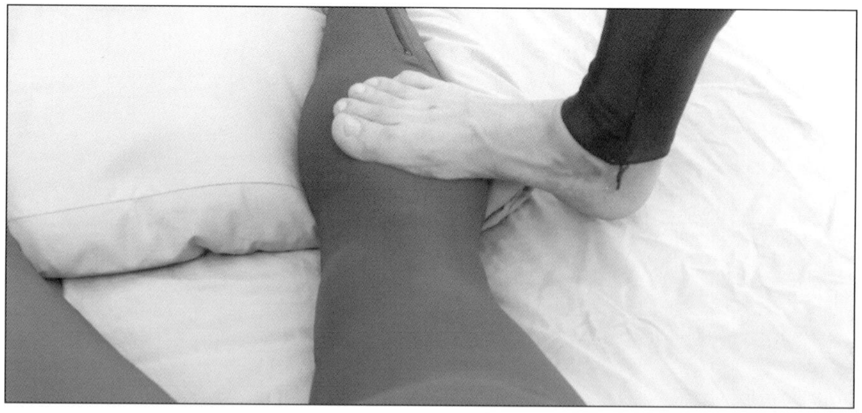

Warm-up or treatment for lateral gastrocnemius.

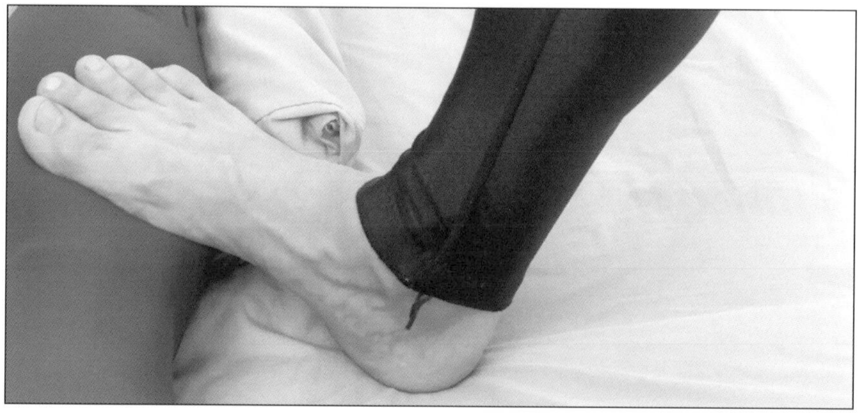

Controlled pressure with heel suported.

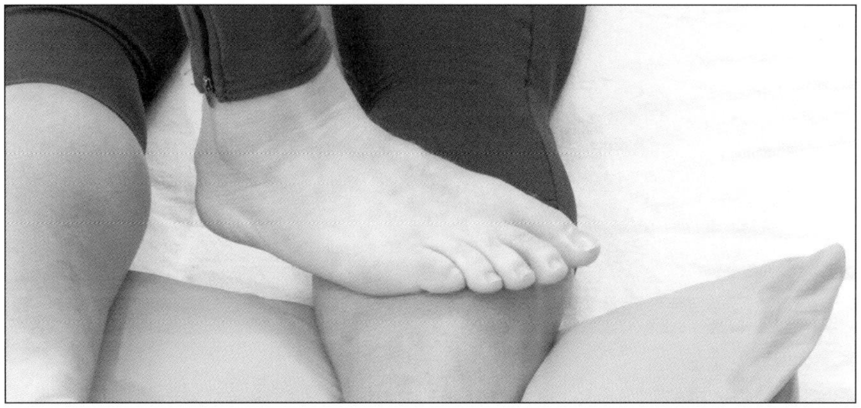

With client prone and ankle well-bolstered, gently warm the twin bellies of the gastrocnemius with foot compressions. Use care – this region is tender on many people.

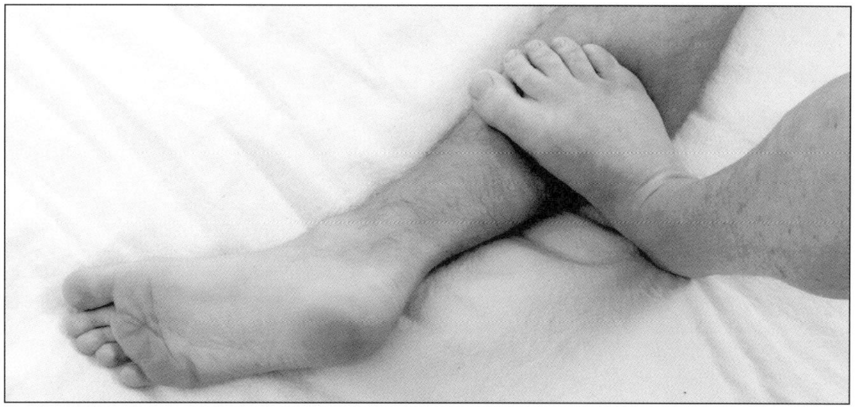

Side-lying warm-up to the distal gastrocnemius.

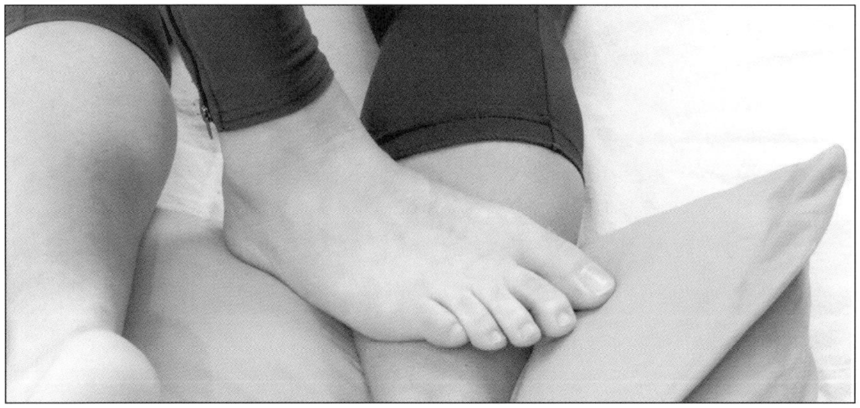

Treat the trigger points with direct pressure from the heel or the ball of the foot.

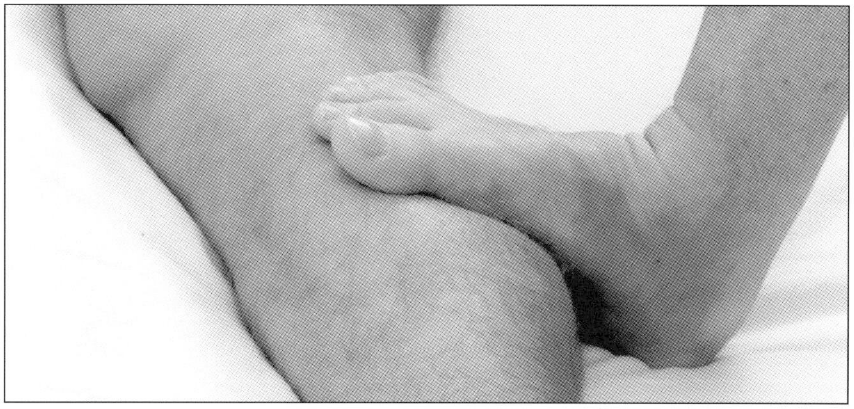

Heel-supported foot lessens pressure, enhances control, and gives you a bit of a calf stretch.

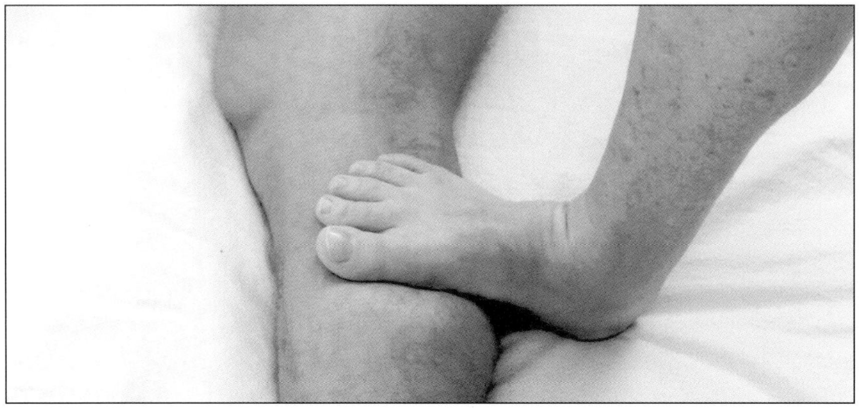

Side-lying direct pressure to the medial head of the gastrocnemius.

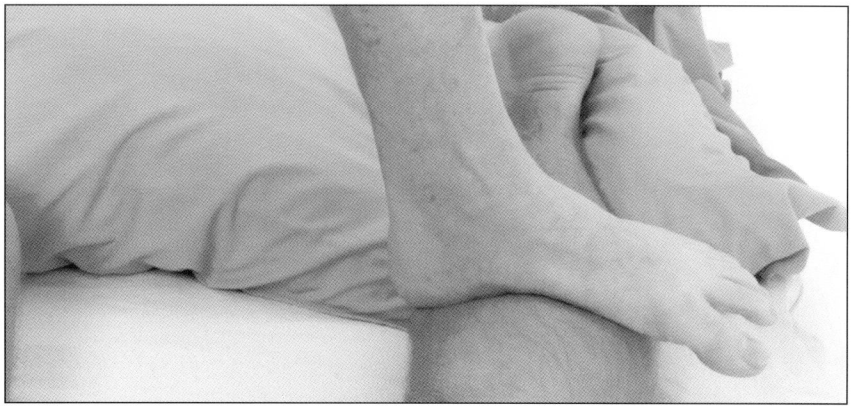

Distal gastrocnemius warm-up.

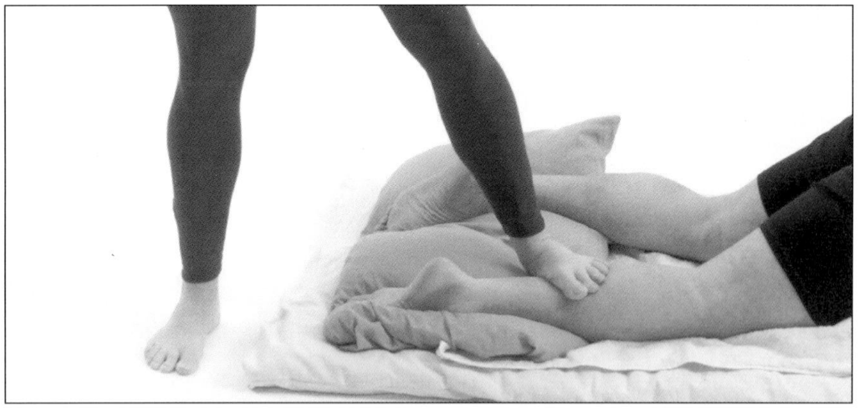

If needed, treat with gentle myofascial stretches.

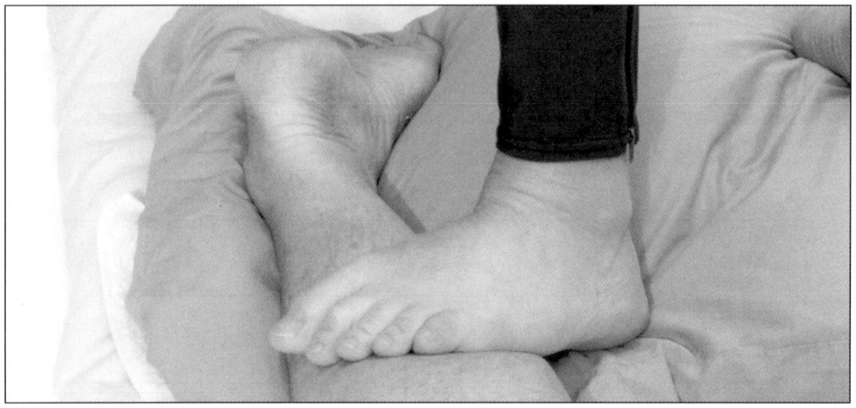

Slight pronation softens contact.

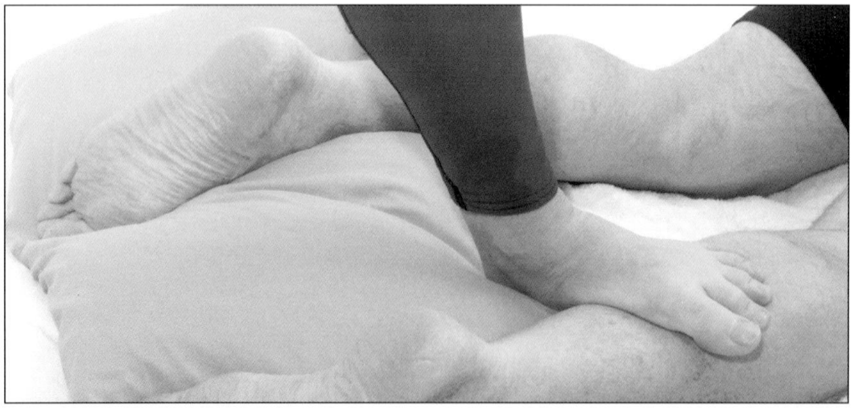

Supported heel plus slight pronation softens contact at arch and first ray.

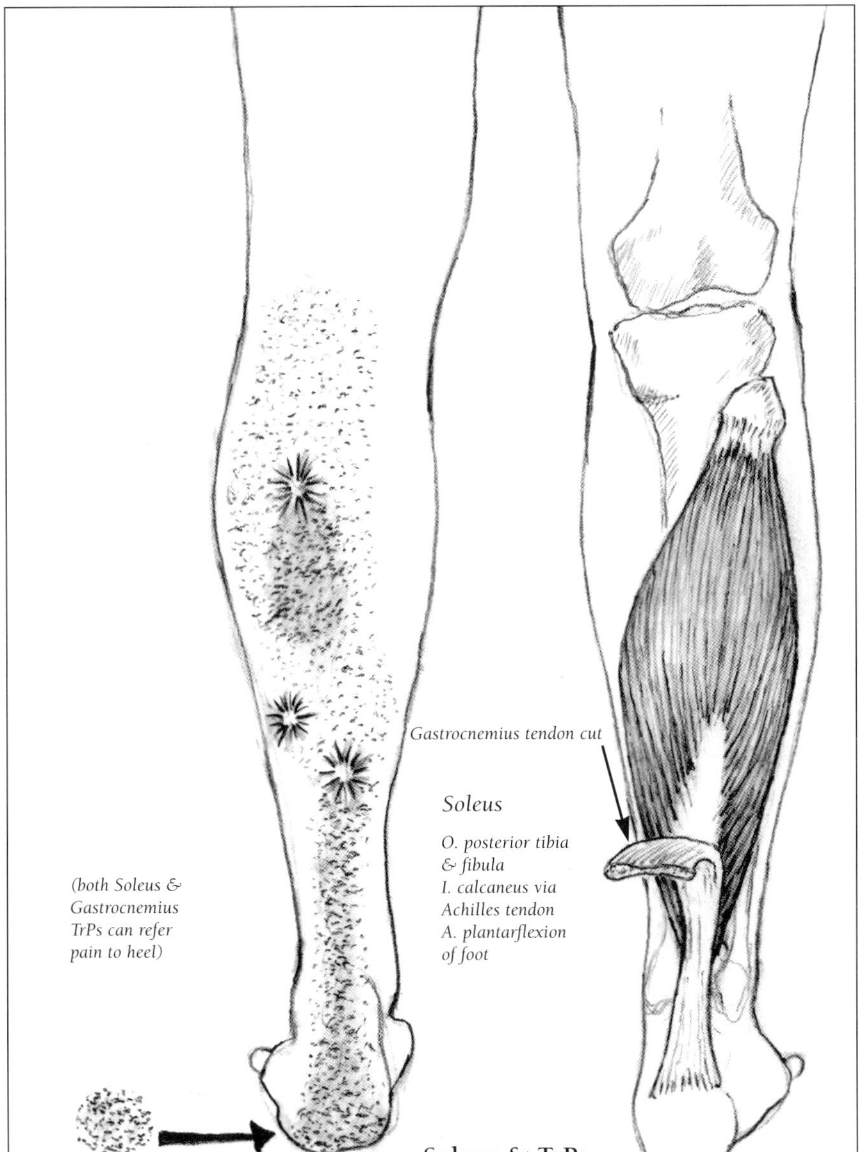

Soleus & TrPs

The soleus, with assistance from the gastrocnemius, is the major plantarflexor of the ankle when running. This muscle also plays a critical role in ankle stabilization when walking or standing. Because of its mechanical effect on venous return from the leg, the soleus is often referred to as the "second heart."

Trigger points in this muscle can refer from the plantar surface of the heel to the ipsilateral (same side) sacrum. Trigger point examination must include both the proximal and distal ends of the muscle. We best accomplish this exam on the distal portion of the muscle using pincer palpation on both sides of the Achilles tendon with the gastrocnemius on a slack. The proximal portion of the muscle is examined with direct pressure.

Soleus trigger points are often caused by overuse in jogging, unaccustomed hill climbing, beach running in soft sand, quick lateral movements and sprints.

The trigger point pain referral pattern can mimic Achilles tendonitis. To circumvent unnecessary cross-fiber treatments on the tendon, always check for referred pain from the soleus first. If there is tendonitis, we use a moderately painful, prolonged cross-fiber friction treatment.

The soleus is held in a shortened position when clients sleep on their backs with their feet held in plantarflexion by the weight of heavy blankets. This foreshortened position perpetuates soleus trigger points.

Cautions

We are putting pressure into the deep compartment of the leg. The peroneal and tibial veins, arteries and nerves are all located here. Go slowly and exercise caution with both pressure and duration.

Much of the soleus lies directly beneath the gastrocnemius. When working on the soleus through the gastrocnemius, caution must be exercised to avoid damage to the distal head of the gastrocnemius.

Check range-of-motion for adequate ankle dorsiflexion. Trigger points in the soleus shorten the normal range. To check, compare with the contralateral leg.

Direct pressure or compressions for tennis leg (in the medial head of the gastrocnemius) in early healing stages can exacerbate the tear by breaching the newly forming scar.

Refer immediately with any of the following warning signs as they can indicate a calf clot or phlebitis (also true with gastrocnemius):
- Temperature difference between the feet or a lack of pedal pulse.
- Deep pain in the calf region accompanied by swelling and pain on walking (sometimes even at rest).
- Calf tenderness, redness, diffuse warmth and foot pain.

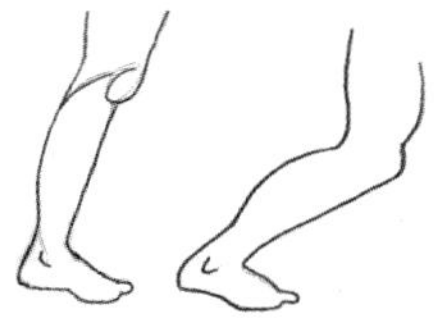

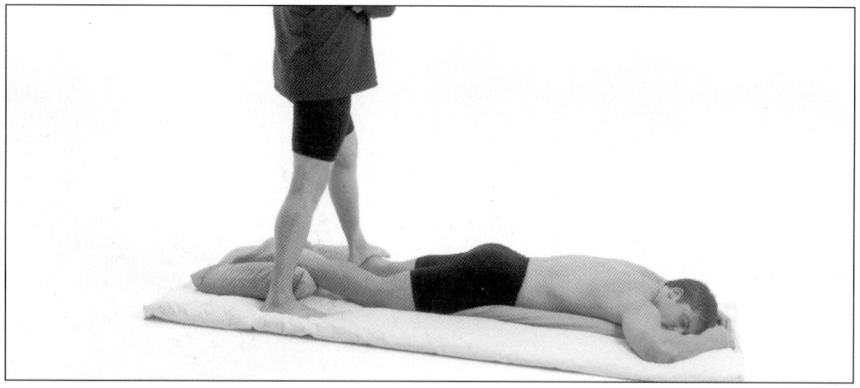

Post exercise soleus soreness is common. Warm the muscle slowly and carefully using foot compressions.

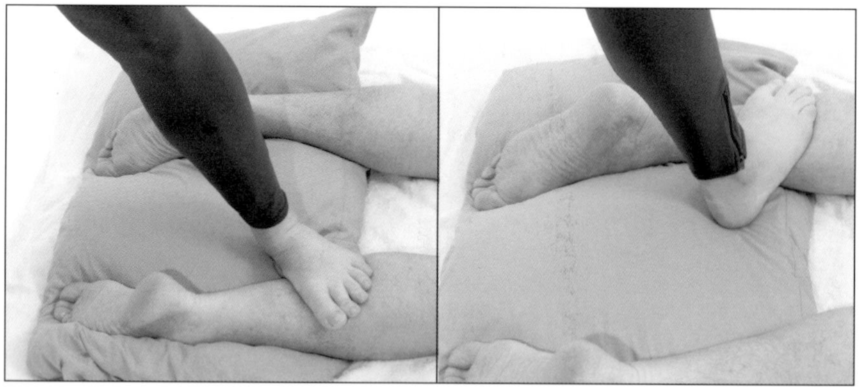

Prone fascial stretch and warm-up.

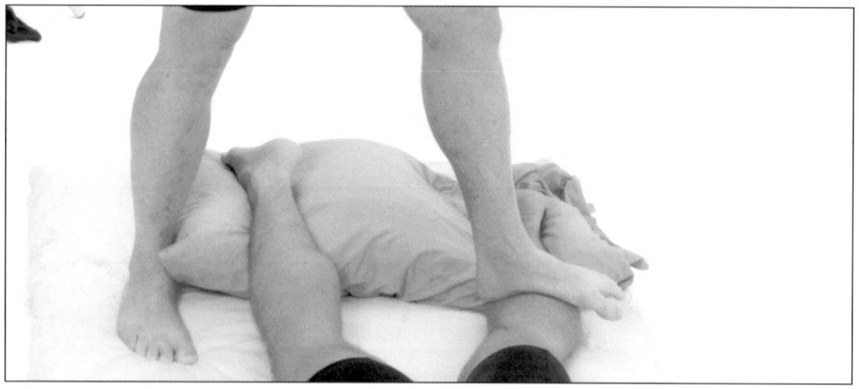

Bolster carefully to avoid stressing knee.

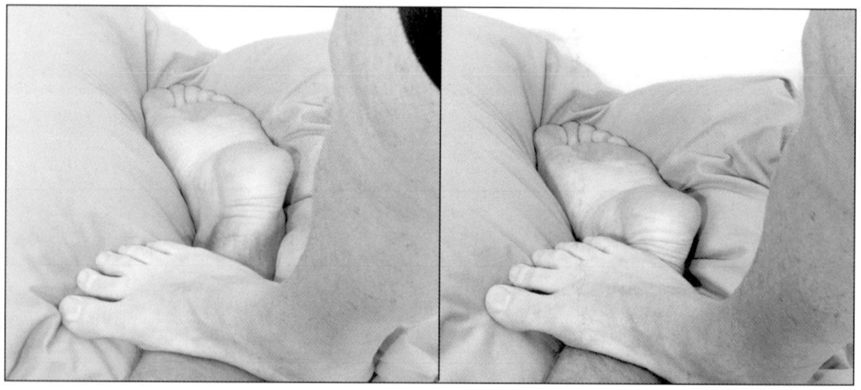

Achilles tendon warm-up.

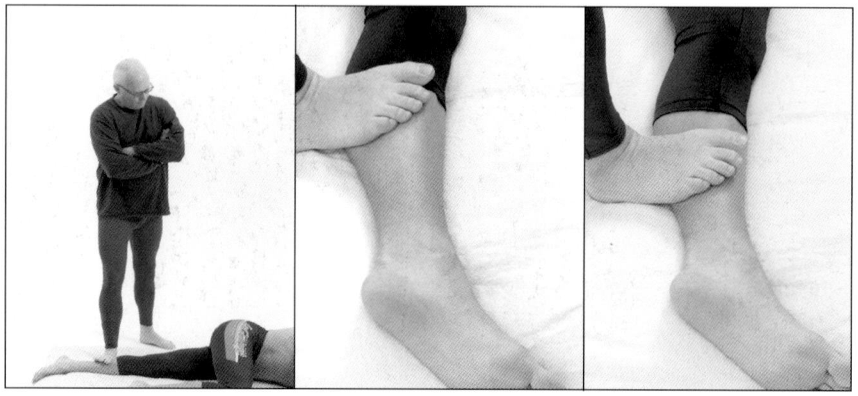

Side-lying soleus warm-up.

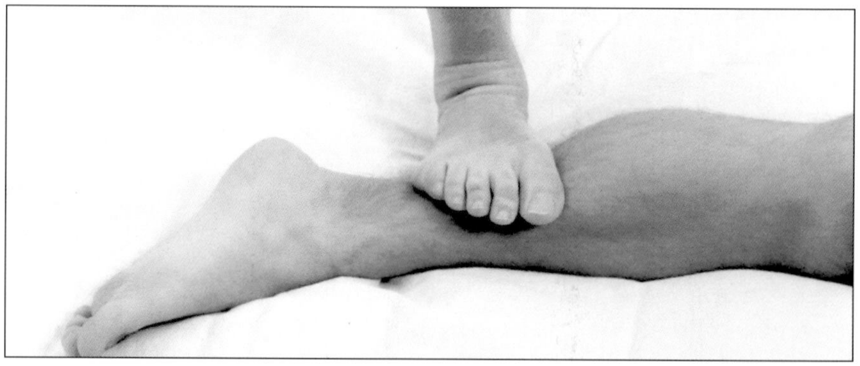

Side-lying Achilles tendon warm-up. Direct pressure to the tendon affects golgi tendon organ to soften muscle. This proprioceptive softening is temporary, but provides good access for treatment and enhances stretching.

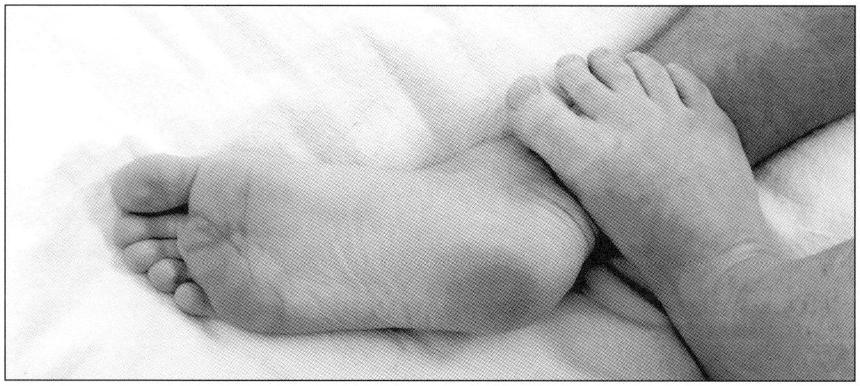

Strong pressure from the first ray is not administered behind the posterior aspect of the medial malleolus. The posterior tibial artery, nerve and vein are all located near the surface.

Table Work

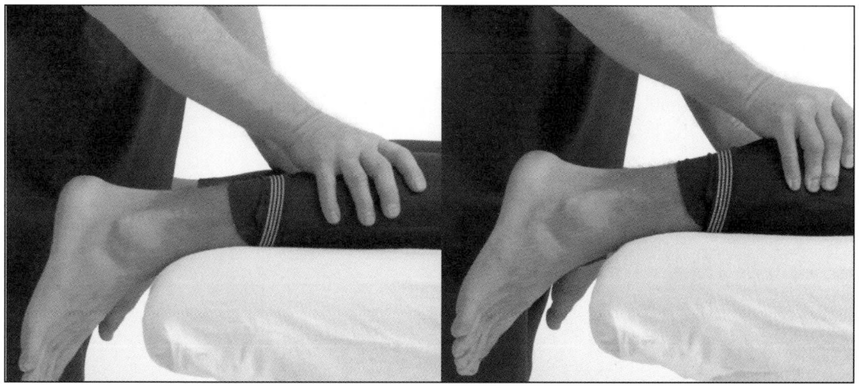

A ruptured Achilles tendon is a bar to treatment. Prior to treatment, assess for tendon integrity. With client prone and ankle past the edge of the table, squeeze the calf to ascertain the integrity of the Achilles tendon. Plantar flexion suggests the tendon is intact. Little or no movement suggests a rupture.

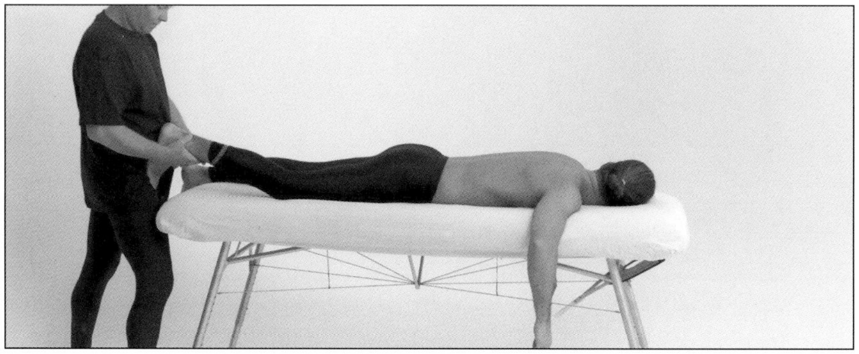

For assessment and treatment of an Achilles tendonitis, put client's foot into slight, passive dorsiflexion.

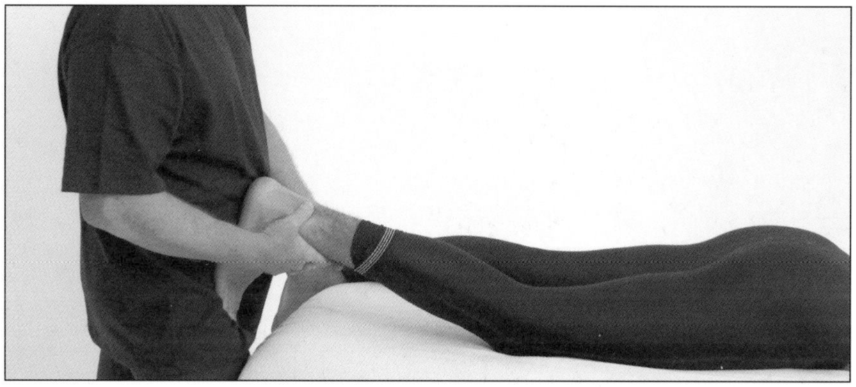

Use the pads of your thumbs to friction the medial and lateral aspect of the tendon searching for the most tender spot.

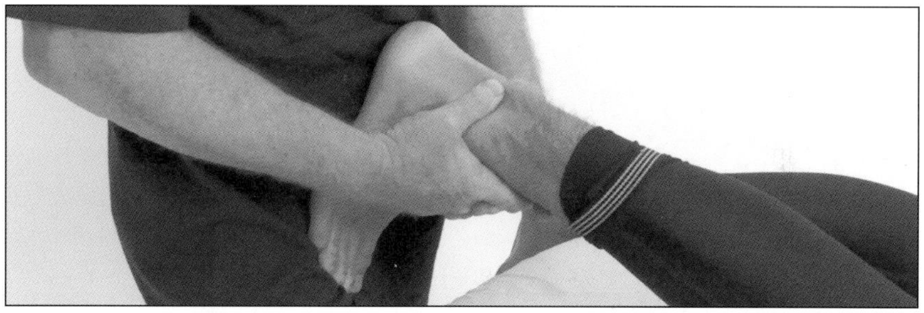

To protect your hands, do not flex and extend your thumbs. The thumbs lock onto the tendon, and the movement comes from your wrist and shoulder. The friction alternates between the medial and lateral side – as one thumb goes up, the other thumb pulls down. The posterior aspect of the tendon is rarely involved and thus requires no friction. Occasionally a ballet dancer will have a tendonitis right at the calcaneal attachment. The other exception is when a stiff heel in a shoe or a boot rubs against and irritates the tendon.

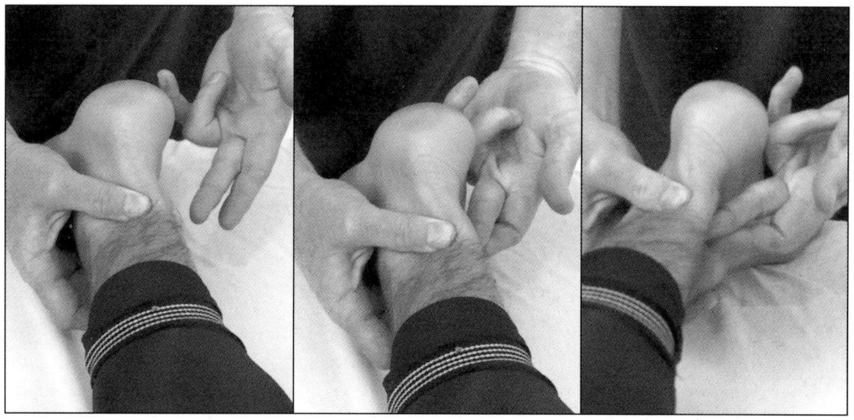

To friction the anterior surface of the tendon, place the foot onto the table in passive plantarflexion and push the tendon medially as far as you can. With your opposite hand lying parallel to the tendon, reach under the inflamed area, push to the ceiling, and half pronate and supinate (alternatively) to create a cross-fiber friction.

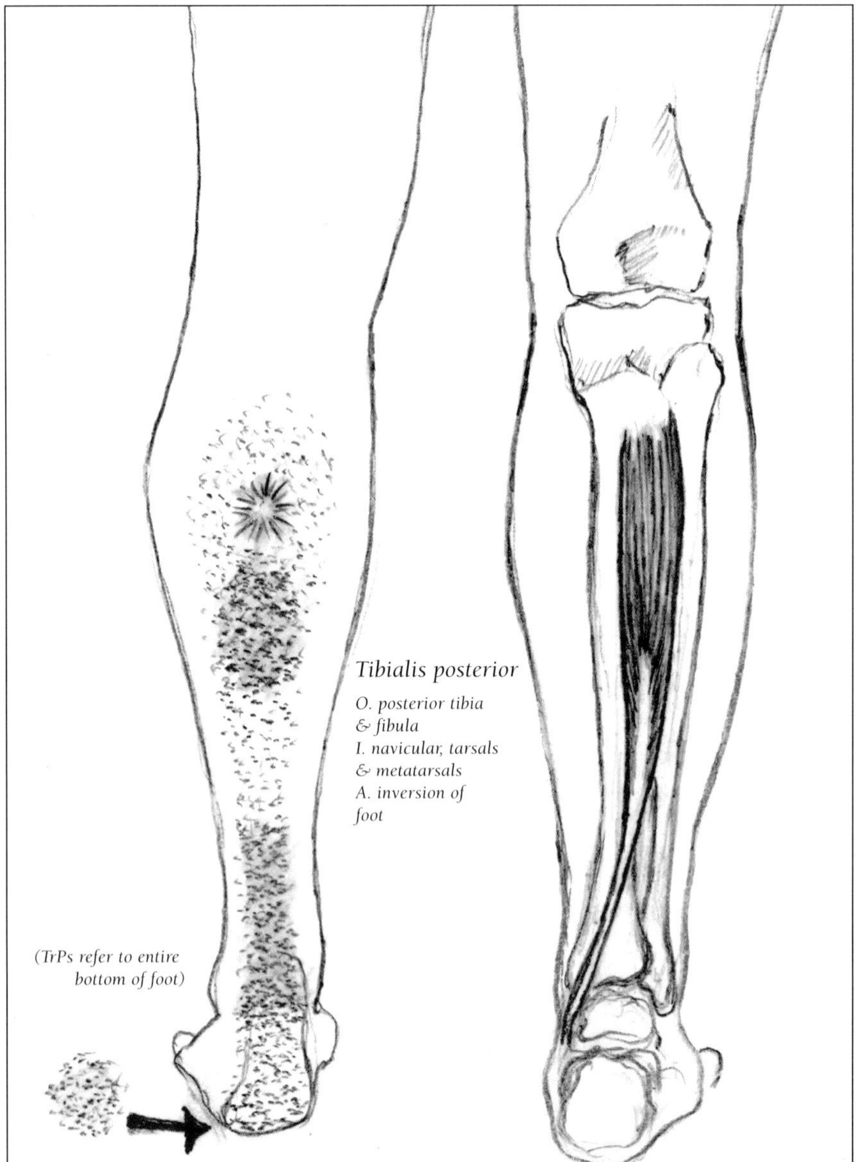

Tibialis posterior & TrPs

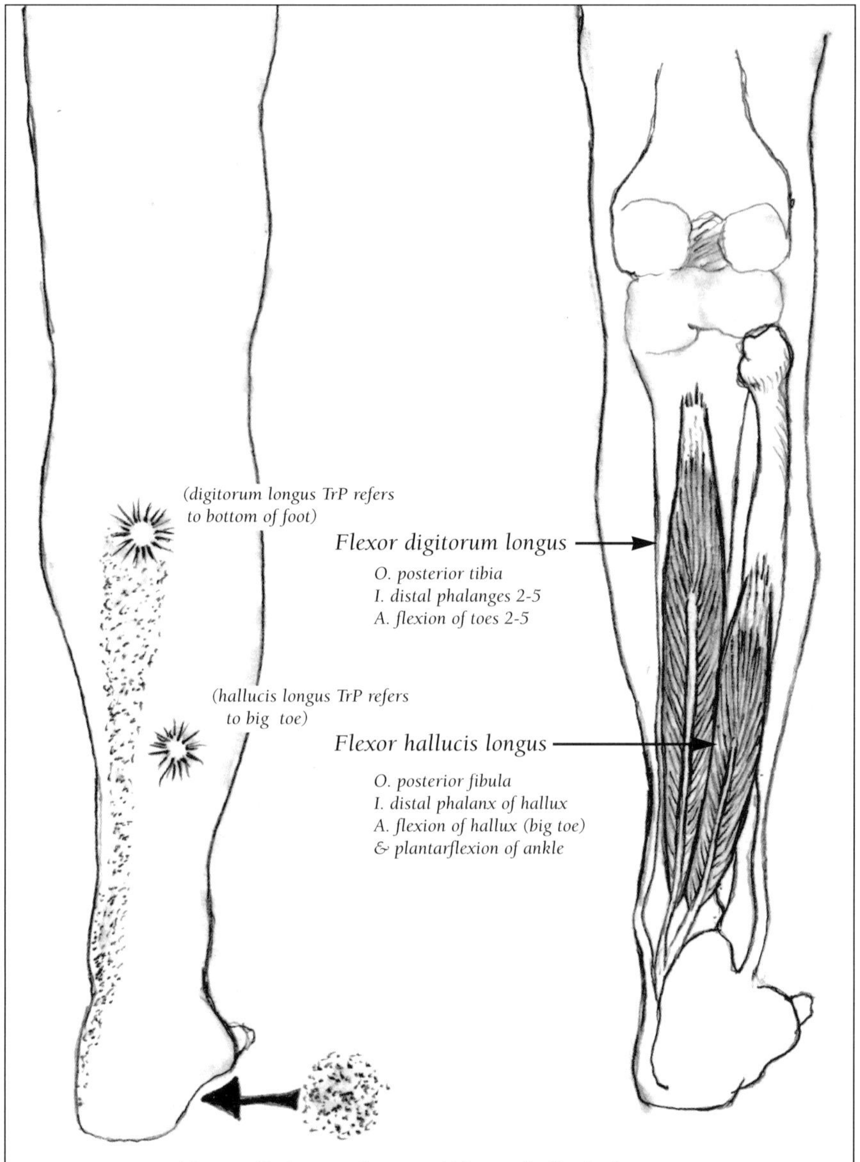

Flexor digitorum longus / Flexor hallucis longus

THE TIBIALIS POSTERIOR, flexor digitorum longus and the flexor hallucis longus form the deep compartment of the leg. These muscles (commonly referred to as Tom, Dick & Harry to facilitate memorizing them for a test) all assist in plantarflexion of the ankle. The flexor digitorum longus and flexor hallicus longus also flex the digits of the foot. The tibialis posterior is an inverter of the foot. These deep calf muscles, with sheathed tendons that wrap around the medial maleolus, are susceptible to tenosynovitis.

The tibialis posterior is often involved in the catch-all phrase "shin splints." Shin splints is the general term for pain on or near the medial or lateral aspect of the tibia. A more descriptive term is medial tibial stress syndrome (syndrome is used because of the difficulty in ascertaining which of the multiple possible causes is responsible).

Shin splints can be caused by hyper-pronation during the stance phase in running. Excessive pull on the muscles of the deep compartment of the leg results in a slight pulling away of the tibial posterior tendon from its bony attachments on the mid third of the tibia. Another cause is an inflammation of the tibial periosteum – a periostitis where the excessive pull or overuse of the muscle causes the irritation.

Our treatment is moderate direct pressure BY HAND along the sore points of the medial tibia. The commonly used long stripping strokes along the medial aspect of the tibia are contraindicated, in our opinion, because they can cause a worsening of the condition.

MODERATE FOOT COMPRESSIONS to the deep compartment through the posterior compartment will relax the muscles, bring additional blood flow to speed tissue healing, and lessen the hyper-irritability of trigger points. Avoid excessive pressure as it will worsen inflammation.

Rest with ice is a major part of the treatment when addressing posterior shin splints in runners. Combined with compressions and direct pressure to trigger points, the prognosis is good. Runners who won't quit running can't expect the same outcome. For exercise-addicts, recommend running in harness at the deep end of a swimming pool. It exercises the runner without any deleterious leg stress.

STRESS FRACTURES

Tibial stress fractures, whether caused by excessive muscular tightness or weakness (there is a controversy about this) need to be medically evaluated. Since the symptoms can be similar to shin splints, good practice suggests referral.

Strengthen the tibialis posterior and other stirrup muscles in hyper-pronators. Some runners or others will prefer to use an arch support to avoid having to create one. The above combination can also serve to preclude or reduce knee, low-back and hip pain.

Compartment Syndrome

Extremely strong or abrupt compressions to the deep compartment can conceivably tear tissue and cause a bleed-out into the compartment. A compartment syndrome can be created. Don't do this. Work moderately on this vulnerable area. To make balance and depth easier to control, keep your heel or ball of foot on the floor while applying compressions.

ACUTE COMPARTMENT SYNDROME

Acute compartment syndrome is a rare occurrence and usually occurs with an injury to the lower leg (tibial fracture and muscular rupture). It can be life-threatening. Lower leg muscles are surrounded by bone, interosseous membranes and other muscles. Any swelling which creates pressure above physiologic levels within these fascial confines is serious.

The pain of the acute compartment syndrome is usually much more than would be suspected with the presenting injury. This pain, along with dystasia (difficulty in standing), is an indicator for a physician to test the compartment pressure. The syndrome is usually in the anterior or deep posterior compartments of the leg.

The acute nature of this problem doesn't diminish with time. If not treated with fasciotomy (a longitudinal slicing of the involved fascia), inter-compartment pressure stays above physiologic limits and results in stasis, necrosis, and then death. We may never see this problem, but, when suspected, it does require an immediate emergency room referral.

CHRONIC COMPARTMENT SYNDROME

Strenuous exercise can result in up to a 20% increase in muscle volume. If the compartment fascia doesn't accommodate this increased pressure, it can lead to stasis, dull pain and dystasia. Fortunately this chronic exertional compartment syndrome is reversible with rest.

The more superficial posterior compartment can also develop this syndrome, often because of "tennis leg" (a tear in the medial head of the gastrocnemius).

Tennis leg supplies a good example of why we should not work fresh injuries. Because bruising often won't be evident for a couple days, we lack a visual sign that the muscle is torn. Any work we do in the affected region could cause additional seepage of blood and interstitial fluids and add to the likelihood of a compartment syndrome. At best, we would exacerbate the injury creating secondary or hypoxic tissue death, and delay tissue healing.

A tibialis posterior trigger point can be mistaken for an Achilles tendonitis. The trigger point refers pain into the tendon. First check for the trigger point in the tibialis posterior. It is easier to treat, and much less painful than the cross-fiber friction required for a tendonitis. The tibialis posterior trigger points can also refer pain to center of the sole of the foot, and are particularly noticeable when walking or running. This reinforces our understanding that just working at the spot that hurts is often ineffective in bodywork.

Another problem that can give a diffuse sense of pain and could be mistaken for Achilles tendonitis is tenosynovitis of the tibialis posterior's sheathed tendon next to the medial maleolus.

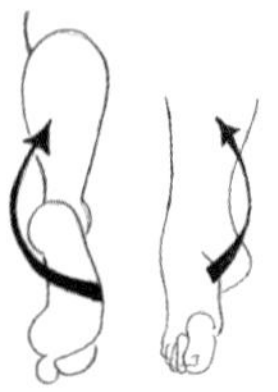

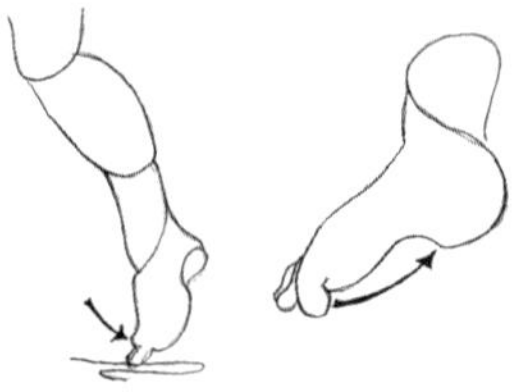

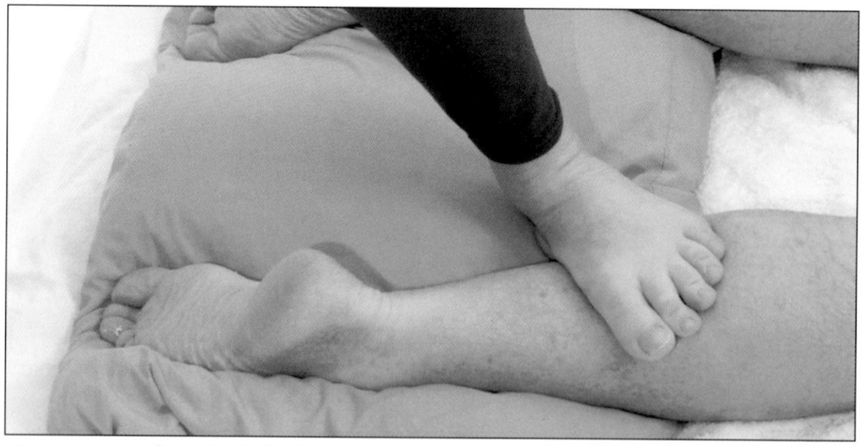

Direct pressure from the ball of the foot to the posterior deep compartment.

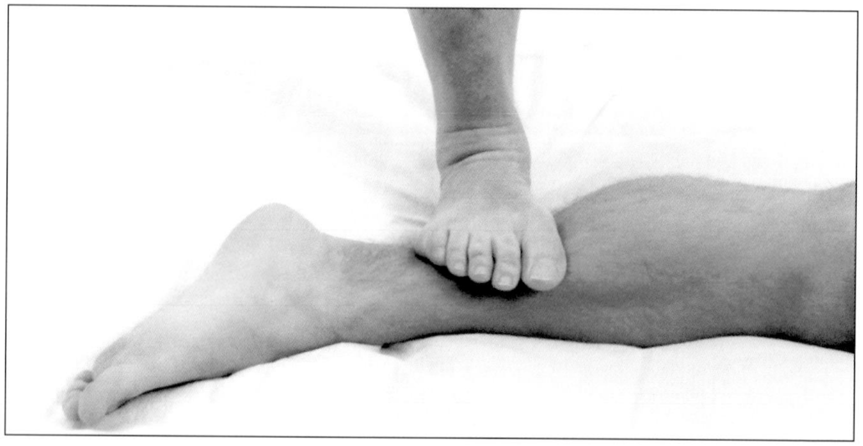

Side-lying, ball of the foot direct pressure to the flexors hallicus and digitorum longus.

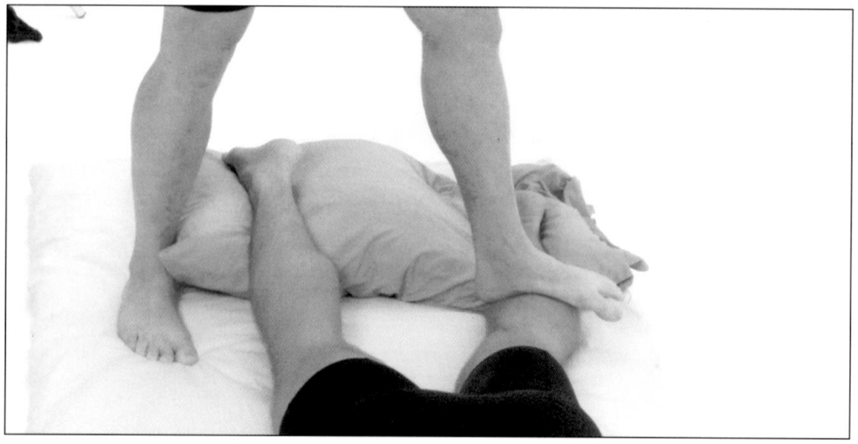

Warm-up for the deep posterior compartment.

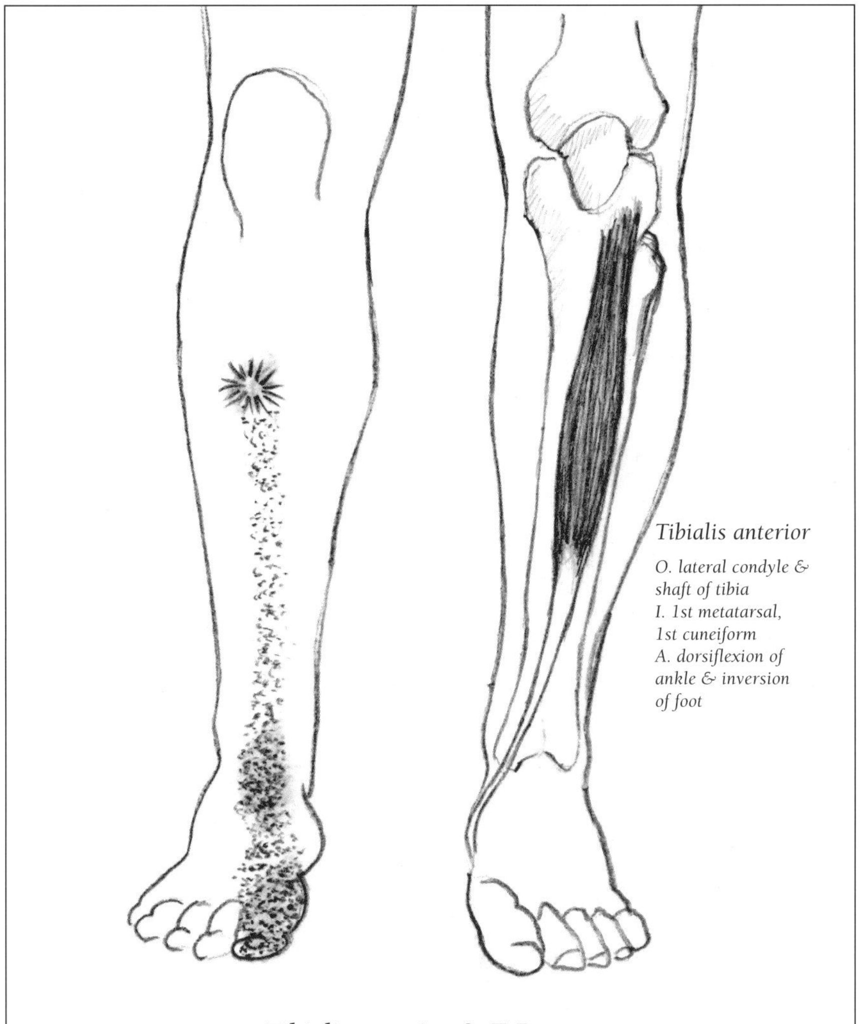

Tibialis anterior & TrPs

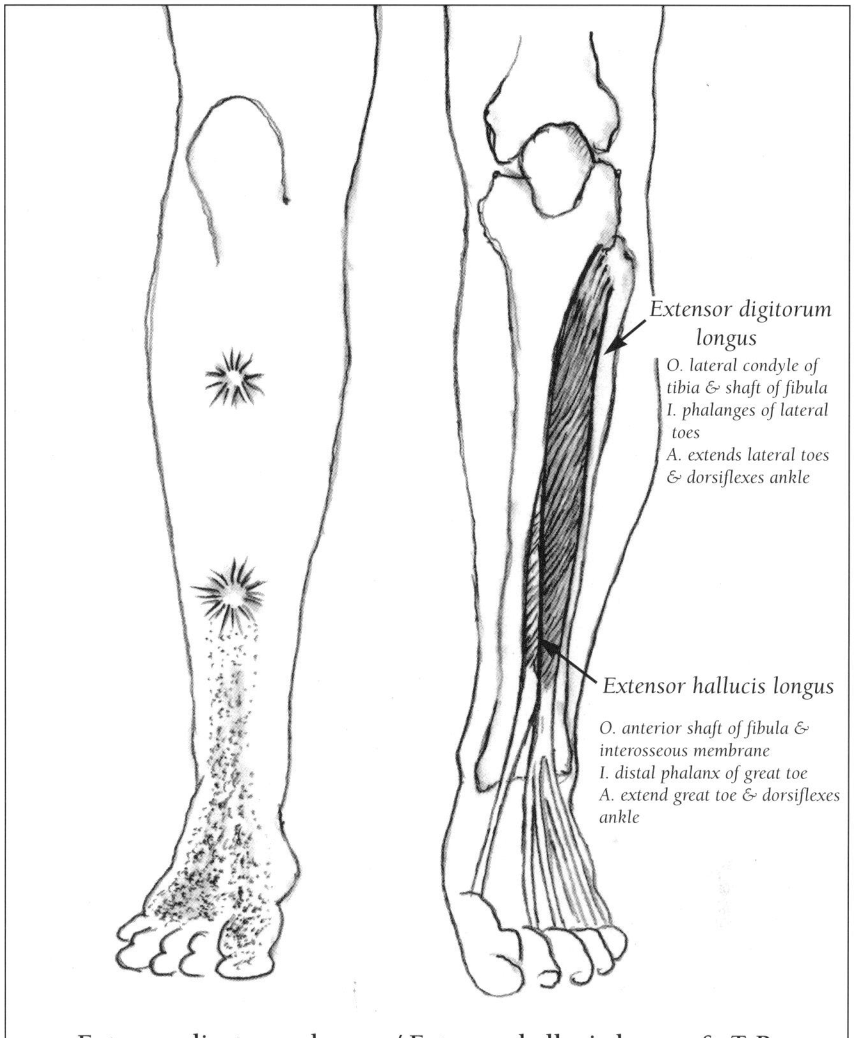

Extensor digatorum longus / Extensor hallucis longus & TrPs

The tibialis anterior, extensor digitorum longus and extensor hallucis longus form the anterior compartment of the leg. They function together to prevent foot slap at heel strike and keep us from stubbing our toes.

Anterior compartment trigger points cause weakness and a clumsy gait. Prolonged ankle dorsiflexion (driving with your accelerator foot in partial dorsiflection for extend periods of time) will create or perpetuate trigger points in some people. We advise these clients to either use cruise control or punch it.

Muscle problems also occur in the musculotendinous juncture. Generally this is a tendonitis and treated with cross-fiber friction.

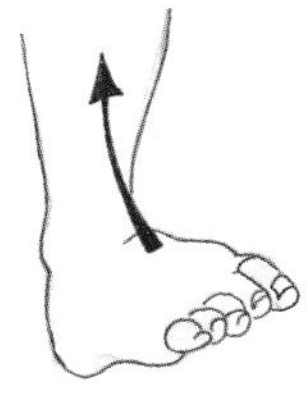

Caution

Occasionally you may see a client with anterior compartment syndrome. This is a potential medical emergency. If the tibialis anterior is hard and woody and the client lacks sensation on the dorsum of the foot next to the big and second toes they could be in real trouble. Scratch this area to check for lack of sensation. If this area is numb, refer for immediate medical evaluation.

Treatment

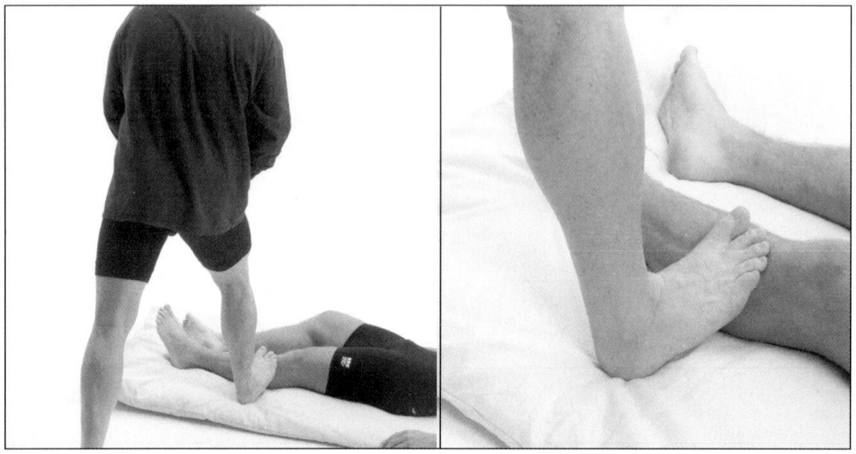

Warm-up to the tibialis anterior with the client prone.

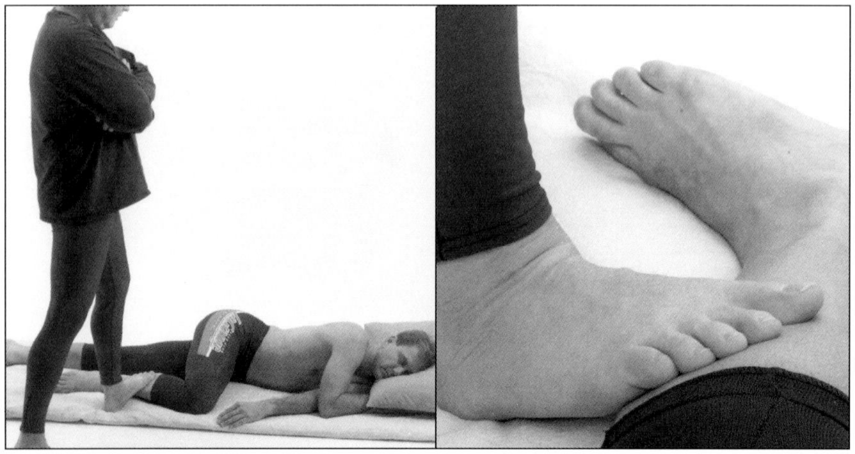

A warm-up or direct pressure to the anterior compartment is best achieved with the client side-lying.

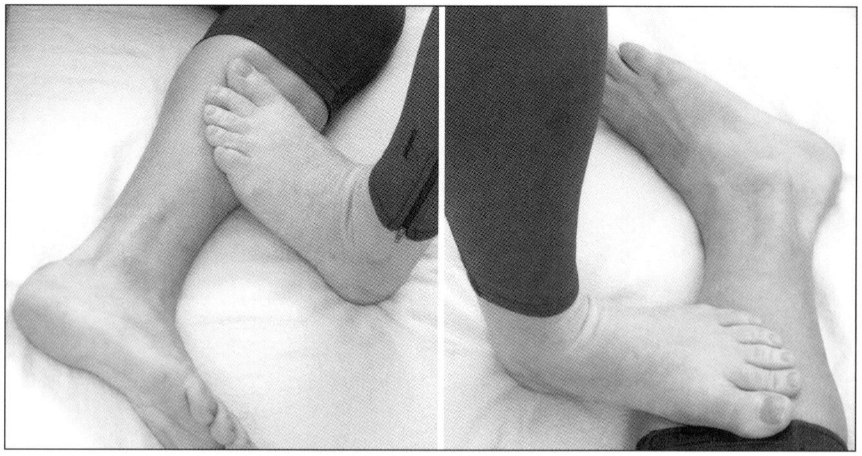

Direct pressure from the ball of the foot (supported by heel) of therapist.

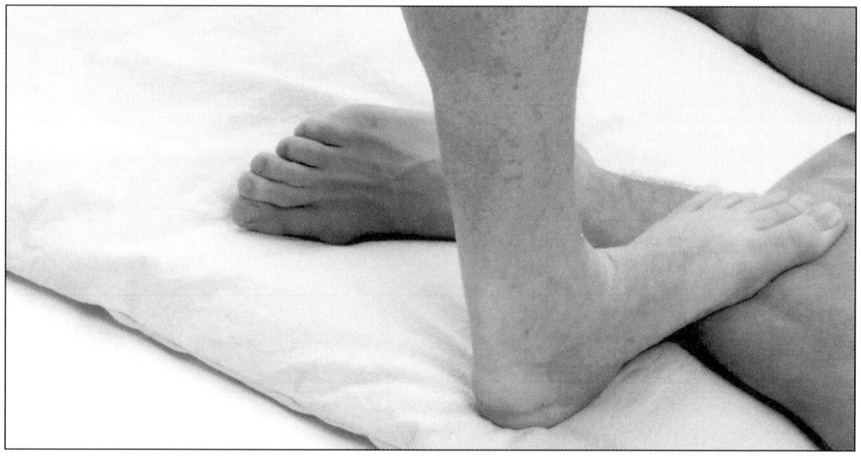

Therapist's heel is supported to give more control over pressure.

Lateral Compartment of the Leg

Peroneus longus and Peroneus brevis

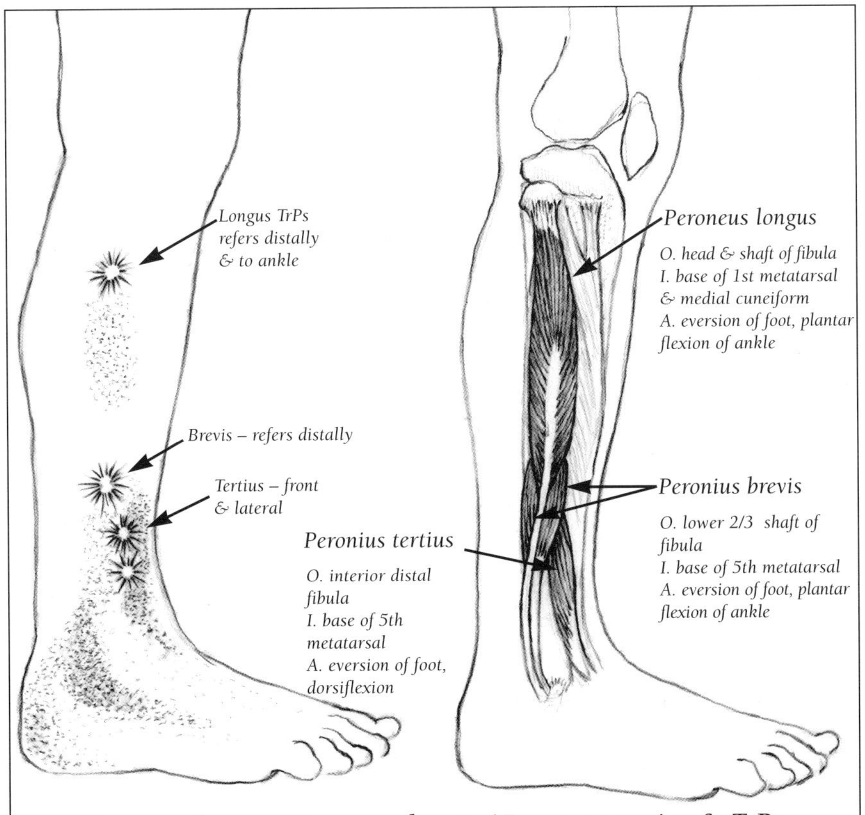

Peroneus longus / Peroneus brevis / Peroneus tertius & TrPs

The peroneus longus and brevis muscles comprise the lateral compartment of the leg. They function primarily as ankle stabilizers and prevent inversion sprains. Runners, hikers on uneven terrain and folks who jump in sport or work utilize these muscles to the max. Interestingly, the interplay between these muscles, ligament reflexes at the ankle, and the proprioceptors at the knee, ankle and foot help to determine how vulnerable you are to inversion sprains and strains.

The most common injury to the ankle is an inversion sprain (an over-stretch to the ligaments of the lateral malleolus). The most common ligament to sprain is the anterior talofibular ligament, followed by the calcanofibular ligament and then the posterior talofibular ligament. While we can prevent adhesions from forming during the healing process, stretched-out ligaments tend to stay stretched. These lax ligaments make future inversion sprains more likely.

Walking barefooted, movement on a variety of terrain and wobble-board strengthening of the stirrup-muscles are effective ways to prevent re-injury. Overly supportive shoes diminish strength and proprioception, and inhibit balance.

Tenosynovitis of the sheathed portion of the peroneus longus and peroneus brevis tendon is not uncommon in conjunction with an inversion sprain.

Treatment

Cross-fiber friction given on a stretch at the site of the lesion (usually from 1 inch above to 1/2 inch below the lateral maleolus) will address the tenosynovitis.

> If the tendon inflammation occurs simultaneously with an inversion sprain, DON'T invert the foot to treat the tenosynovitis. It will exacerbate the ligament pull. Simply press into and stretch the tendon either above or below the lesion and cross-fiber friction the lesion with your client's foot in a neutral position.

Trigger points in the belly of the peroneus longus or brevis often refer pain to the general region of the lateral malleolus and can mimic a tenosynovitis. With sufficient stimulation, a local twitch response will differentiate trigger points from tenosynovitis of this muscle.

Don't use prolonged compression on the peroneus longus just below the head of the fibula because of the superficiality of the deep or superficial peroneal nerves. Compressing these nerves against the fibula can cause burning or prickling sensations around the ankle. Prolonged application of ice can also damage this nerve.

Direct pressure to the trigger points in these muscles will address referred pain, entrapments, and loosen the muscle enough to assist a peroneal tenosynovitis healing. Following direct pressure and stretches, client self- stretches and strengthening will help prevent the recurrence of the problem.

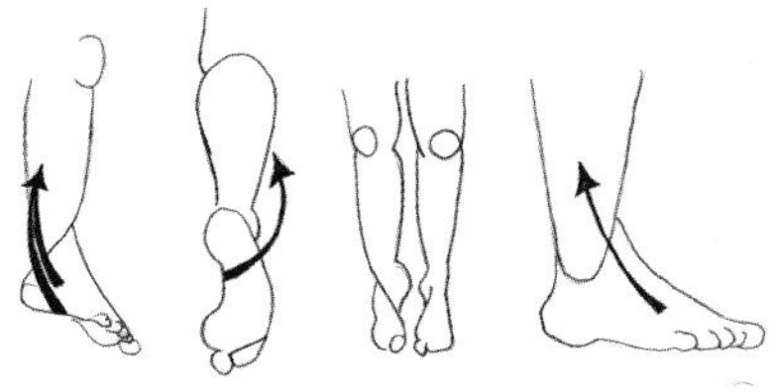

Swelling around the ankle indicates a sprain. Swelling helps to differentiate pain experienced from a sprained ankle and the pain associated with a trigger points referral (usually from tibialis anterior) into the ankle region.

Caution

Internal joint problems cause internal swelling and are experienced, in part, as restricted dorsiflexion and plantarflexion. Tight stirrup muscles (tibialis anterior; peroneus longus; tibialis posterior) can also cause a restricted range of motion, but aren't usually painful. When this painful, swollen, restricted range of motion exists, it's time for a medical referral.

Lateral compartment syndrome, while less common than anterior compartment syndrome, is a possibility. Again, this calls for a medical referral.

Entrapment of the three peroneal nerves creates symptoms similar to the trigger point referrals. If relief is not immediate with deactivation of the trigger points, refer for competent medical evaluation.

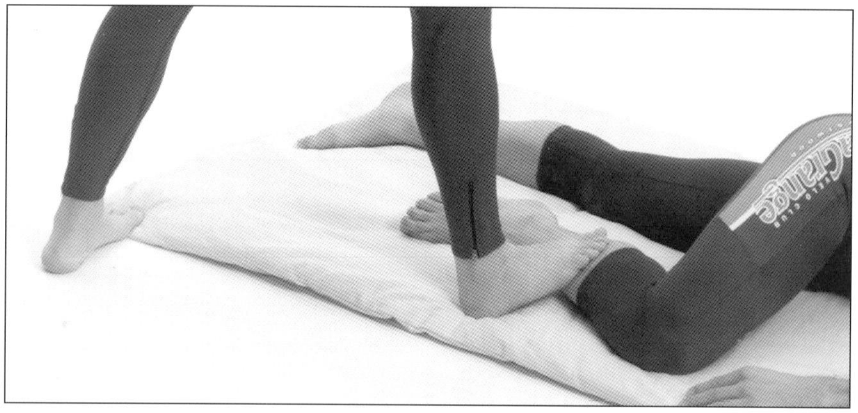

Warm-up to the anterior and lateral compartment of the leg.

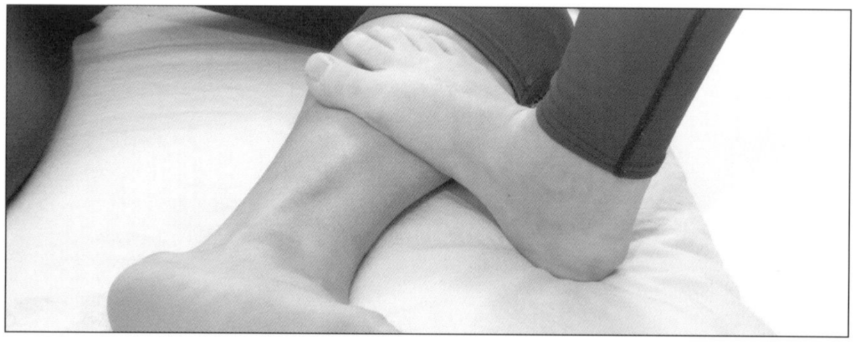

Side-lying warm-up for the lateral compartment.

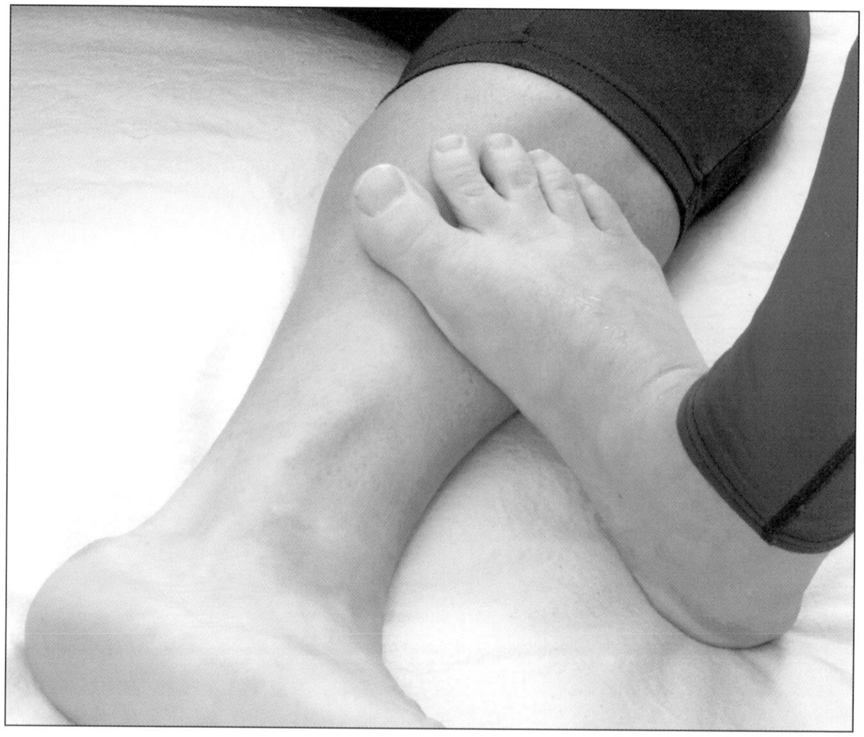

Direct pressure from the first ray into the anterior portion of the lateral compartment.

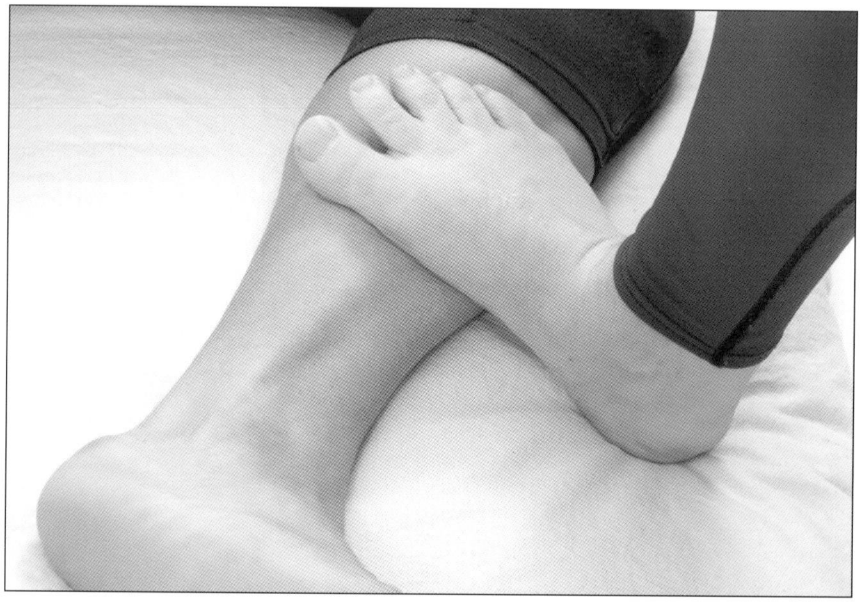

Direct pressure into the peroneus longus and brevis muscles.

Selected Foot Muscles

Plantar Flexors and Abductors of the Foot

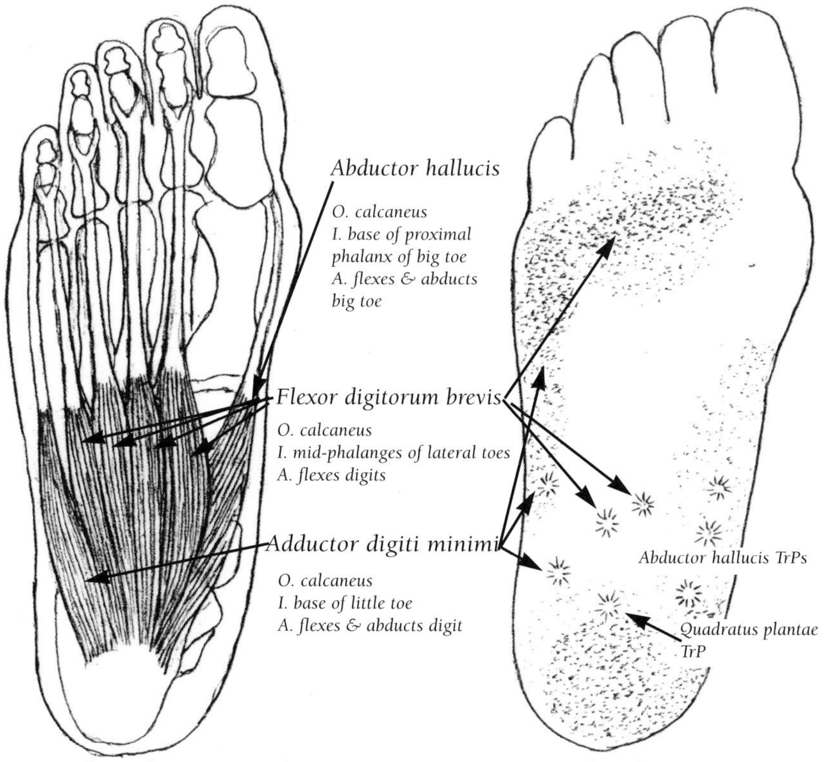

Selected Foot Muscles & TrPs – Deep / Superficial Intrinsic

It's quite amazing that there aren't more problems associated with the intrinsic musculature of the foot. The trigger points we do find hurt during ambulation, but occasionally they also refer pain at rest. Rigid shoes and walking on flat surfaces generally decondition the foot and its proprioception. Our modern habits have taken the foot far from its evolutionarily designed environment.

The One-Foot Test

A good test for foot proprioception is to balance on one foot, then close your eyes and see if you immediately topple or sway excessively. This exercise gives you a good sense of how much you rely on visual clues for balance. We often have clients practice this technique on alternate feet to enhance their balance and prevent sprained ankles. In conjunction with the one-foot test, we also recommend walking barefoot on uneven surfaces, and doing yoga postures with eyes closed.

Caveat

If you bump your head, don't blame us. Practice in an open space.

Treatment

1. With the client side-lying (easier access to the plantar surface of the foot) or prone (with a pillow or bolster placed at the ankle to protect the ankle joint), warm the foot with gentle compressions.

2. Search the plantar, medial and lateral surfaces with thumb or finger to locate jump response.

3. Use heel, first ray or lateral edge of the foot to apply direct pressure to the trigger point.

4. Complete treatment with further compressions; active and passive stretches.

Self-treatment with direct pressure using golfballs and rolling pins is recommended by Travel and Simons – we prefer tennis balls. All work well in conjunction with strengthening, and stretching.

Proper shoe fit for both hypo- and hyper-mobile feet is an important consideration. If possible, it is better to retrain the intrinsic and extrinsic muscles of the foot rather than rely on orthotics or hyper-stable shoes. We think these devices further weaken affected muscles. However, most clients won't take the time to strengthen, so shoe devices do have their place.

Caution

Avoid strong, direct pressure beneath the medial malleolus as the posterior tibial artery courses beneath the flexor hallucis longus tendon.

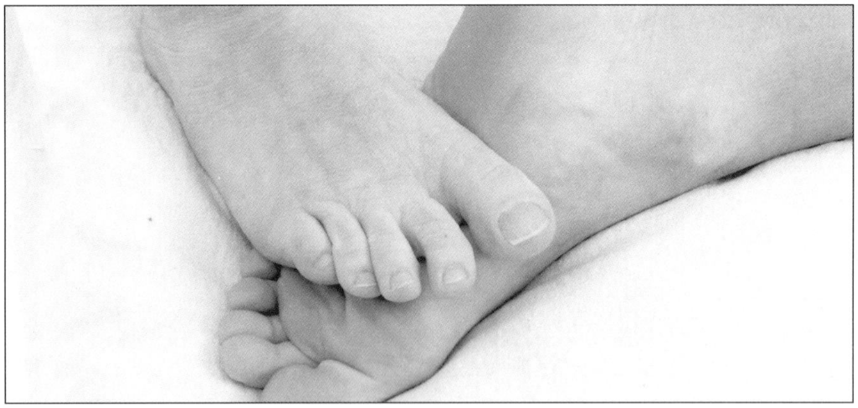

Direct pressure from the first ray to the plantar surface of the foot.

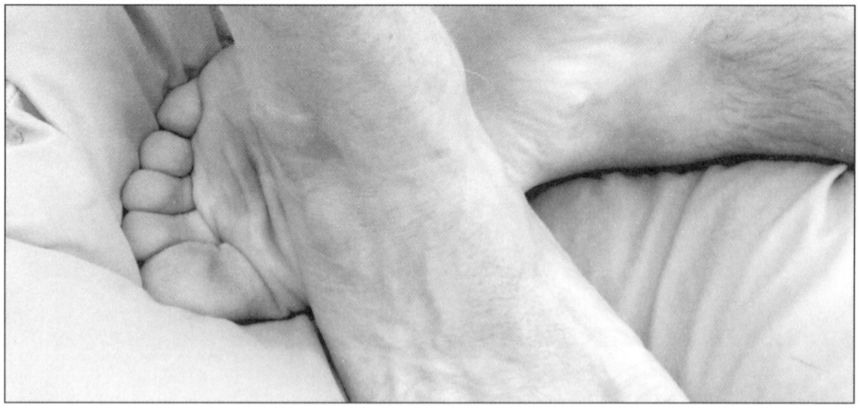

Direct heel pressure into the ball of the foot.

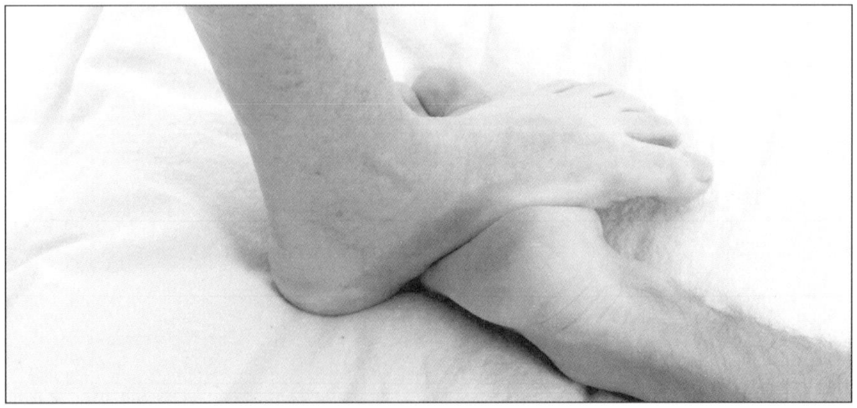

Side-lying warm up, "arch to arch."

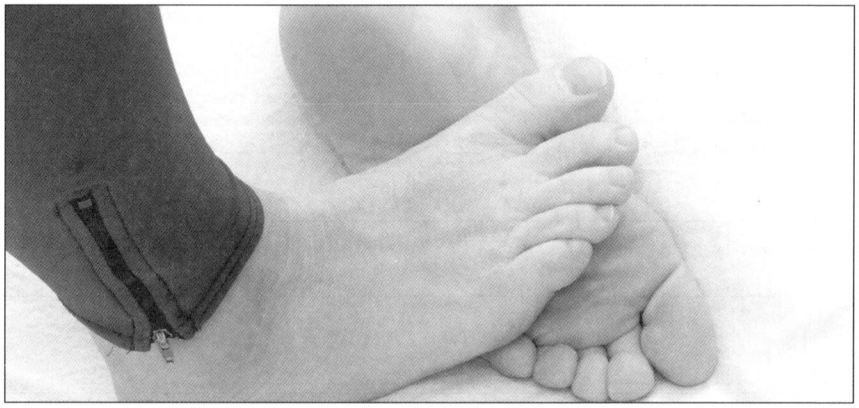

First ray pressure into the plantar fascia.

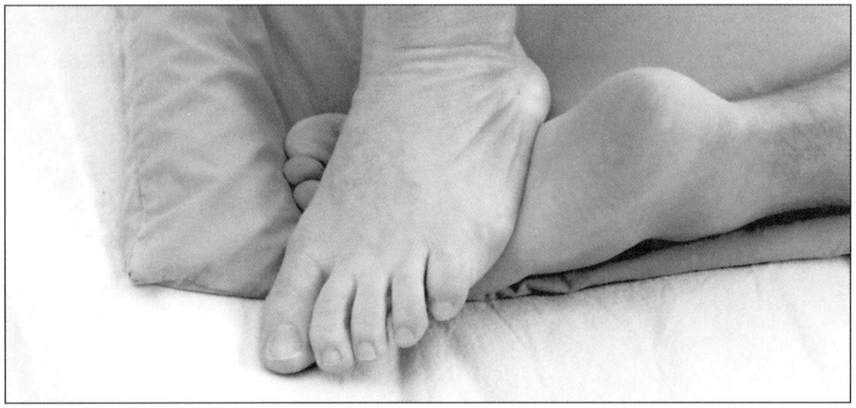

Prone warm-up.

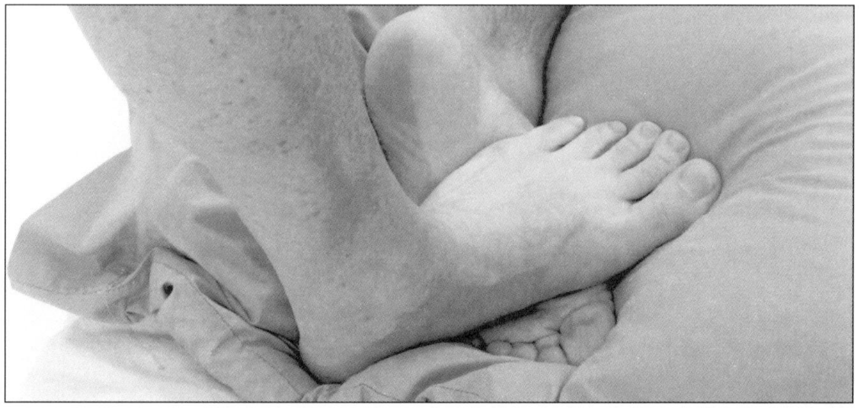

Clients with stiff, high arch cavus foot must have sufficient foot and ankle support to avoid pain or injury with compressions to the foot. A side-lying approach works best for these clients.

CHAPTER 12

Arm and Hand Pain

MUSICIANS, desk jockeys, laborers, bodyworkers and watchmakers have common afflictions. This section addresses their problems – ones we see on a regular basis.

Hand and wrist pain that originates in the extensors and flexors of the wrist and fingers is addressed first. Carpal tunnel, the problem everyone thinks they have, has been a real rarity in our practices. We're sure it exists, but probably in much fewer numbers than is supposed. The supinator often relates to tennis elbow and is easily treated with direct pressure from a heel.

For bodyworkers, we offer an effective treatment for sore, fatigued and painful thumbs (adductor and opponens pollicis), and a helpful friction massage protocol for preventing and aborting osteoarthritis.

Caveat: Wrist and hand pain can be referred from many sources. If you don't find culpable trigger points in the forearm, look to the scalenes, serratus anterior, and infraspinatus.

We close with the pectoralis major and minor. Pecs play a key role in proper shoulder mechanics and, while their referral is primarily local, their trigger points can also refer into the arm.

Before You Begin

Safe, effective arm and hand treatments are enhanced by first reading the *Indications, Client Intake, Contraindications, Deep Compressive Massage, Endangerment Sites, Trigger Points, Cross-fiber, Fascial Release, Stretching* and *Hydrotherapy* sections.

Note the specific procedural notes and cautions. They will help you effectively treat your client without harm. Protocols and guidelines are included to help you know when to treat and when to refer.

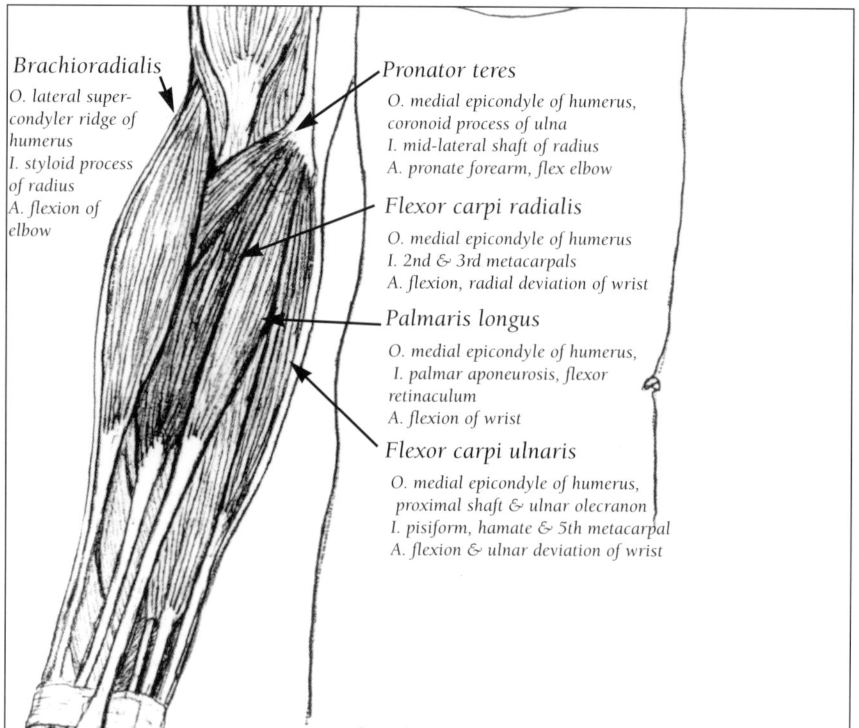

Superficial Forearm Flexors

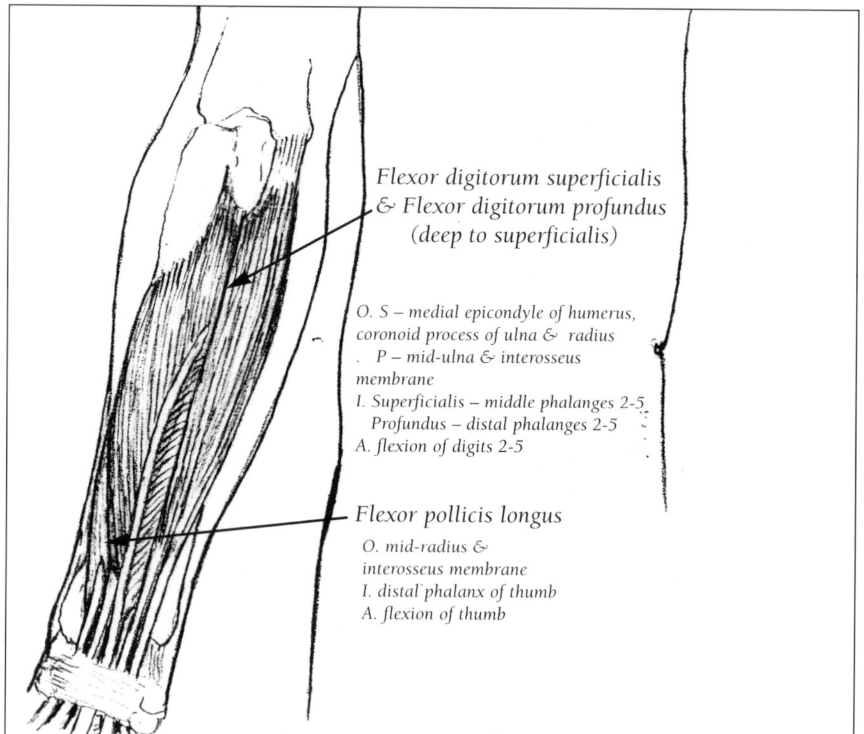

Deeper Forearm Flexors

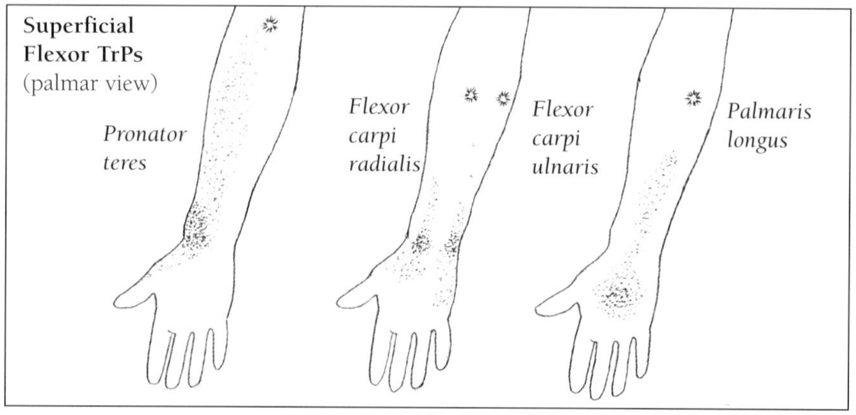

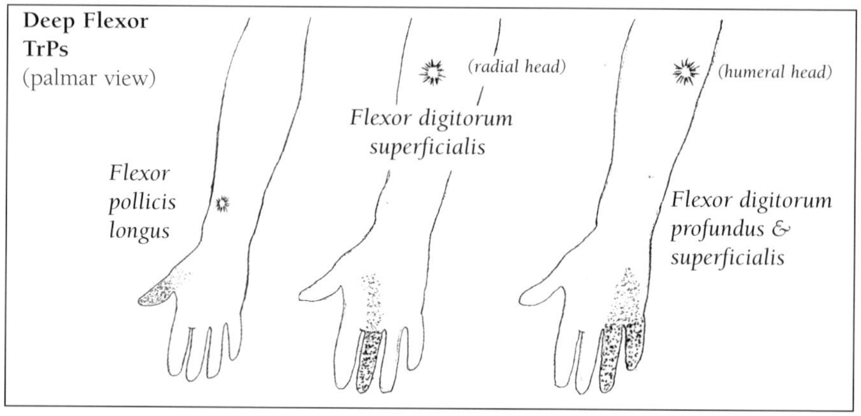

REPETITIVE TASKS that we moderns engage in leave our wrists and fingers vulnerable to injury. Unbelievably, some of the worst chronic extensor injuries we've seen have come from computer operators changing to a new mouse! Eradicating trigger points in the finger and forearm flexors can release nerve entrapments that cause both pain and weakness.

Symptoms from trigger points in the pronator teres, wrist and finger flexors and extensors, and lateral epicondylitis (tennis elbow – usually a tendonitis of the extensor carpi radialis brevis near the lateral epicondyle of the humerus) are the most common complaints. If these trigger points are recognized and addressed, and with perpetuating factors modified, complete relief can occur in a matter of a week or two.

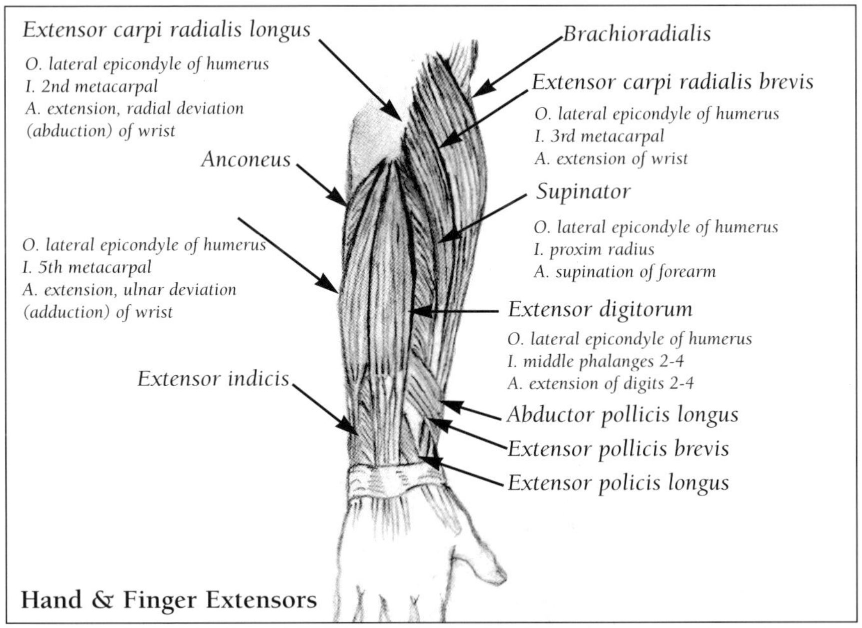

Hand & Finger Extensors

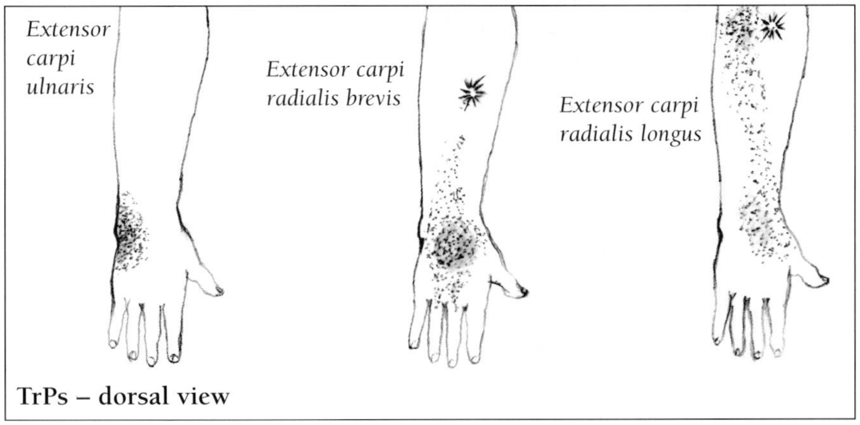

TrPs – dorsal view

PERPETUATING FACTORS

Dr. Travell, when writing her classic *Myofascial Pain and Dysfunction – the Trigger Point Manual*, found a break every 15 to 20 minutes ensured her own physical well-being. She got up, moved around and stretched. When thoroughly engaged by a sedentary task, we can stay focused much longer than is good for us. Dr. Travell used an alarm clock to interrupt the intense focus that comes with writing.

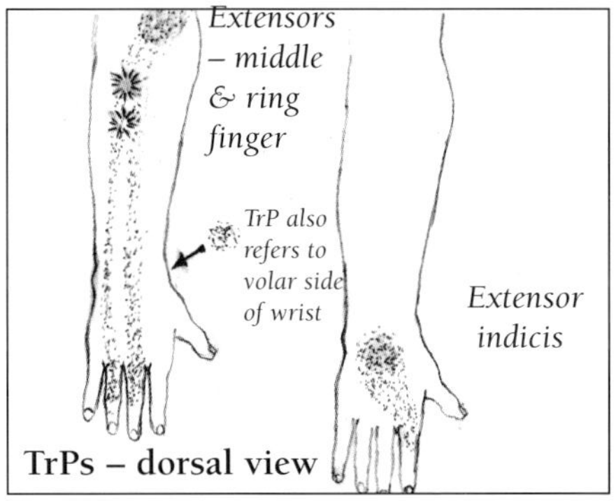

TrPs – dorsal view

Carpal Tunnel

In our practices, clients occasionally complain of carpal tunnel syndrome (often self-diagnosed). We find that in a majority of our clients, the source of the symptom (pain or pins and needles in the wrist, hand, thumb and fingers) is most likely to originate from trigger points in the anterior and middle scalenes, the infraspinatus, or in the finger flexors or extensors in the forearm rather than from compression of the medial nerve at the wrist.

In actual cases of carpal tunnel, where the carpal bones are pushing against the median nerve, or the sheathed flexor tendons at the wrist are enflamed and swollen, we refer. Acupuncturists have had some good results needling the inflamed tendon sheaths to reduce the swelling and thereby create more space for the median nerve through the carpal tunnel. Alternatively, in some cases, surgical release is an answer.

Tennis elbow is an area of mild contention. Some authorities say that it is a tendonitis, primarily of the extensor carpi radialis brevis, while others suggest that it is the result of forearm supinator trigger points. Both result in pain in the same general area, with the supinator trigger points also referring pain to the dorsal web of the thumb.

We use direct ischemic pressure on the extensors, flexors, pronators and supinators to eliminate trigger points first, and follow with cross-fiber friction, usually to the extensor carpi radialis brevis. The cross-fiber, by its very nature, can be more painful than direct pressure.

Tennis elbow may take three weeks of friction massage and ice to clear up. If, however, your client is a concert pianist and an avid tennis buff, it could take a year to heal an extreme tennis elbow.

Use friction for the inflamed tendons and have clients use ice following each treatment, especially for post-treatment pain. With trigger points, use direct pressure and follow with moist heat to prevent post-treatment soreness.

In many cases, very brief friction treatments will re-initiate the body's own healing response. This is different from the mechanical effect that is attributed to prolonged cross-fiber friction. If the brief treatment (30 to 60 seconds) isn't sufficient, give longer friction treatments, but only for 2 or 3 minutes maximum. If that doesn't create substantial improvements in 3 or 4 treatments, refer.

Following the cessation of pain, give several more light friction treatments to the tendon and compressions to all the forearm muscles. When the treatment is successful, the pain goes, and it's time to stretch and strengthen before resuming normal use.

Dr. Cyriax described an average course of treatment as comprising 8 to 12 visits on alternate days. Our experience has shown that in many cases positive changes will occur with half this number of visits using 2 or 3 minute treatments instead of his initially recommended 20 minutes (now 10 minutes).

As the initial scar forms in a muscle belly, a rapid diminution of pain will occur. If we resume heavy use too soon, this green (incompletely matured) scar tissue tears, resulting in excessive scar formation, which increases the possibility of adhesions and nerve entrapments.

Treatment: Extensors

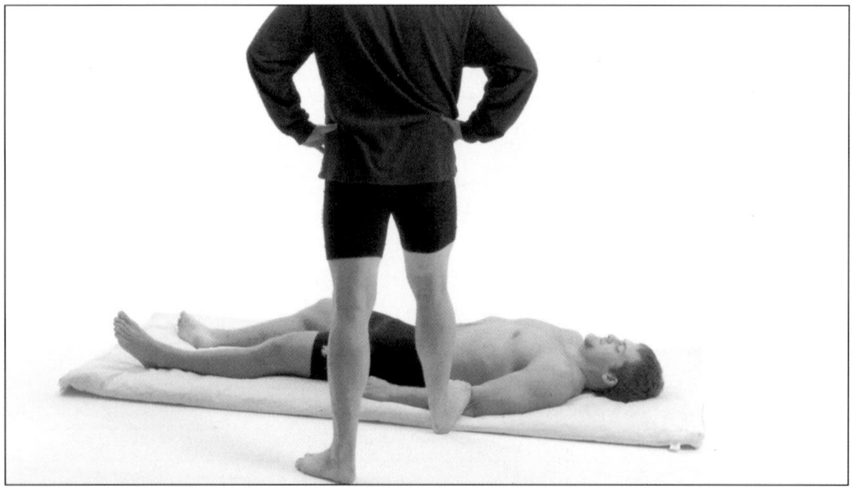

Warm-up from a soft foot. The pressure is below the elbow and into the wad (extensor carpi brevis, extensor carpi radialis longus and the brachioradialis). The heel is not supported on the mat and the pressure is straight down and moderate. The therapist has the majority of his weight on his support leg.

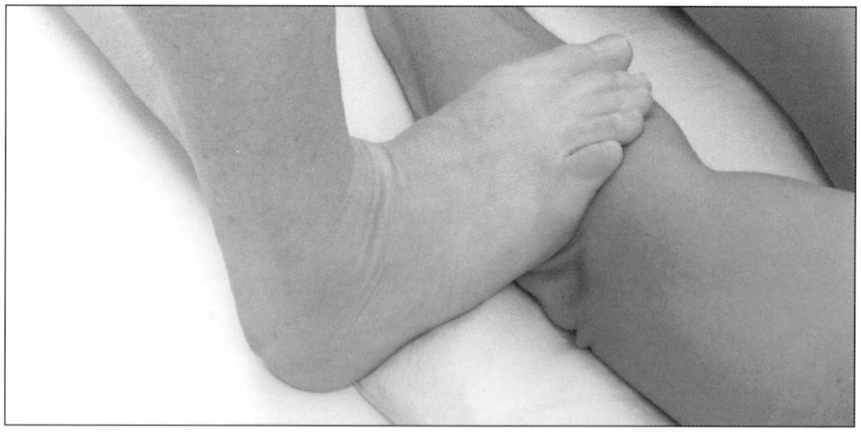

Direct pressure from the first-ray into the extensor carpi ulnaris and the superficial extensor muscle for the ring finger.

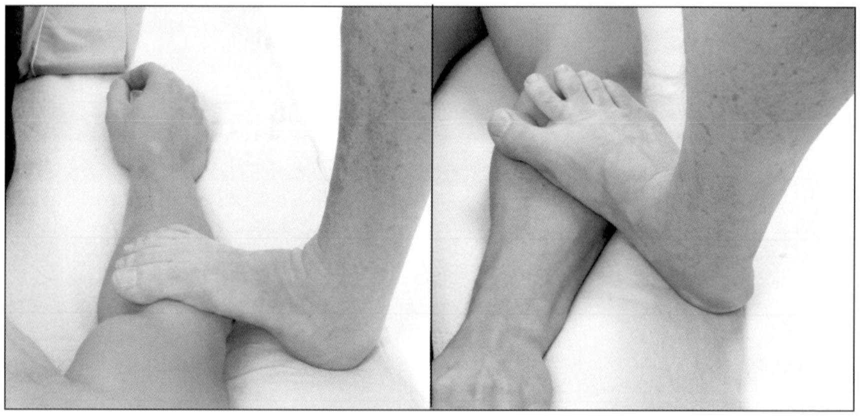

Therapist's foot is slightly inverted to give direct pressure with the first ray.

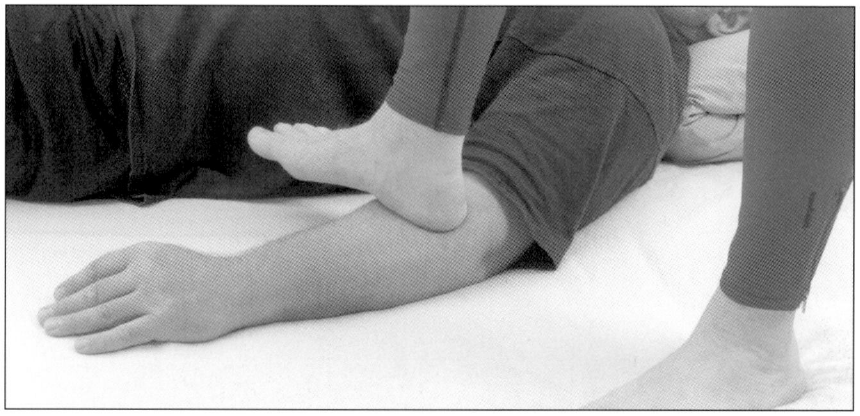

Direct pressure administered with the heel.

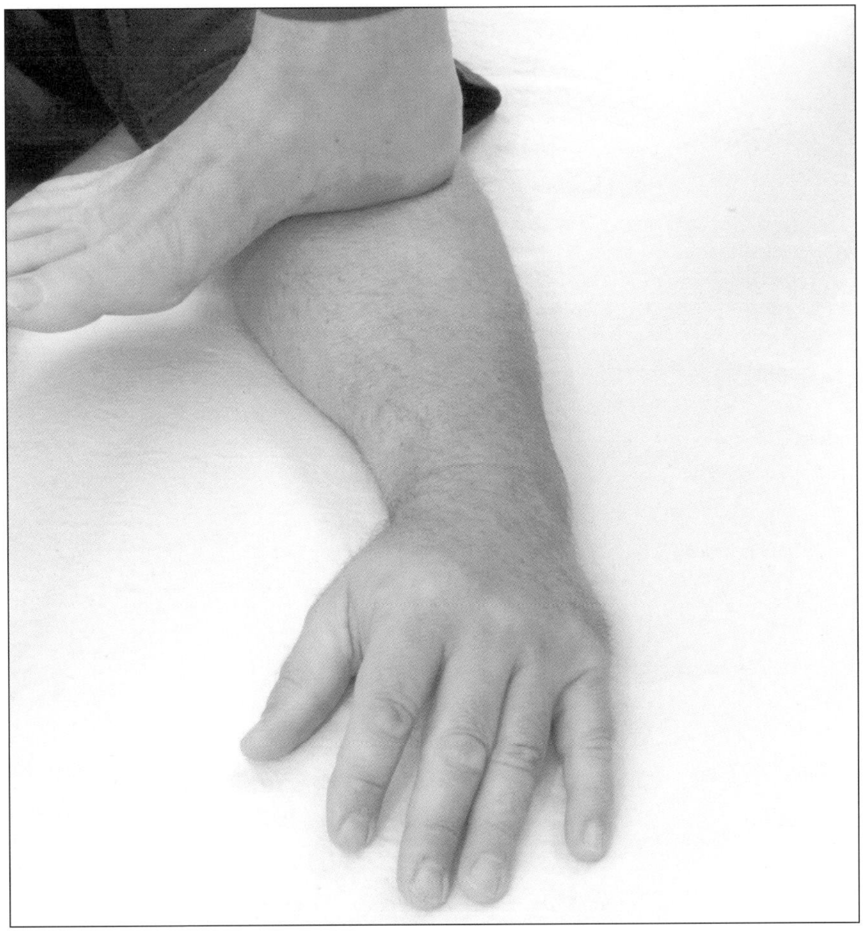

Direct pressure into WAD to eliminate TrPs.

Treatment: Flexors

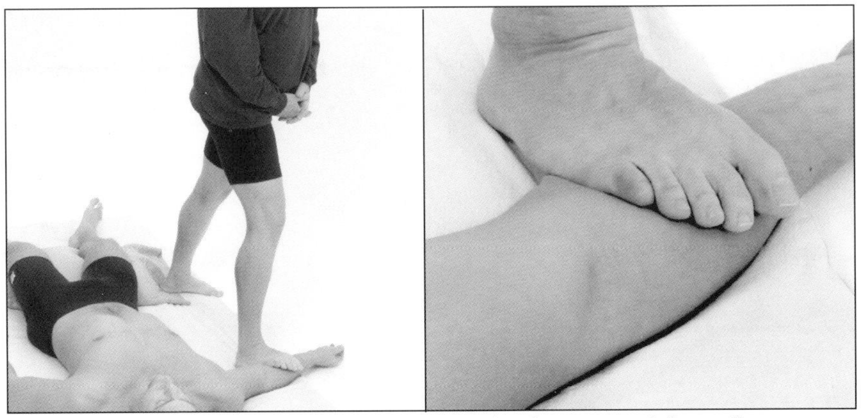

A warm-up compression for the bulk of the muscles for wrist and finger flexion – just below the medial epicondyle.

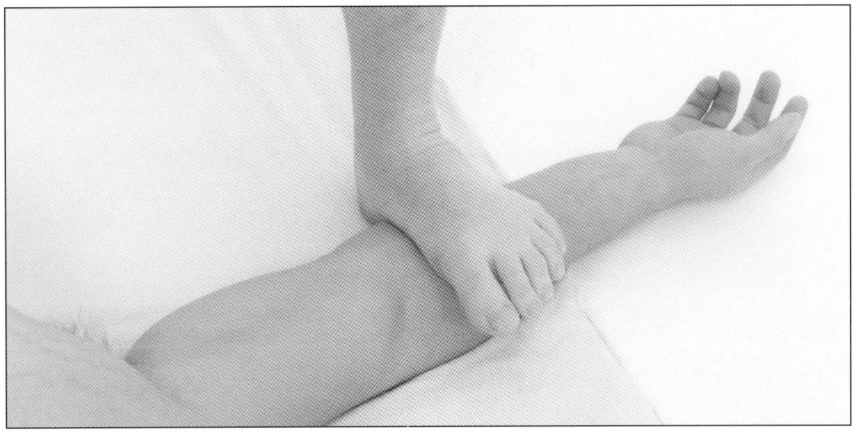

Compression from a relaxed foot.

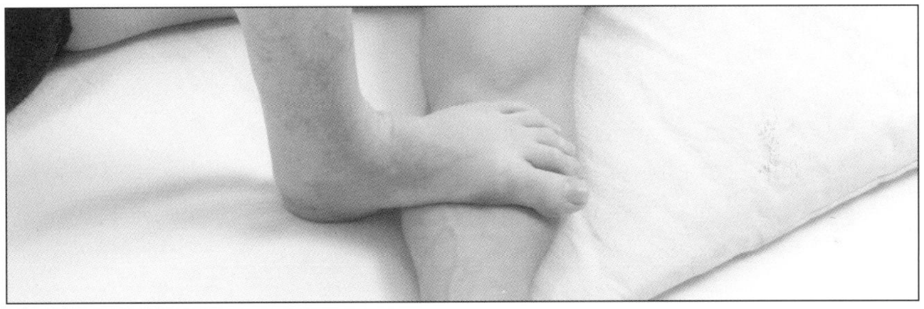

Slightly evert your foot for an increase in direct pressure from the lateral edge. With several clients we have encountered the strange phenomena of a referral pattern (of the superficial finger flexors) that extends out past the ends of the client's fingers – analogous to phantom limb pain.

Treatment: Pronator teres

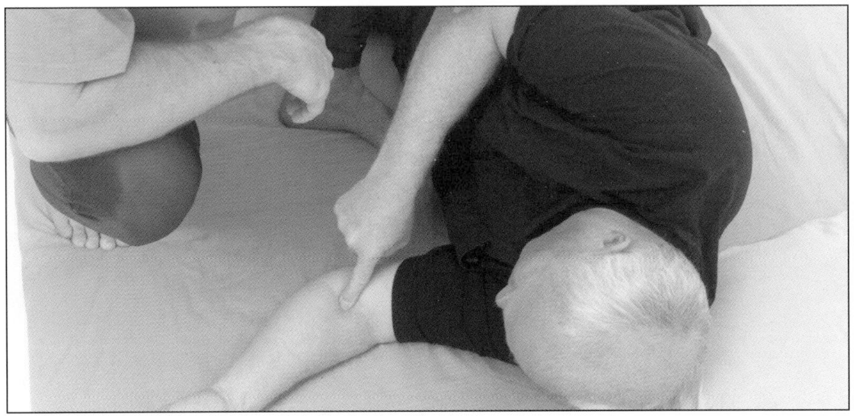

The pronator teres is right here.

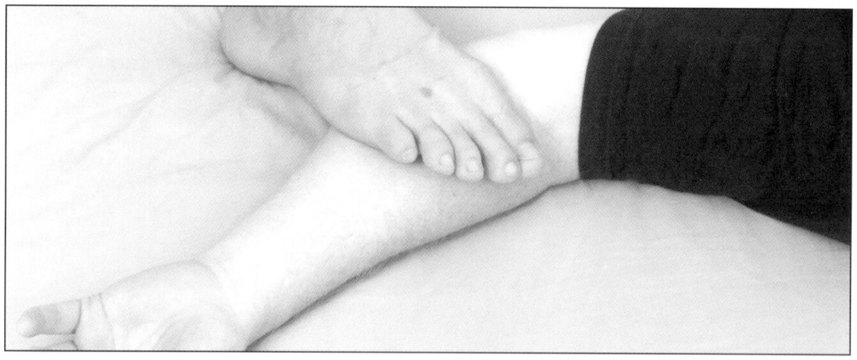

Use the ball of your foot to warm muscle bellies before treating TrPs with direct pressure.

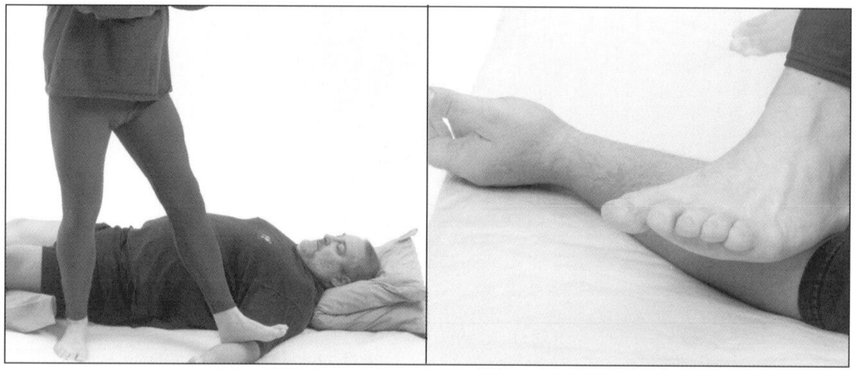

Invert your foot for more pressure. Press into the pronator teres and the flexors of the pinky and ring finger.

Table/Hand Treatment

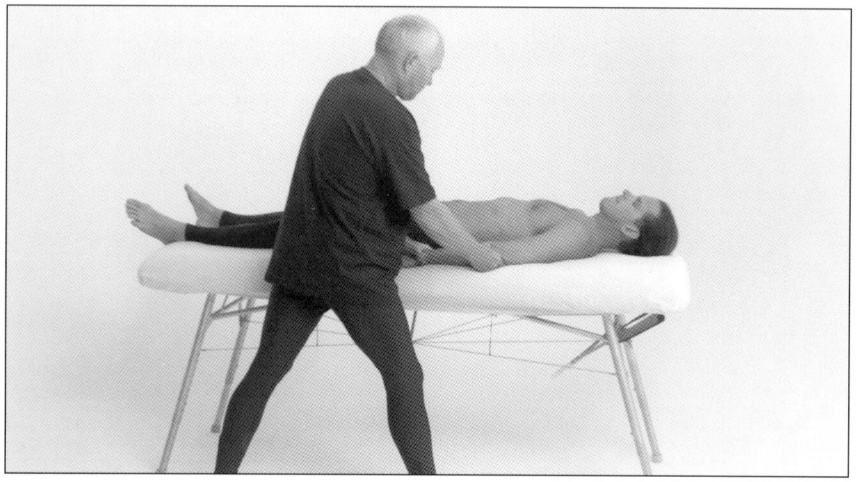

Tennis elbow examination with cross-fiber friction to find the exact site of the lesion.

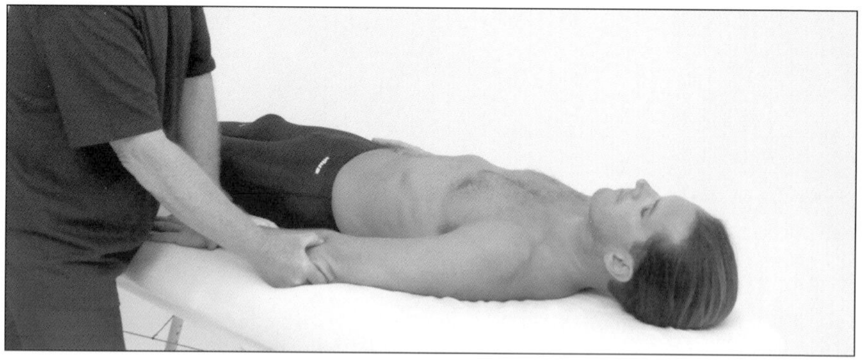

Friction across the approximately 1 inch long extensor carpi radialis brevis tendon, any part of which can be the exact site of the lesion.

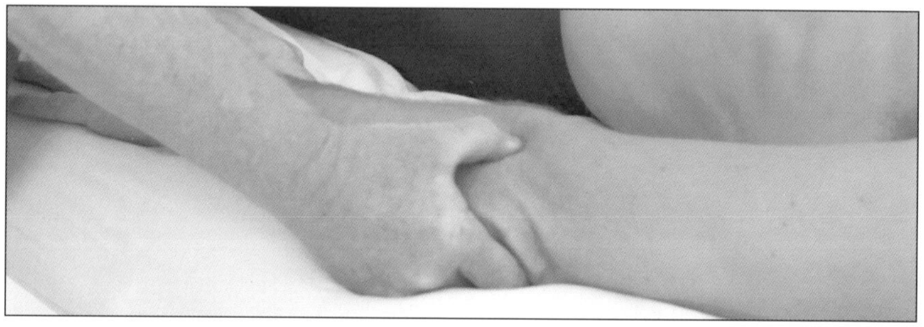

Once you've found the lesion, friction by supinating and pronating your wrist. The thumb is locked without any flexion or extension within the thumb itself.

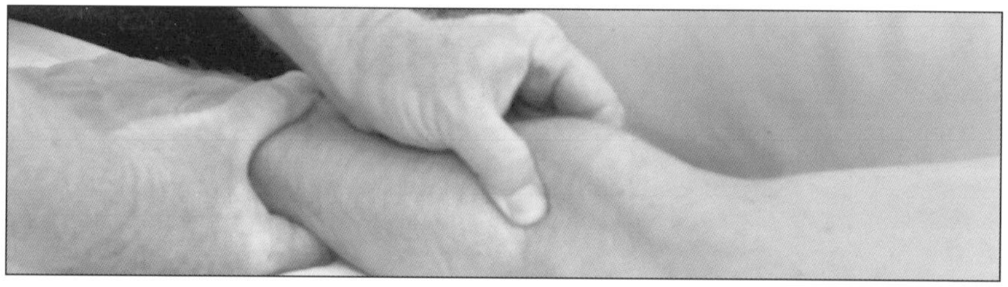

Pincer palpation to the WAD to eliminate TrPs concomitant with the tendonitis.

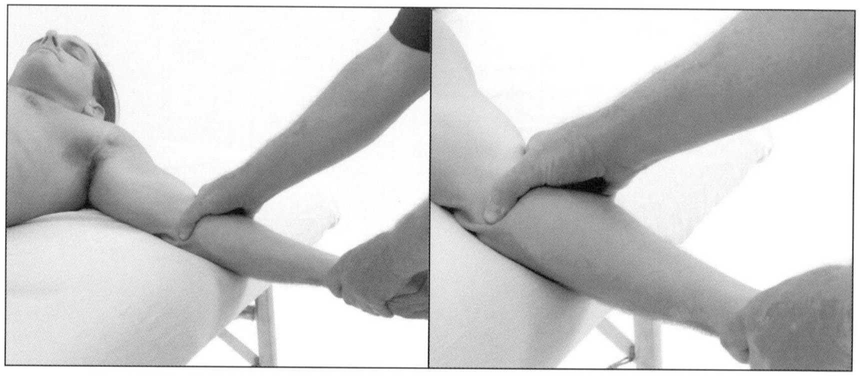

Golfer's elbow, a tendonitis of the common flexor tendon, is examined just below the medial epicondyle. The lesion, the most painful spot in the tendon, is then frictioned across the grain.

SUPINATOR

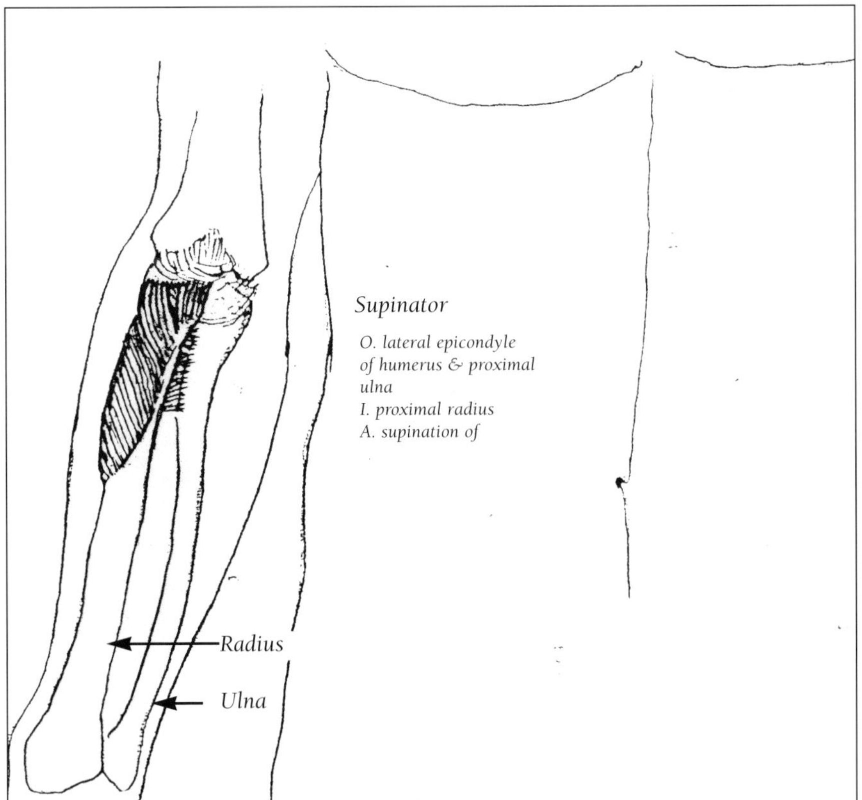

Supinator

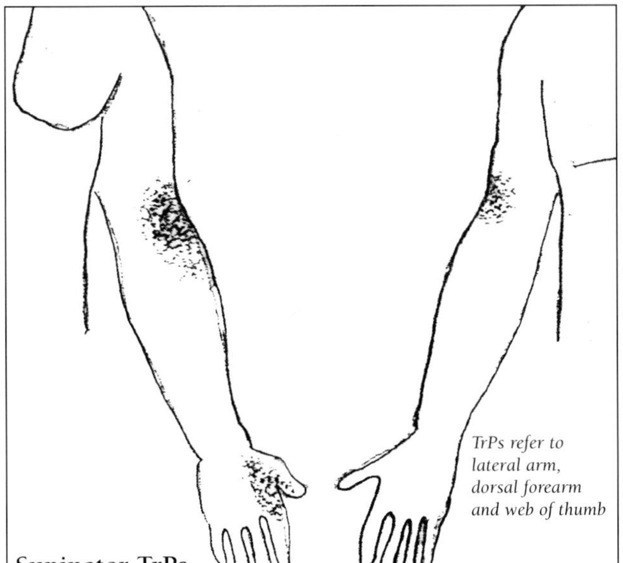

Supinator TrPs

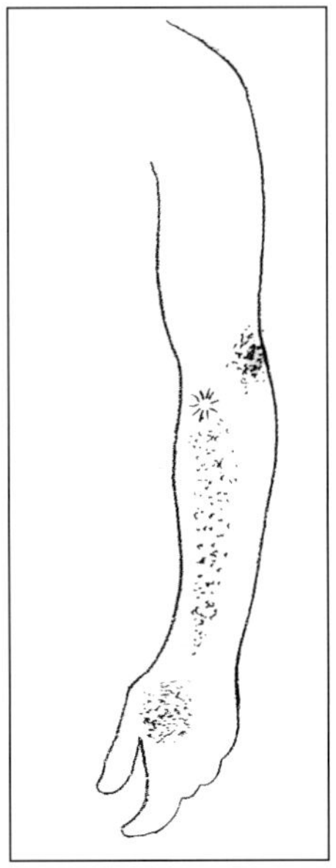

SUPINATOR TRIGGER POINTS can present as tennis elbow. The client's pain pattern feels identical to that of a tendonitis in the extensor carpi radialis brevis and longus. In our treatment of lateral elbow pain, the supinator is always examined.

When supinator trigger points are severe, pain will be referred into the webbing between the thumb and the back of the index finger. Place the clients arm palm down, plant your heel on the floor, and use the ball of your foot to direct pressure into the supinator.

Palpate the surrounding muscles and treat where necessary. This is particularly true when dealing with the WAD (extensor carpi brevis, extensor carpi radialis longus and the brachioradialis), and wrist, finger and forearm flexors.

Compression injuries to the ulnar, radial and median nerve are all possible when working deeply in the forearm. Avoid compressing major nerves. Any client feedback indicating a numb, electric, tingling, funny-bone kind of feeling means it's time for you to get off the nerve.

Treatment

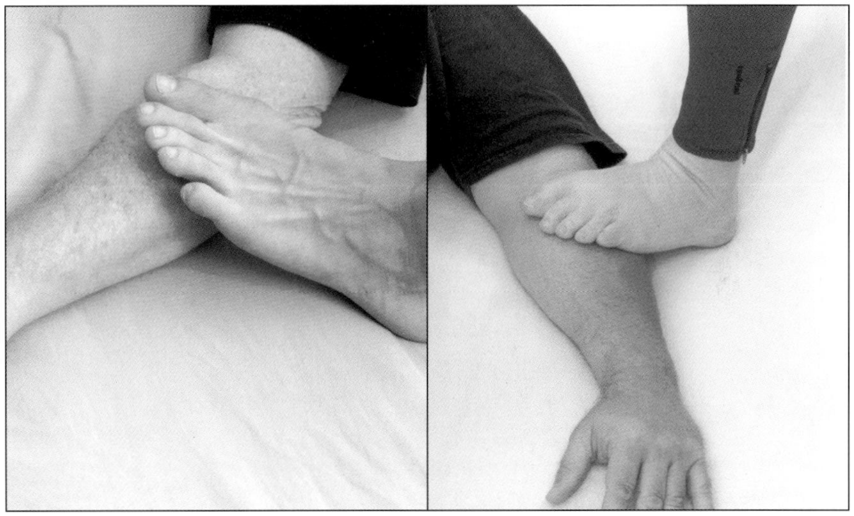

Direct pressure from the first ray into the belly of the supinator.

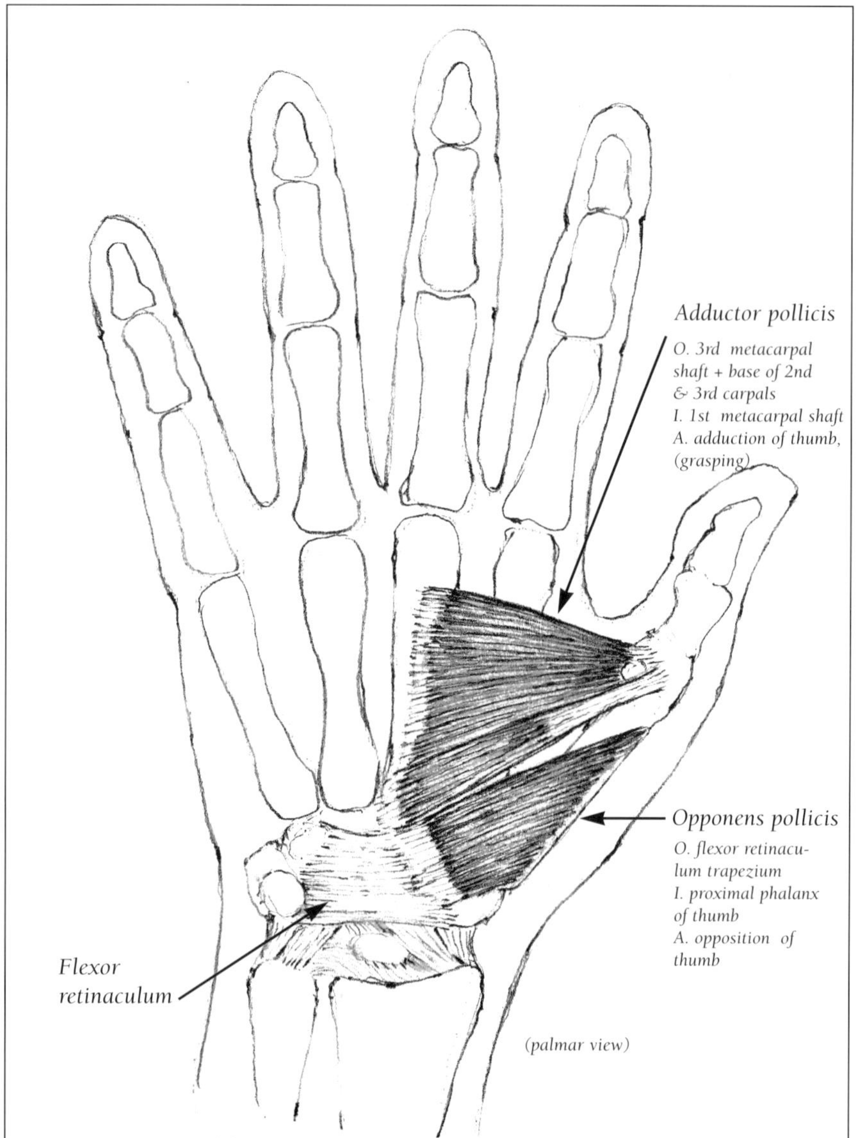

Adductor pollicis / Oppenens pollicis

The thousands of pincer palpations and kneading strokes given by massage therapists can create "overuse" injuries. The adductor and opponens pollicis muscles are particularly vulnerable. Fortunately trigger points, whether in massage therapists or others engaged in hand-intensive work, respond quickly to pressure. As therapists, we can deeply appreciate the relief that prolonged deep compressions give these overworked muscles.

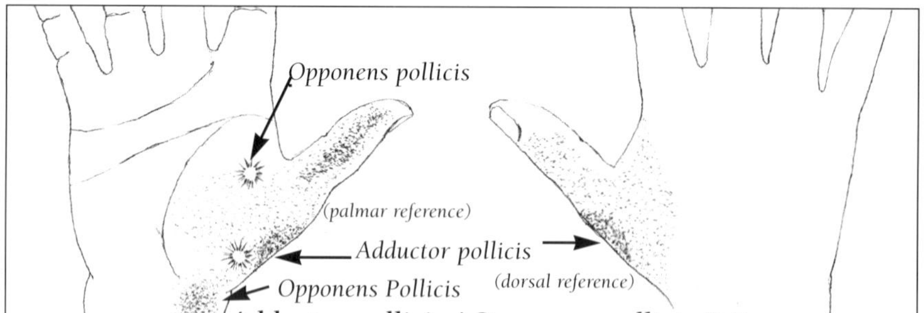

Adductor pollicis / Oppenens pollicis TrPs

Between these two muscles is the tendon of the flexor pollicis longus. This long thumb flexor tendon becomes particularly sore from kneading strokes, pincer palpation and friction massage. To locate tendon, palpate firmly in the middle of the thenar eminance while client flexes and extends thumb. Friction and direct pressure here relieve the ache and treat or prevent a tendonitis, or, even worse, a trigger thumb.

We have developed a potent "heel-on-thumb whammy" that gets the pressure up there where the strong and active benefit. Sink in slowly and rely on duration to complete the treatment.

Clients who continuously use their hands – artisans, politicians, queens or laborers – can also benefit greatly from a self-stretch program. This protocol is most useful when used intermittently throughout the day.

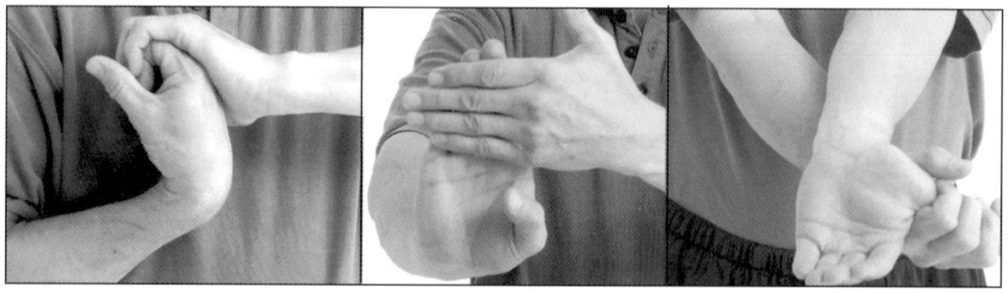

Wrist and finger extensor stretch. Wrist and finger flexor stretch. Opponens pollicis stretch.

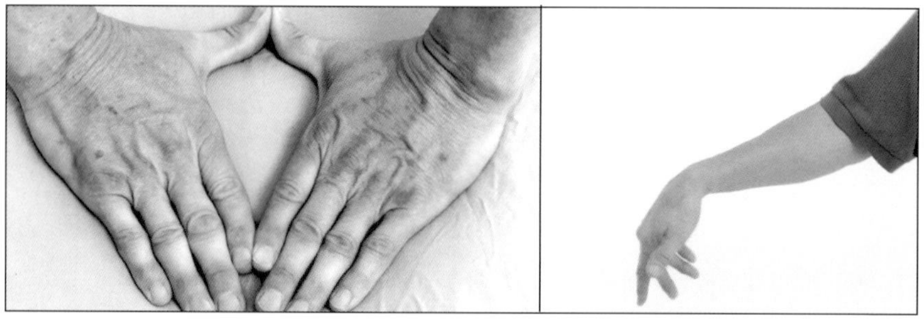

Adductor pollicis stretch. "Flutter" for finger and wrist joints. Shake limp wrist and fingers rapidly for 20 to 30 seconds…good one for drummers, piano players, violinists etc.

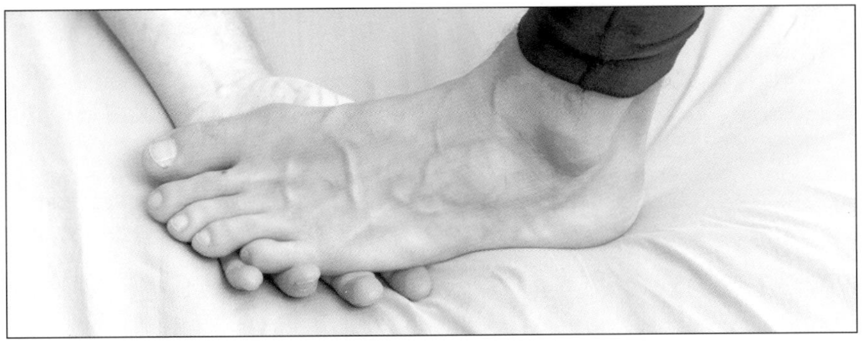

Prolonged pressure from a soft foot leads to relaxation. Stay off the wrist.

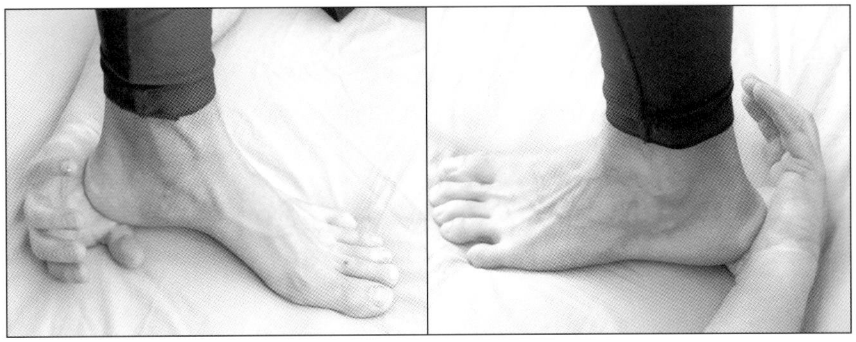

The "whammy." Client is supine with hand rolled into supination.

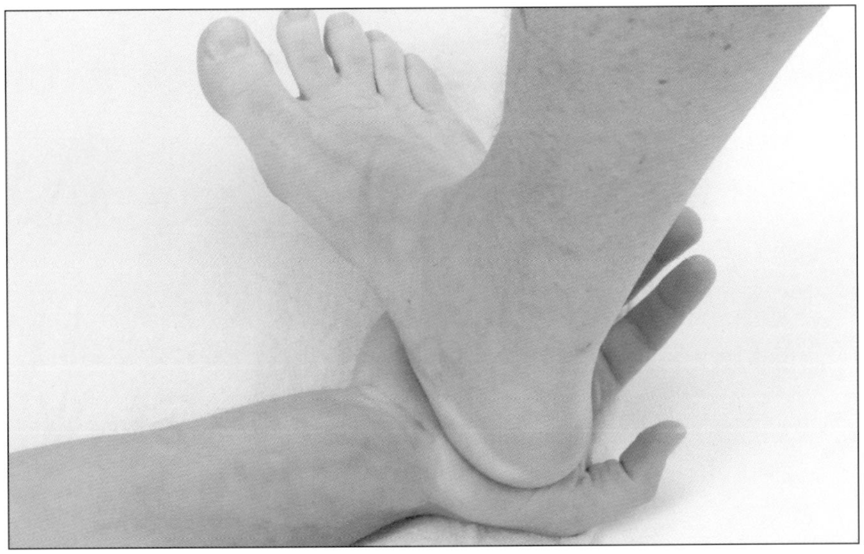

Heel pressure to the thenar muscles. Pressure is applied gradually with the support leg carrying most of the therapist's weight.

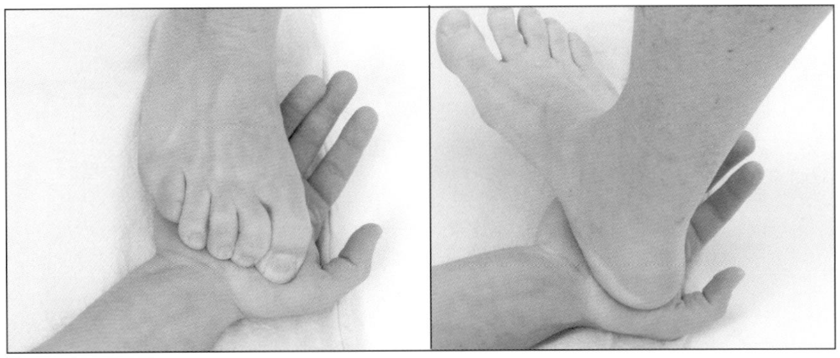

Direct pressure of the long flexor tendon and opponens pollicis from therapist's flexed big toe and heel.

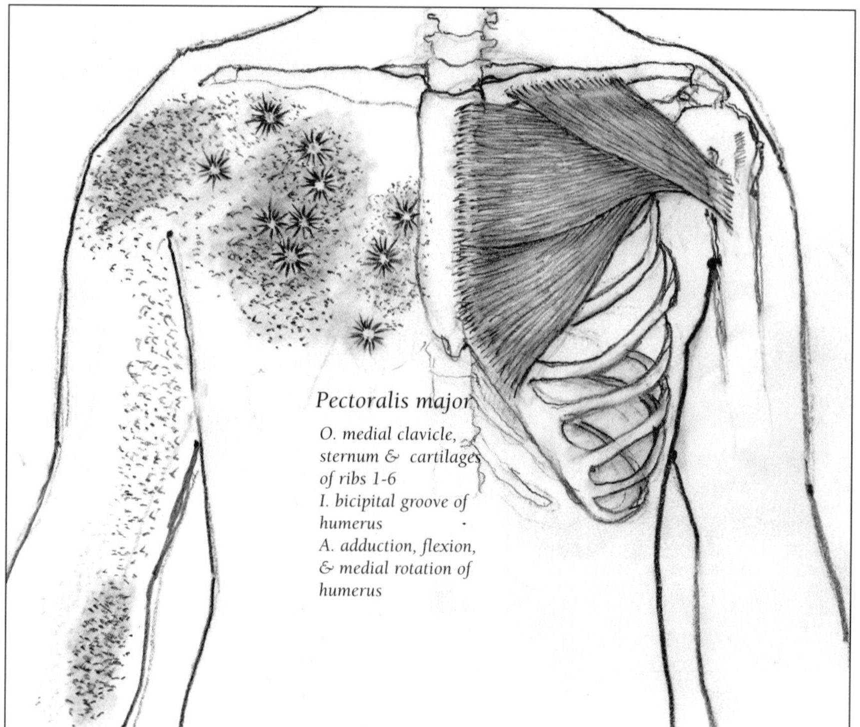

Pectoralis major & TrPs

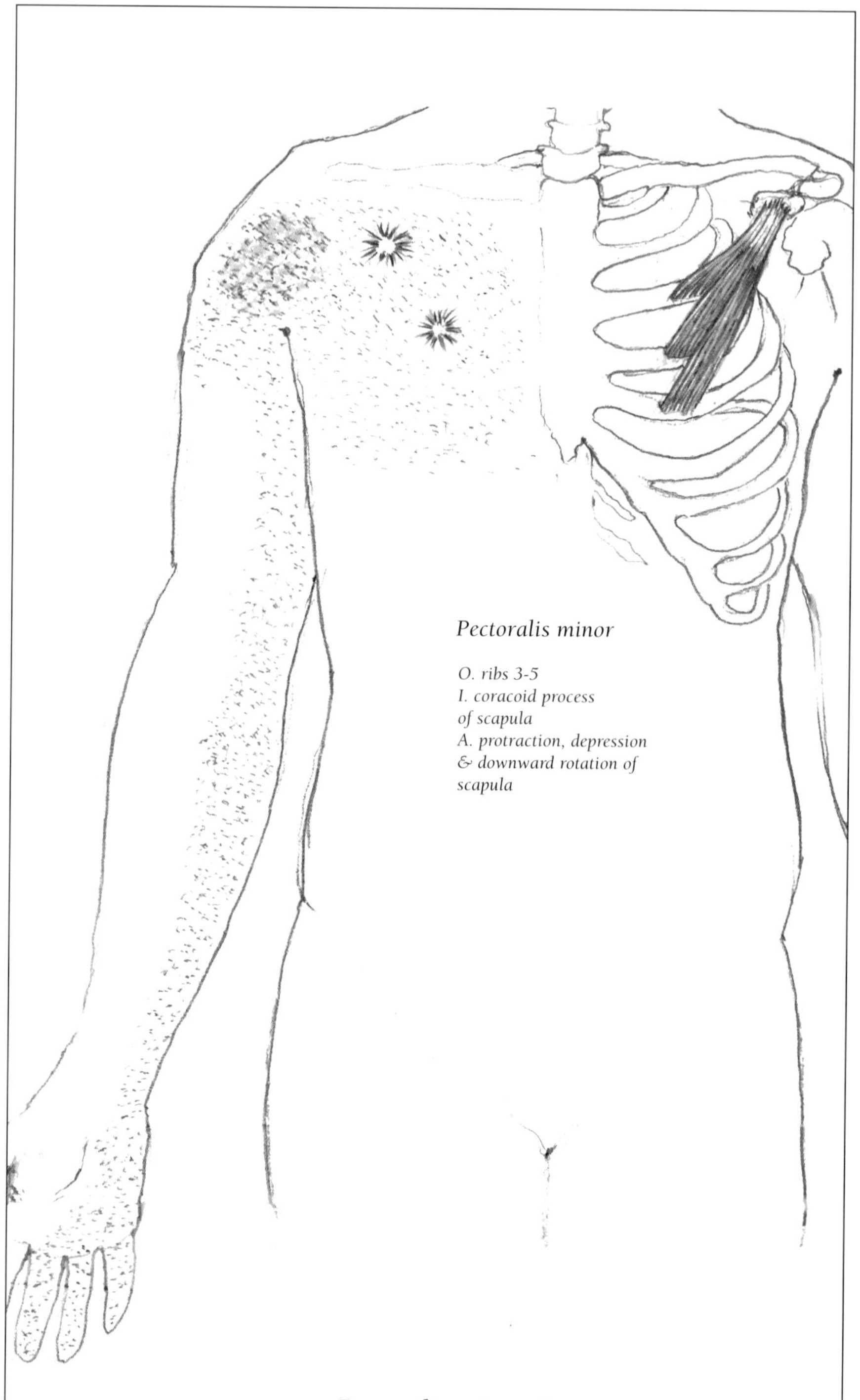

Pectoralis minor & TrPs

CLIENTS CURSED WITH HEAD FORWARD, stooped shoulder, internally rotated humerus and a generally woe-be-gone posture need help. A good beginning point is treating pectoralis major trigger points. The pecs are thick, strong and quick to hypertrophy (think bench-press). The problem is that bench-press-built pec major muscles easily overwhelm, stretch and inhibit the often underdeveloped, antagonistic mid-traps and rhomboids.

Use pincer palpation to examine for trigger points for the bulk of the pec major. Treat all trigger points with pincer palpation or direct pressure. On heavily muscled clients, we use the heel to eliminate these trigger points. Avoid the delto-pectoral groove, and use care not to compress breast tissue.

The second part of this protocol is a stretch for the pectoralis major combined with training the client to do a daily door stretch for home care. Balancing the shoulder girdle requires strengthening the mid-traps and rhomboids. Scapular retractions are an effective exercise. Scapular

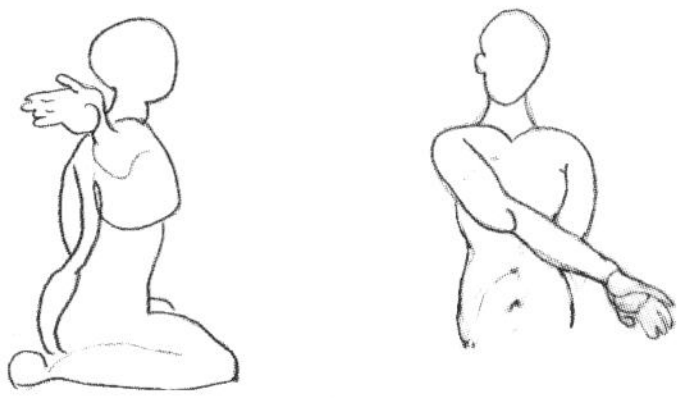

winging can be addressed with push-ups to strengthen the serratus anterior. Occasionally there will be trigger points in the serratus anterior muscle that will need to be eliminated before the strengthening program can begin.

Direct pressure to the serratus anterior on a side-lying client by hand or foot (determined by size and strength) will clear the trigger point. This muscle needs good tonus, but extreme development leads to chronic scapular protraction and even more rounded shoulders.

When balancing the shoulder girdle with resisted exercise, care must be taken to stretch both pecs and the scapular retractors. Over-development of both the anterior and posterior musculature can create a vice-like effect on the upper torso. All strengthening programs should include adequate stretching to maintain balance.

The pectoralis minor serves primarily as a scapular stabilizer. Trigger points here can refer all the way to the hand and mimic a thoracic outlet syndrome. It is not unusual for a short, tight pec minor to compress the brachial plexus and axillary artery.

Treat pec minor trigger points with either direct pressure or pincer palpation (pincer palpation is done with the thumb beneath the belly of the pec major and the fingers on top of the pec major). Remember, over-training the pec minor and major can create severely inwardly rotated shoulders.

When harboring trigger points, the left pectoralis minor can be the source of "mock angina." It refers pain to the heart. Don't second guess on this – refer for medical evaluation.

When the pectoralis minor or major has a trigger point, look for associated trigger points in the anterior deltoid, scalenes, and sternocleidomastoid (SCM). The SCM and scaleni assist with forced inspiration.

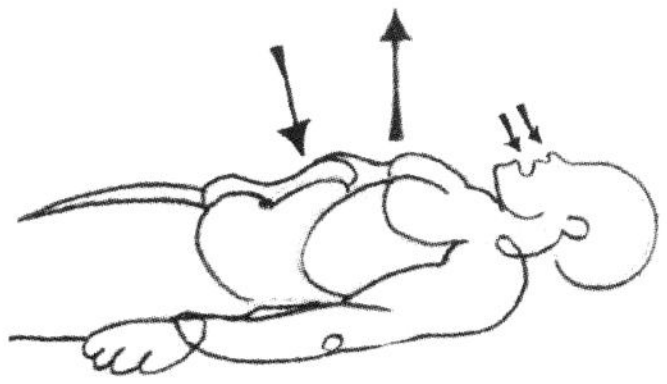

Client paradoxical breathing (covered in the "What To Do" appendix) can contribute to trigger points in neck muscles.

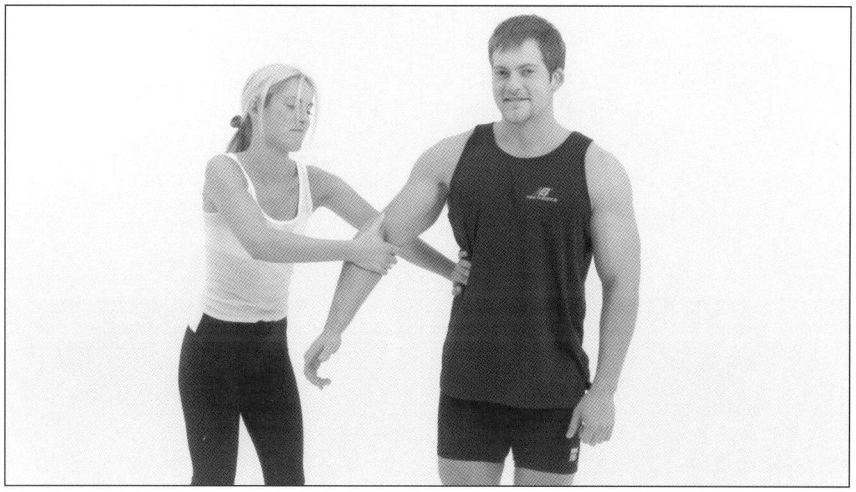

Client adduction of their arm against therapist's resistance tests for tendonitis and muscle belly tears in the pectoralis major, latissimus dorsi, and teres major and minor. Note that the therapist offers resistance above, not below, the elbow joint. This precludes stressing non-contractile tissues (ligaments, bursae and joint capsule) in the elbow joint.

Treatment

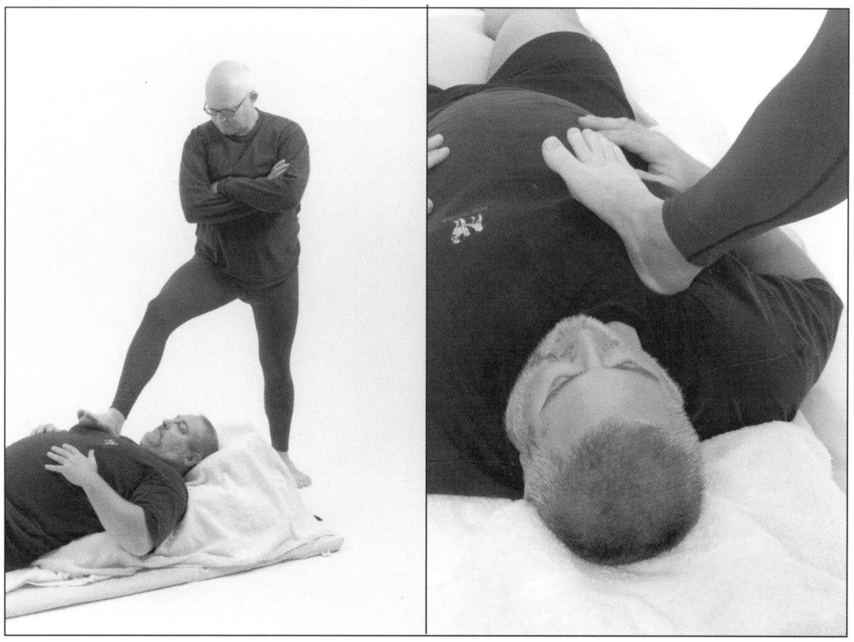

Use of foot on big guy's pecs.

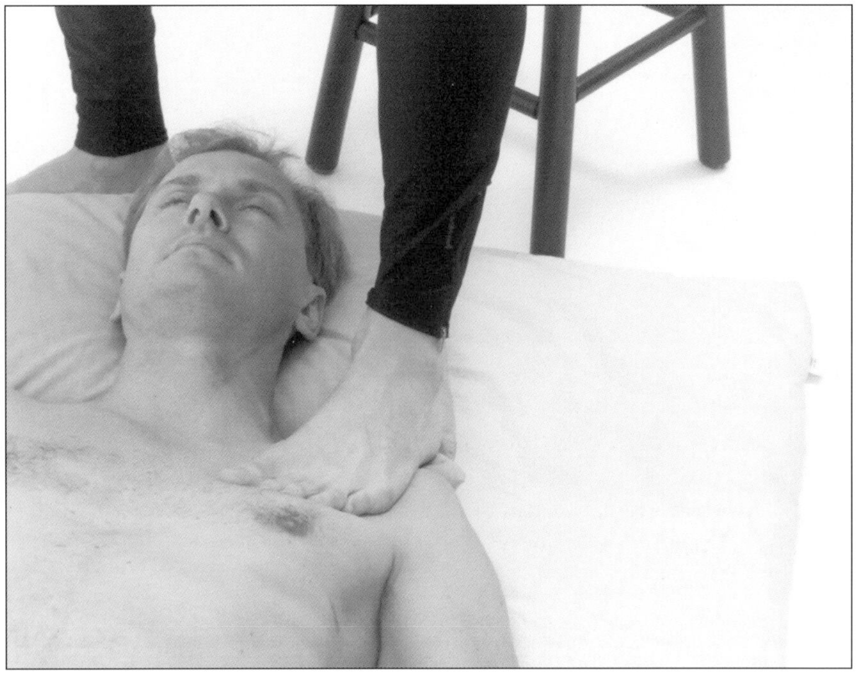

Using seated position to warm pecs.

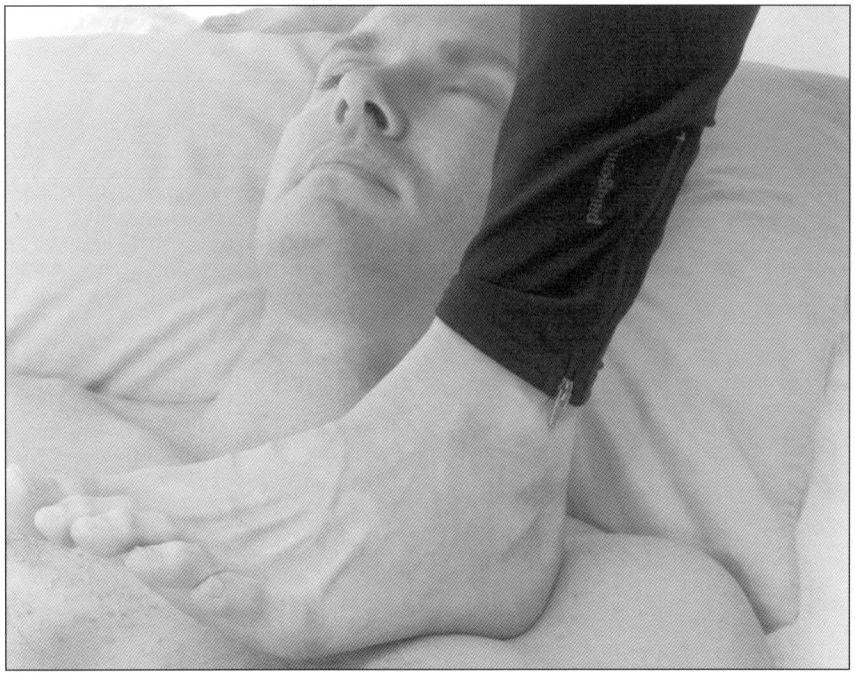

Caution when compressing over the delto-pectoral groove. Pincer palpation is not only a good substitute, but preferable for most clients.

CHAPTER 13

Neck, Mid-back and Torso Pain

THIS SECTION ADDRESSES the common problems suffered by people who live in front of computers. Whiplash victims and headache suffers will also benefit greatly.

We begin with the levator scapula's relationship to neck pain and restricted rotation.

Next we address the latissimus dorsi pain suffered from lifting cuddly little objects out of car seats or highchairs, followed by common problems in the mid-traps, serratus posterior inferior and the rhomboids.

This section concludes with the upper trapezius, housing what Travell and Simons call Trigger Point #1 (the most common trigger point). We've found the upper trapezius to be the primary muscular source of headaches.

Before You Begin

Safe, effective neck, mid-back and torso treatments are enhanced by first reading the *Indications, Client Intake, Contraindications, Deep Compressive Massage, Endangerment Sites, Trigger Points, Cross-fiber, Fascial Release, Stretching* and *Hydrotherapy* sections.

Note the specific procedural notes and cautions. They will help you effectively treat your client without harm. Protocols and guidelines are included to help you know when to treat and when to refer.

Levator Scapula

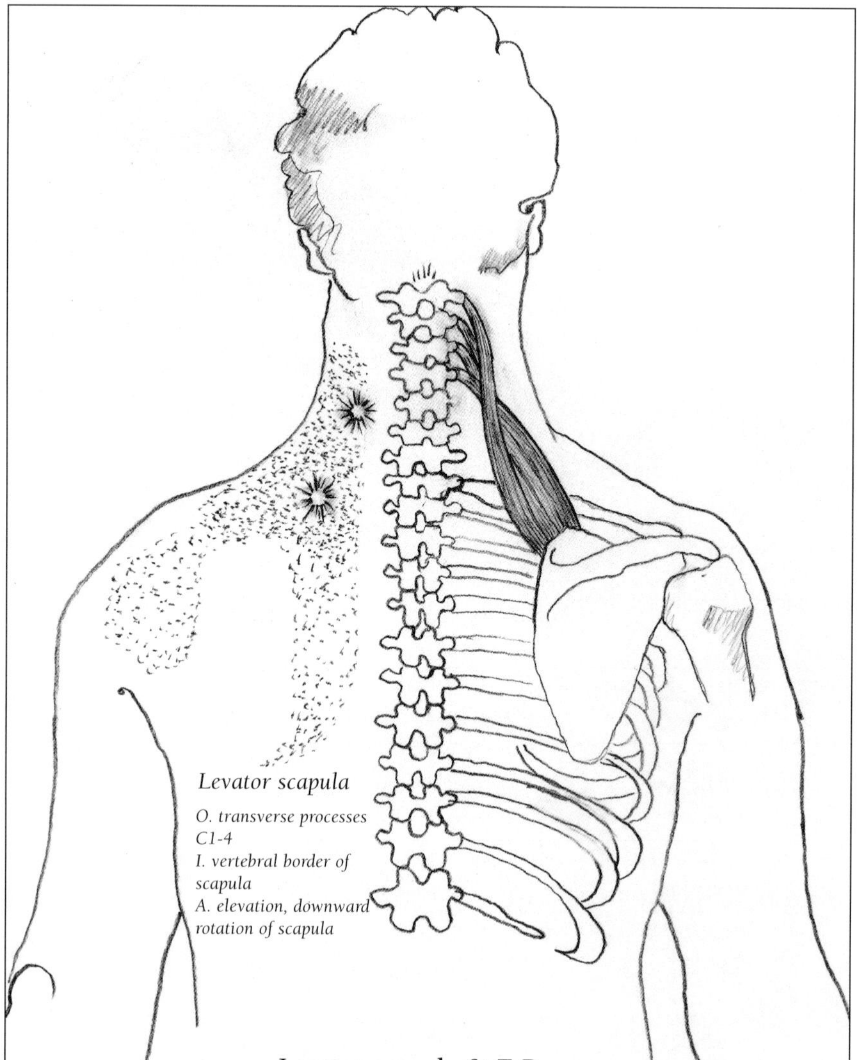

Levator scapula & TrPs

THIS MUSCLE IS MONEY-IN-THE-BANK to message therapists. Pain and restriction on neck rotation are often due to trigger points in the levator scapula. Hotel pillows, a cold breeze on the back of an uncovered neck, phone cradling and other prolonged postural distortions are primary causes of this problem. Referred pain from the levator scapula is located between the superior angle of the scapula and the base of the neck.

Levator scapula trigger points are often painful – squeeze slowly. Your hands will often fatigue quickly holding this muscle, so limit the treatment to 5 to 10 seconds. When seated, have the client turn their head from side to side. If there is an improvement, and there usually is, complete your treatment with barefoot compressions.

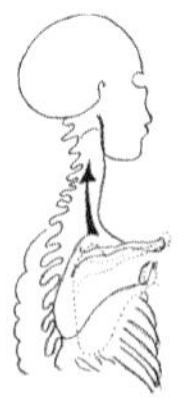

Levator Protocol

Client prone with their head turned to the comfortable side or in a face cradle. Elevate humerus above 90 degrees and, using pincer palpation, grasp the muscle belly next to its scapular attachment. If the upper trapezius is included in your grasp, release it to narrow your grasp to the levator. Then, using both hands, squeeze firmly enough to enter a therapeutic range.

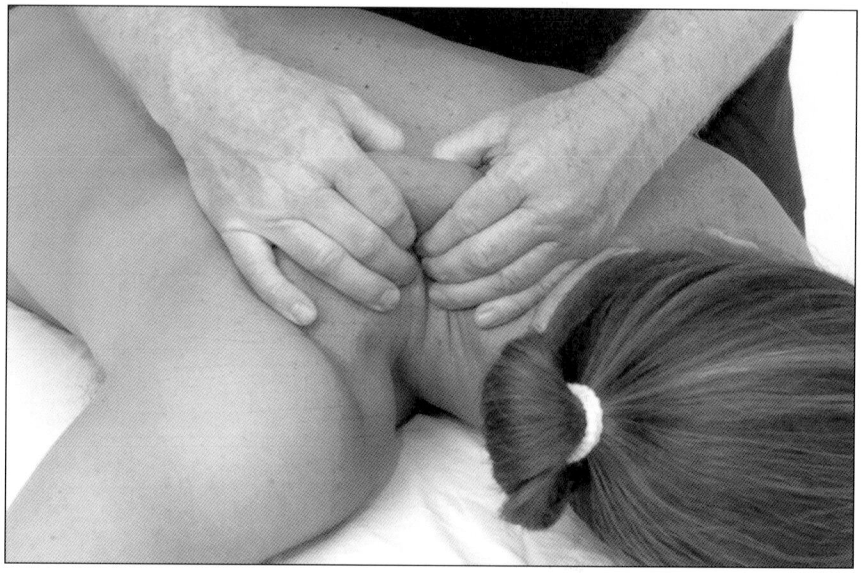

Note that upper trapezius is essentially excluded from the pincer grip.

Big Guy Variation

Place client side-lying with head bolstered safely. Using direct heel pressure while seated is highly effective for the more muscular folks. With pressure progressing from light to moderate, compress the trigger point and hold for 30 to 60 seconds.

Work up the belly of the muscle to the second major trigger point (usually located at the angle of the neck), and hold for another 30 to 60 seconds. Using the pincer grip, palpate through the muscle. Note the reduced level of tonus and pain, and have your client rotate their head again. A dramatically increased pain-free range of motion should result.

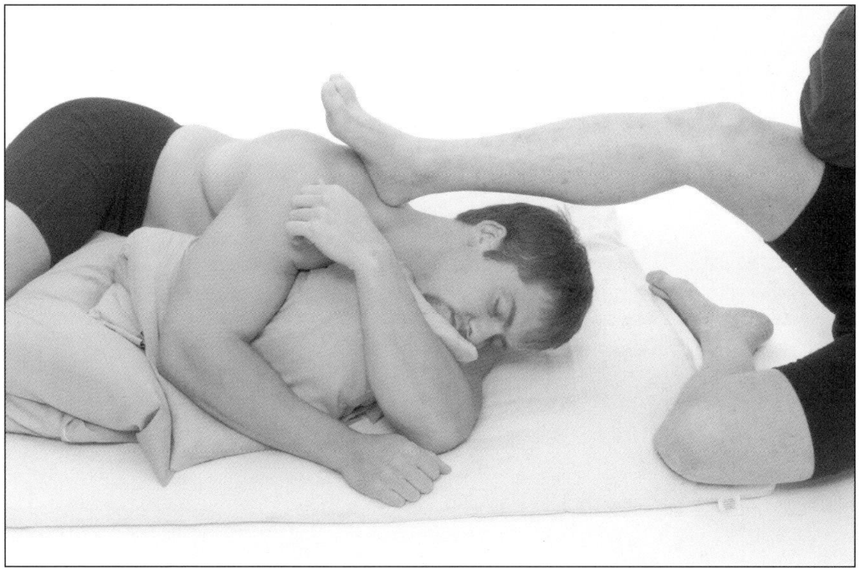

Direct pressure slightly above the levator attachment at the superior angle of the scapula. In our experience, this is the location of the second most common TrP in this muscle.

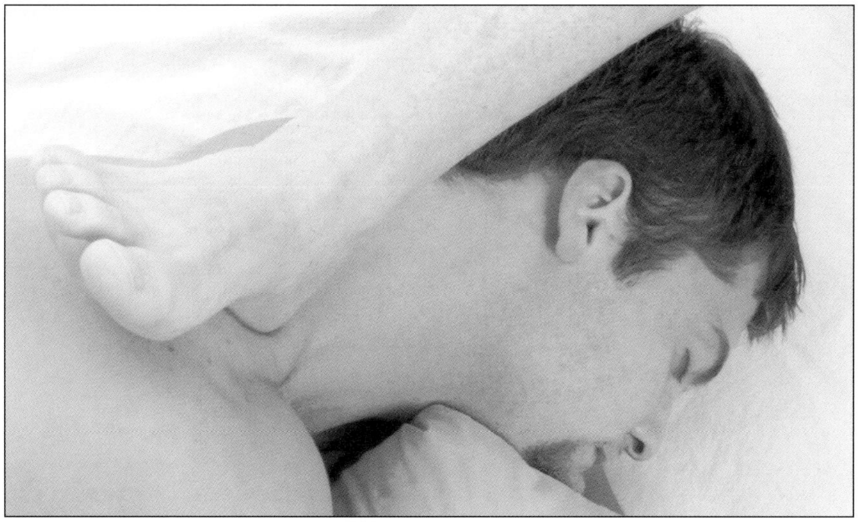

Stretch after treating TrP with direct heel pressure.

A scenario for creating levator problems: Enroute boredom moves you to the hotel bar. You meet someone you'd like to know much better. While waxing witty and urbane, you turn your head to face this person seated beside you. Meanwhile the air-conditioner blows a cold stream on your head and neck. By the next morning, vivid dreams, the hotel pillow, cold drafts and strain have taken their toll – a stiff neck. The immediate solution is a trigger point treatment to the levator. The long term solution – wear a scarf and sit facing your companion.

As with most muscles, the levator needs exercise – weight training and stretching. This combination will go a long way toward developing the bulk and resilience needed to avoid forming or firing trigger points. Thin, deconditioned muscles are highly susceptible to overuse syndromes.

POST-OP STORY

Our client had submitted to 8 laminectomies. Believe it or not, he earned his living working on a computer. Daily Swedish massage gave him several hours of relief from his chronic neck and shoulder pain, but no more. We tried prolonged direct pressure to his levator scapula and the superficial paraspinal muscles in the upper thoracic region. This treatment provided him with pain-free functioning for days rather than hours. An important point here is to treat both the presenting problem and the surrounding musculature, i.e., both synergists and antagonists.

Office workers sometimes have to wear a scarf or high collar to protect the levator scapula from chilling under the air-conditioner. People with this problem need to pay particular attention to computer work-station ergonomics.

SPECIAL CAUTION

Healthy clients can be minimally bolstered at their necks to create a moderate lateral stretch. To avoid possible arterial spasm, basilar insufficiency or other cervical damage, clients with hypermobile cervical vertebra should be bolstered to prevent any extreme stretch.

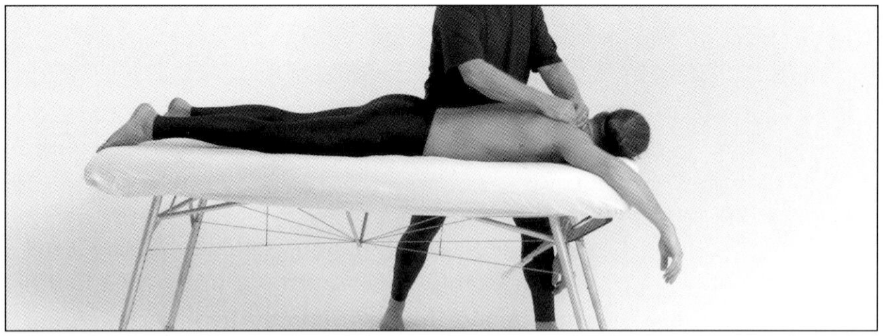

Reach across body to pincer palpate levator scapula TrPs.

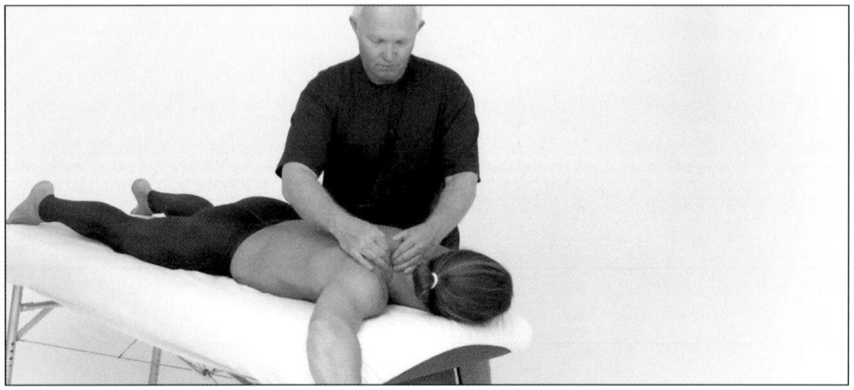

Use two hands to lift and squeeze the bulk of the muscle.

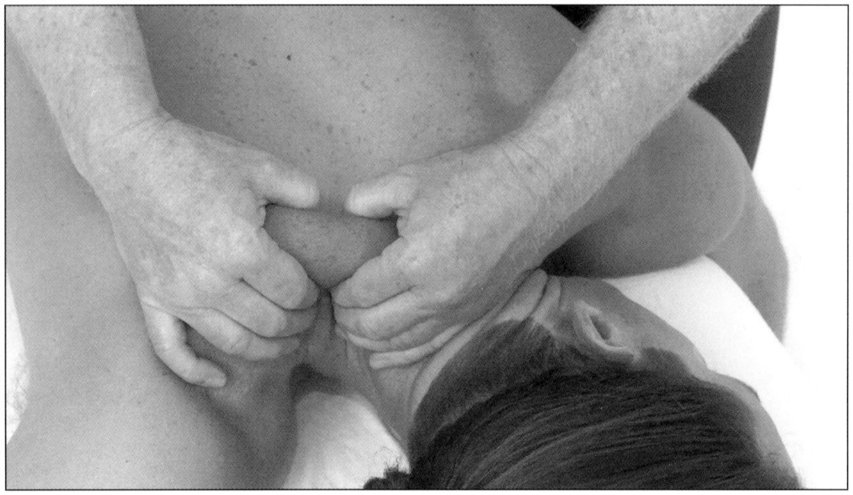

It is easy to squeeze beneath the muscle. To be effective – as with the trapezius – you must squeeze the thick, full middle of the muscle.

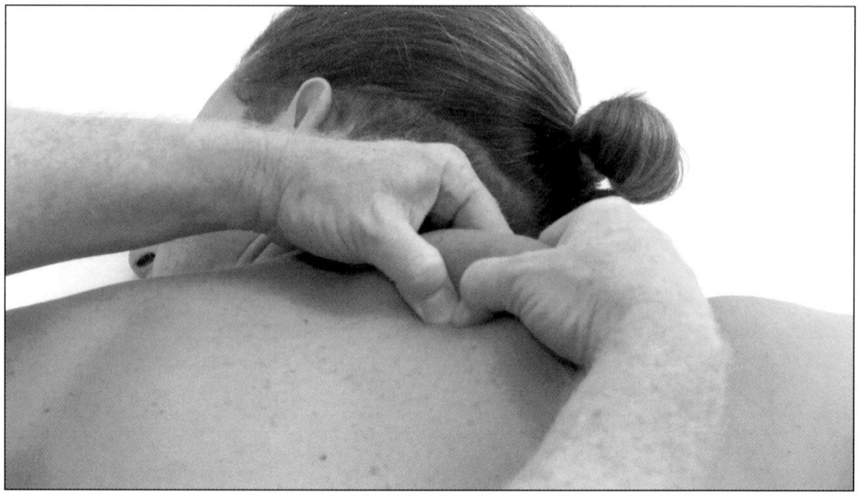

This is just squeezing skin and subcutaneous fat – useless as a trigger point treatment.

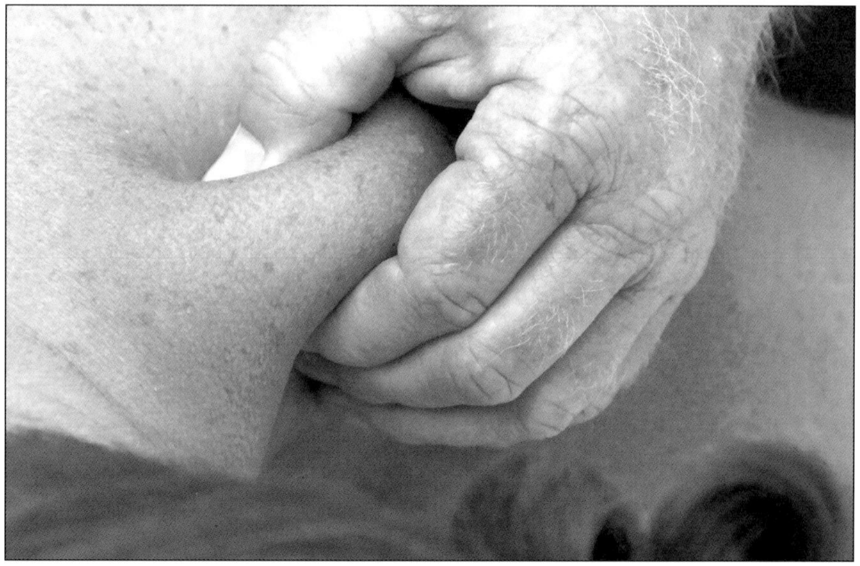

This grip is on the muscle belly. Firmly squeeze between the thumb and index finger.

Latissimus dorsi

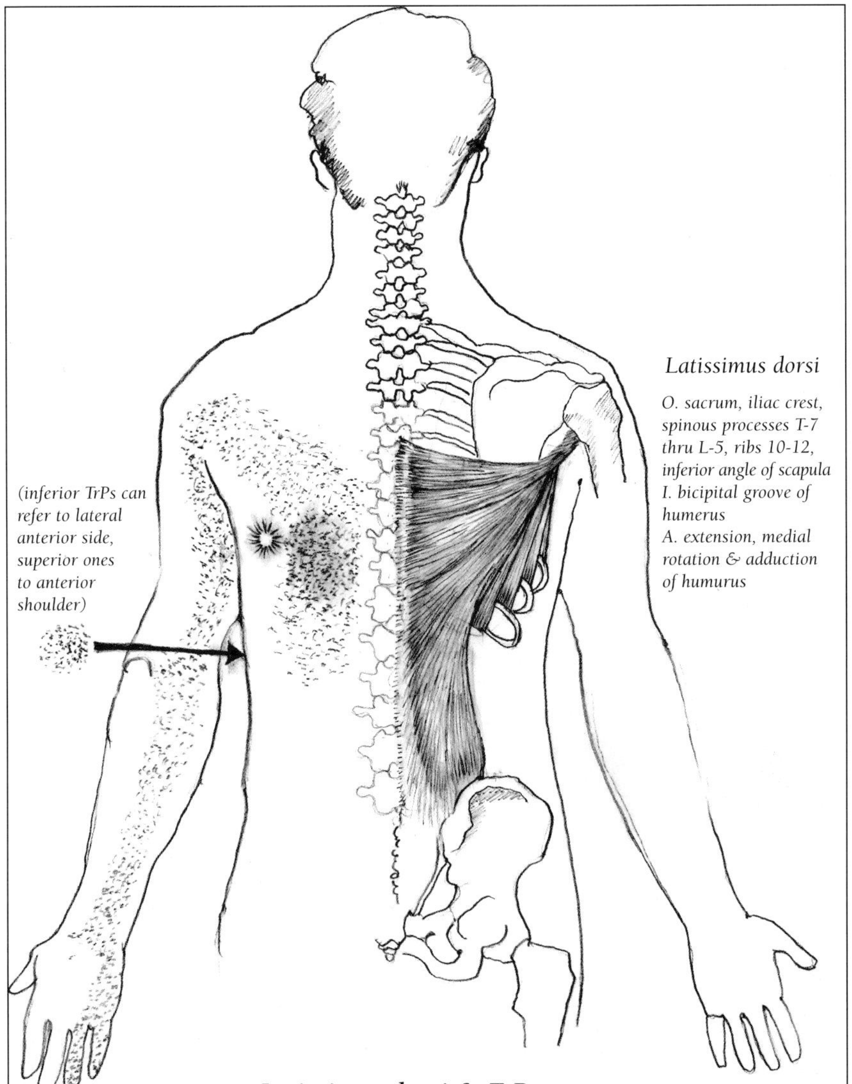

Latissimus dorsi & TrPs

Trigger points keep many muscles from fully stretching. If your client can't bring their biceps up next to their ears with a raised straight arm, a trigger point shortened or tight latissimus dorsi is usually responsible. Accompanying mid-thoracic pain is often present.

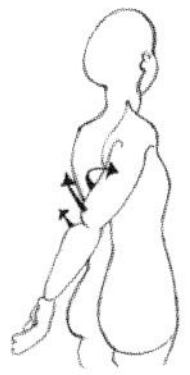

Trigger points in the latissimus dorsi muscle are often created or reactivated by pull-ups or lat-pulls. Holding or lifting heavy weights (including children) out in front of the body also create or fire this trigger point. Every muscle has a story – the lats have many. Lifting kids out of cribs and car seats are two very common examples of precipitative events.

To access the latissimus dorsi, use pincer palpation at the posterior axilla to find the tender (jump sign) point. Bolster your clients and treat them side-lying with direct pressure from your heel to the trigger point.

Treatment

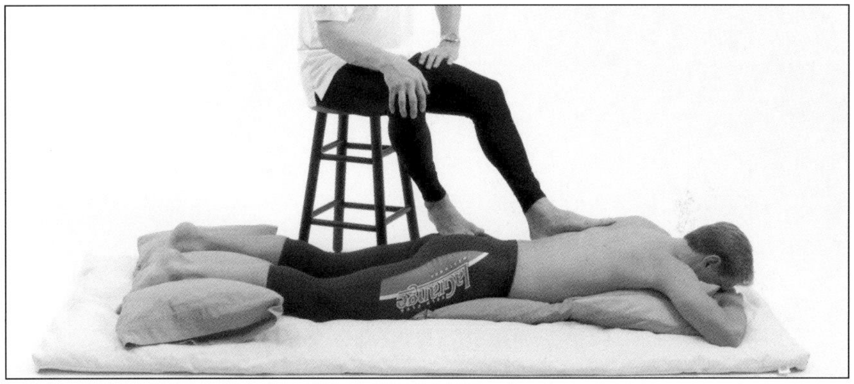

This is one trigger point that you can often work while seated on a stool. Adequate pressure for most clients is created with just the weight of your leg.

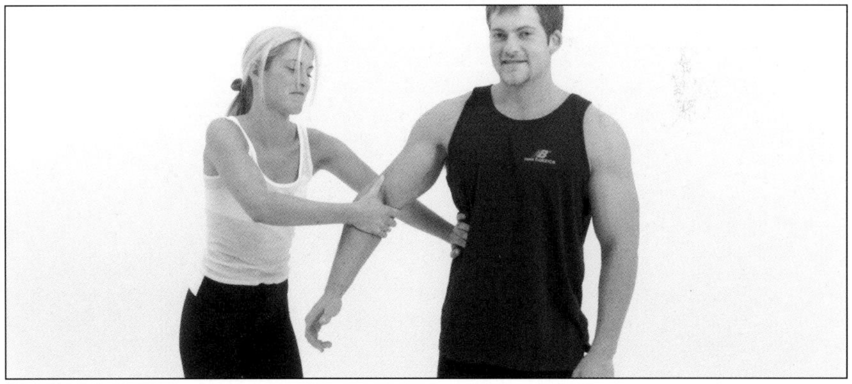

Functional assessment (MTFA test). Client adducts their arm against therapist's resistance to test for tendonitis and muscle belly tears in the latissimus dorsi, pecs, lats and teres. Note that the therapist offers resistance above, not below, the elbow joint. This precludes stressing non-contractile tissues (ligaments, bursae and joint capsule) in the elbow joint.

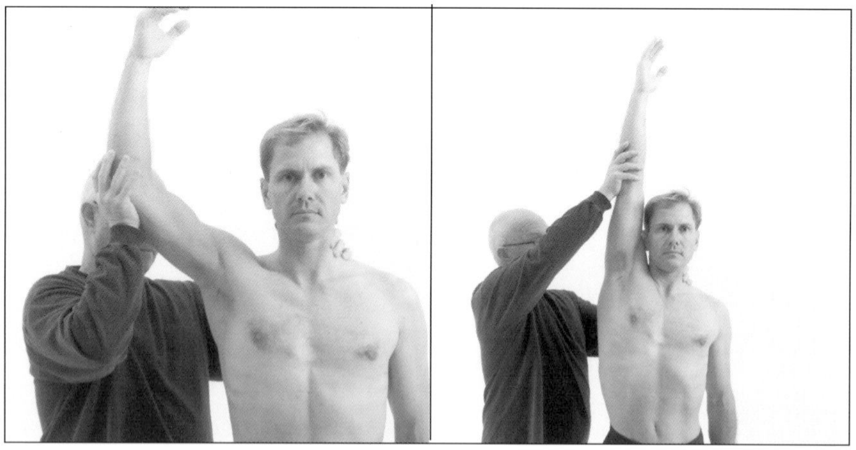

Administer a CRAC stretch: Resistance is offered followed by client actively elevating the humerus (bringing the biceps to the ear) to stretch the lat.

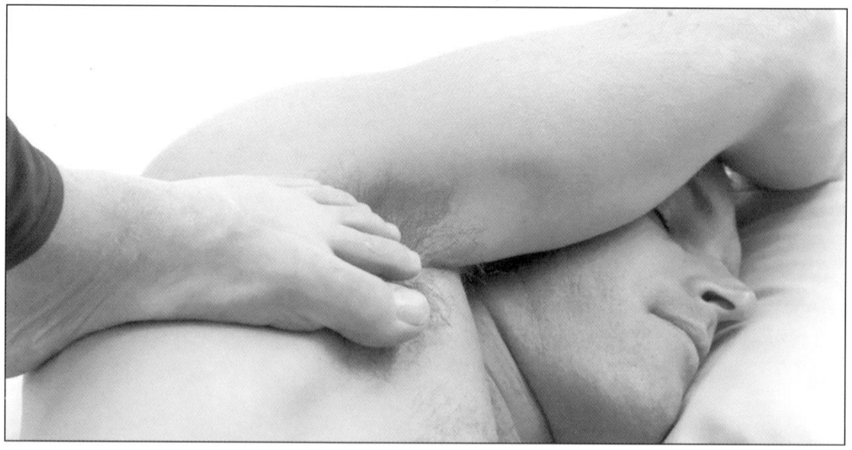

Gentle fascial stretch for latissimus.

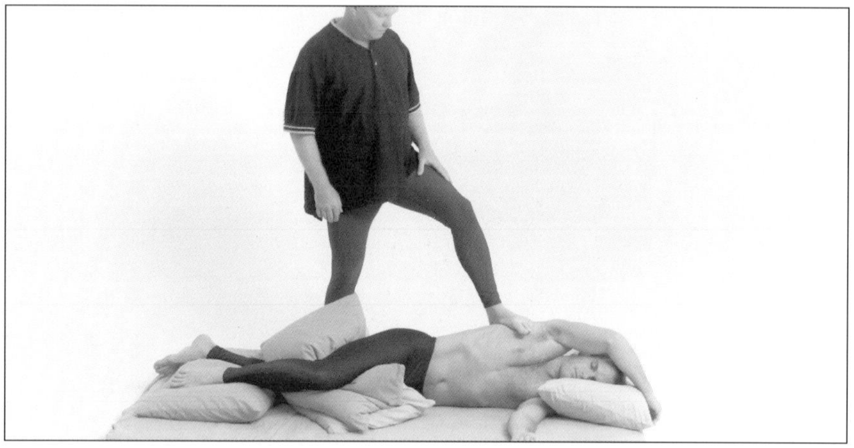

The side-lying warm-up of the latissimus dorsi.

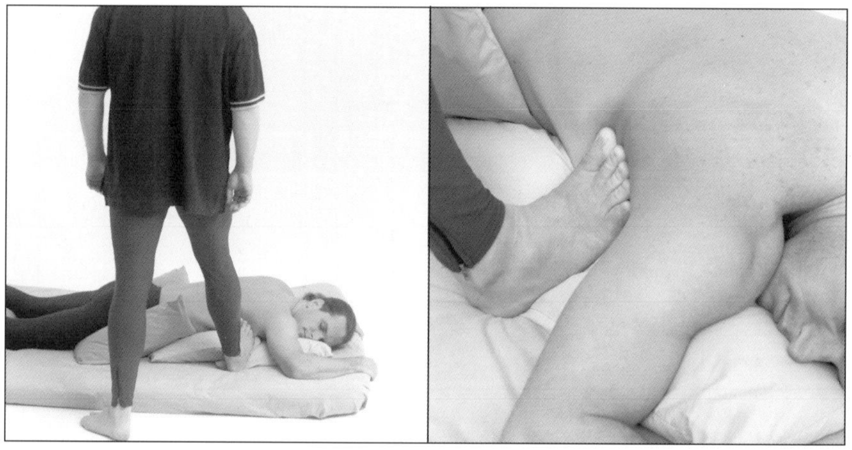

Direct pressure with the ball of the foot to the lateral edge of the latissimus dorsi. Notice the relaxed foot.

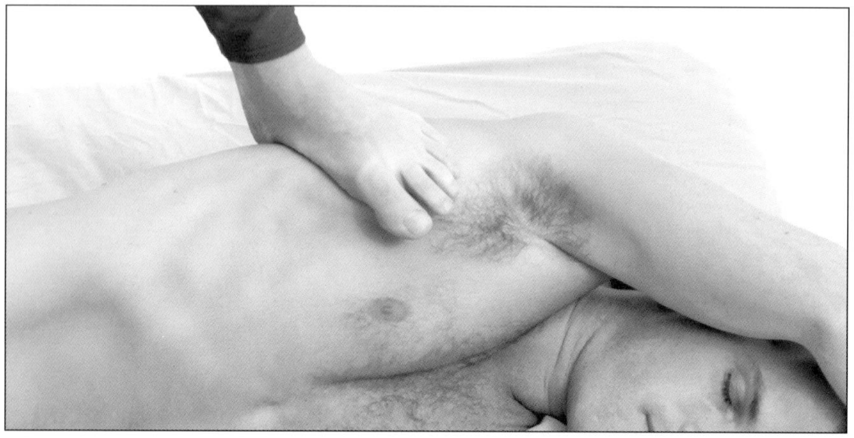

Close-up of latissimus compression. Note relaxed foot.

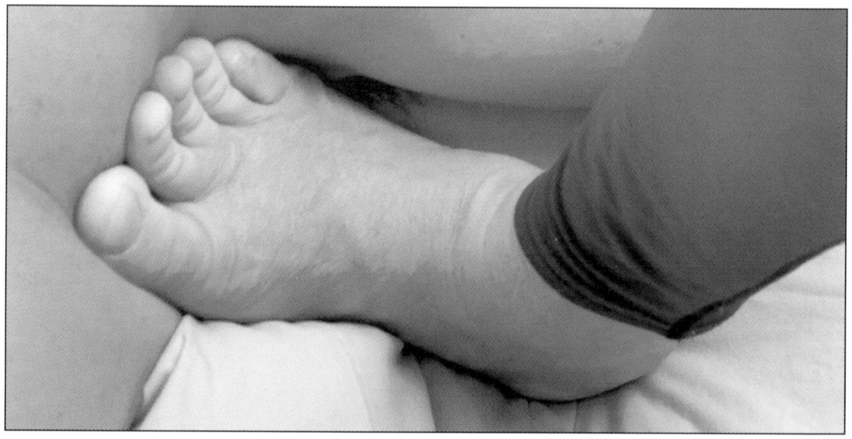

Fascial stretch – in and down.

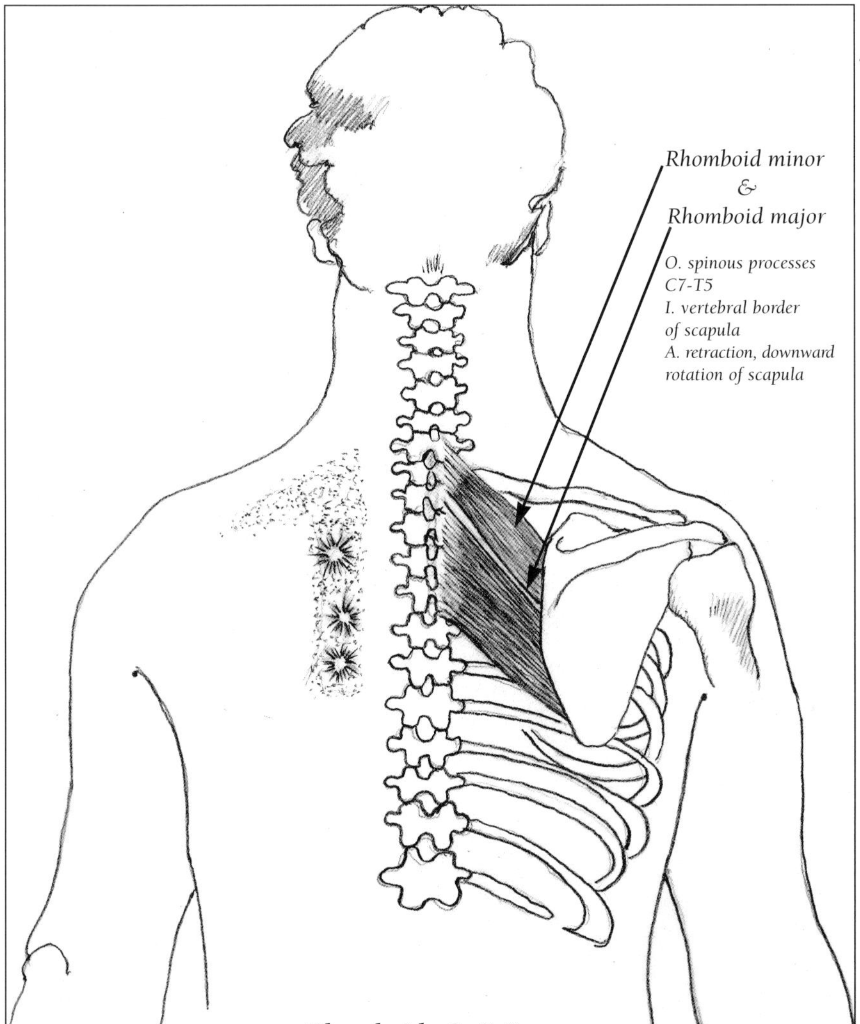

Rhomboids & TrPs

WEAK, OVER-STRETCHED rhomboid and mid-trapezius muscles promote painful trigger points. These trigger points often create the mid-back pain so common to students, office workers and others who labor in a hunched position. Normal shoulder mechanics are also interrupted and can lead to rotator cuff impingement.

Thin, weak muscles are much more susceptible to trigger points. These latent triggers tend to line up along the vertebral border of the scapula. The typical massage approach of rub, rub, rub next to the winged vertebral border of the scapulae is particularly ineffective in providing long-term relief.

While easy to treat with direct pressure, these trigger points may return over and over to cause mischief. Lasting relief comes with your client stretching the pectoralis major and minor and strengthening the mid-traps and rhomboids. This will help balance the shoulder girdle, help avoid rotator cuff impingement, and help properly position the head and neck.

To complete the cure, perpetuating factors and ergonomics must be addressed.

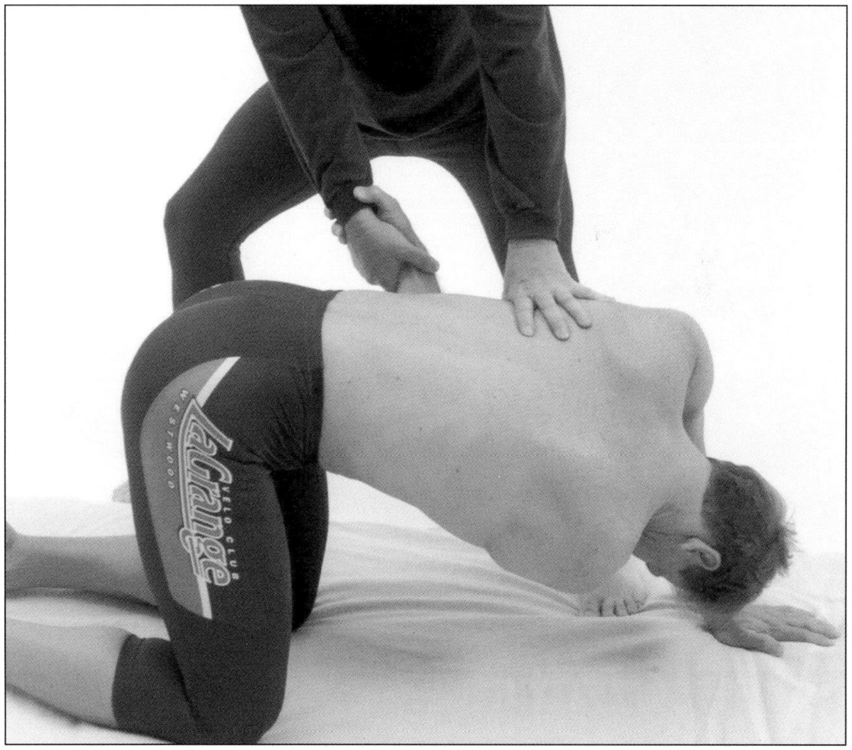

Add a mild mid-trap and rhomboid stretch (post-strengthening) to help prevent post-exercise soreness and the rekindling of trigger points during the initial strengthening period.

ENTREPRENEUR'S STORY

A dynamic, aggressive, entrepreneurial client was plagued by mid-trap pain. She required 3 visits weekly simply to function. Although young, her posture was becoming kypotic and round-shouldered from countless agitated hours spent with the phone braced between her shoulder and her ear. She usually wrote frantically with the opposite hand.

The trigger points were easy to find and treat, but the cure wouldn't hold. Only after the time she spent slumped with the phone glued to her ear was shortened, the thin, weak muscles strengthened, and a hand-freeing headset acquired, did she get well. Postural awareness also became an important part of her staying pain free.

Apparent rhomboid minor and levator scapulae pain that does not respond to treatment may come from the serratus posterior superior muscle. Examine the serratus posterior superior when the pain lies primarily beneath the rhomboid minor and levator scapulae. Clients often feel a deep ache under the superior portion of the scapula. Serratus posterior superior pain will feel deeper than mid-trap pain. We treat these trigger points with a well-placed heel into the muscle with the client side-lying and their scapulae protracted.

Treatment

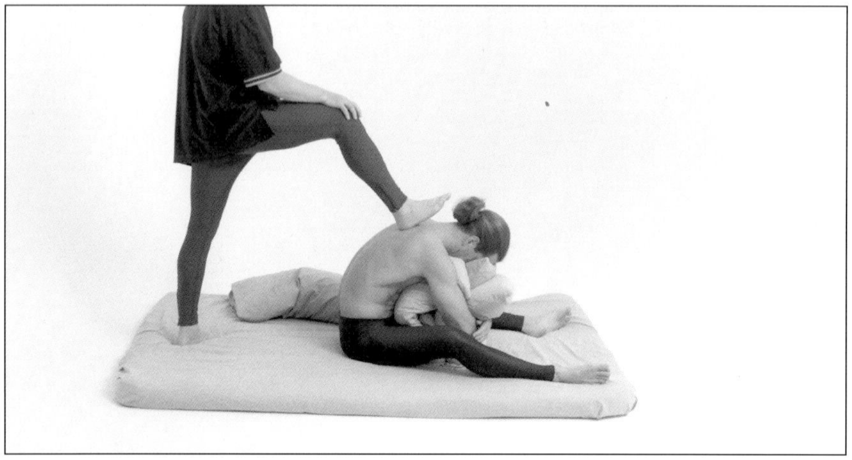

Trigger point treatment for the mid-traps and rhomboids. Well-bolstered client in forward flexion with protracted scapulae gives us great access to mid trap and rhomboid trigger points. Usually only moderate direct heel pressure is needed.

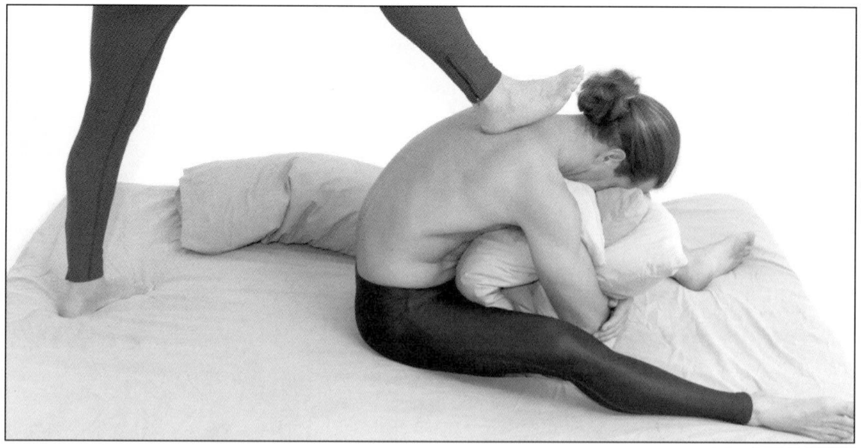

Client should be well-bolstered to prevent a torso collapse that interferes with diaphragmatic breathing. Therapist angle of attack is down and forward.

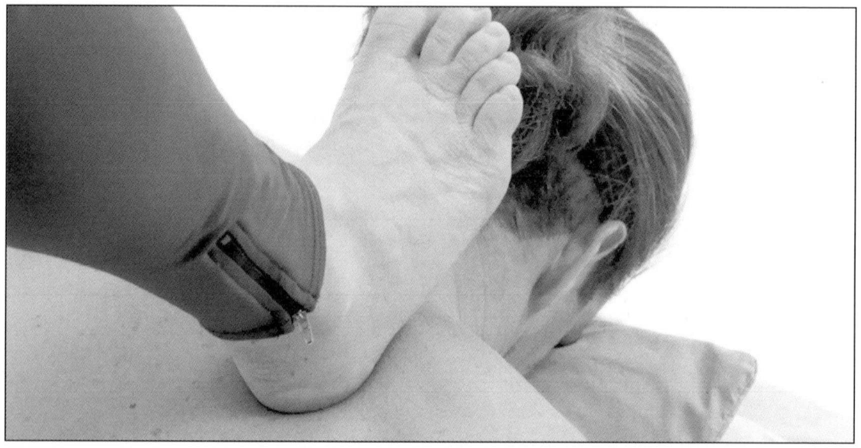

Avoid direct pressure to the vertebral border of the scapula and the spinous processes.

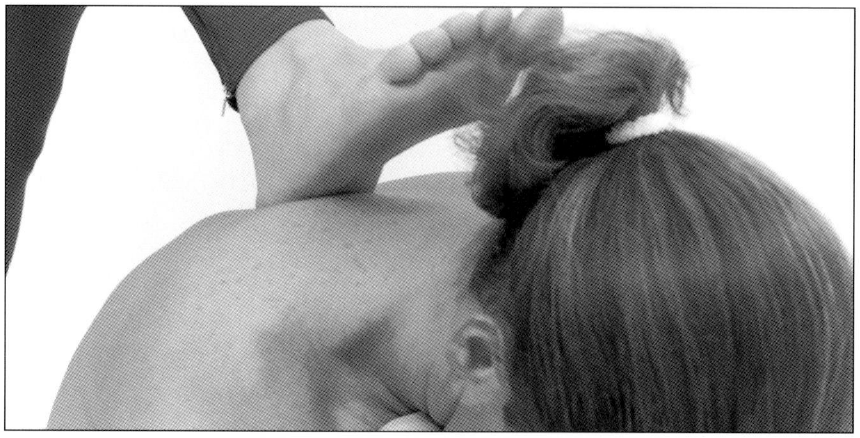

Abundant pressure from a relaxed foot.

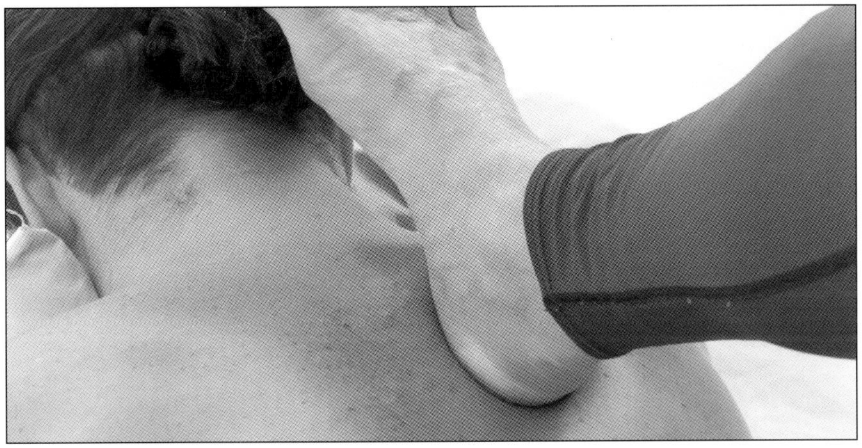

Need we say more?

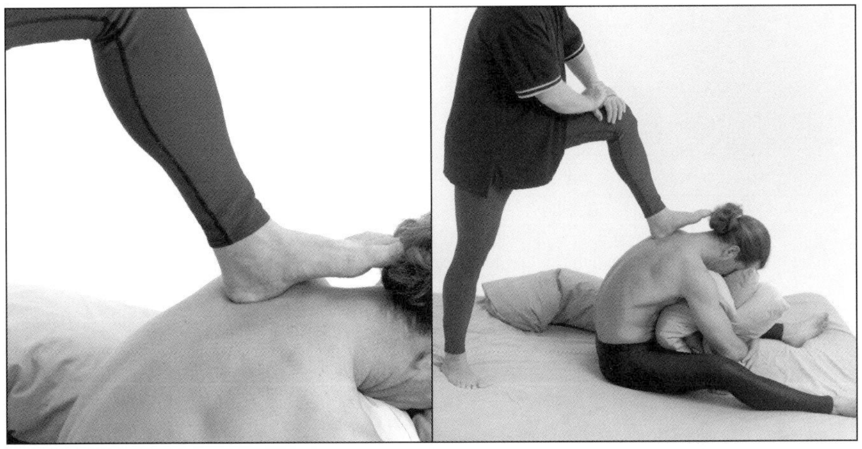

Lean slightly forward to increase pressure.

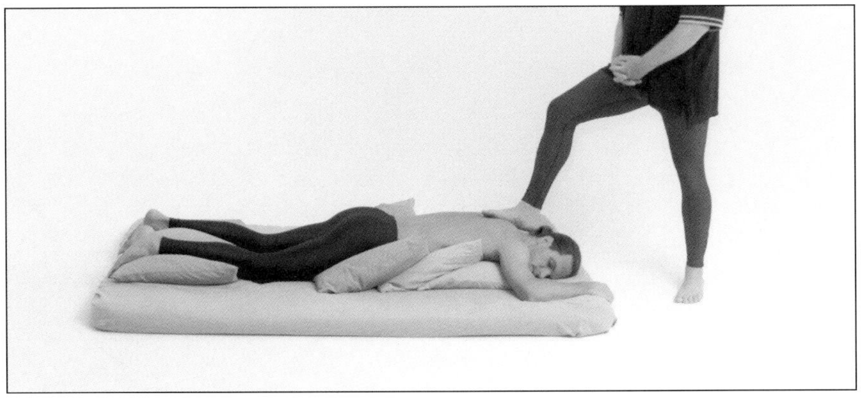

Use the lateral edge of your foot to address mid-trap and rhomboid trigger points when the space between the spinous processes and the vertebral border of the scapula is narrow. Bolster the chest with a pillow to ensure scapular protraction.

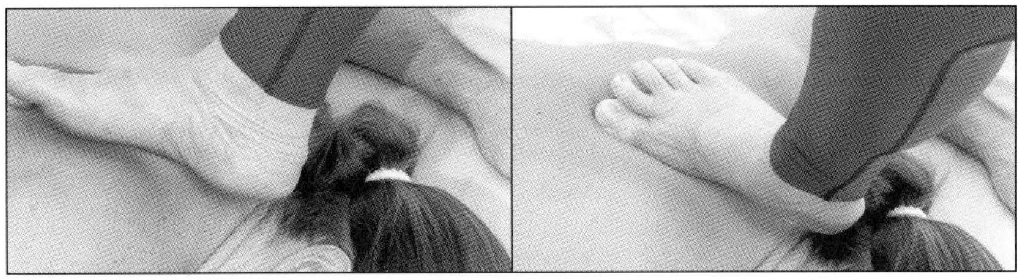

Clients face should always be turned away from therapist's foot. The medial edge of the foot can also be effectively used for TrPs close to the spinous process.

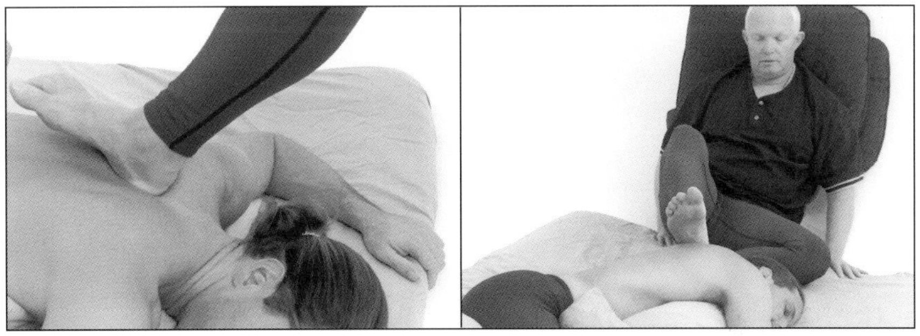

The heel, as always, is our strongest tool for direct pressure. Side-lying approach to the mid-traps and rhomboids.

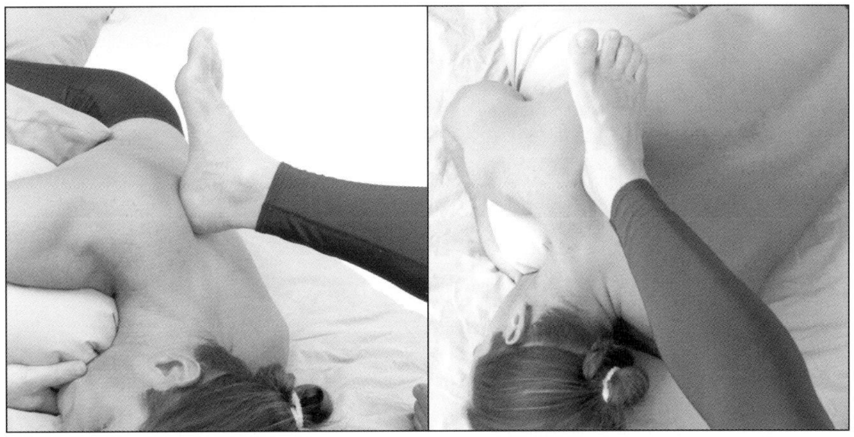

Use direct heel pressure with a slight stretch from lateral twist. Side-lying client should be relaxed and rolled slightly forward into their supporting bolster.

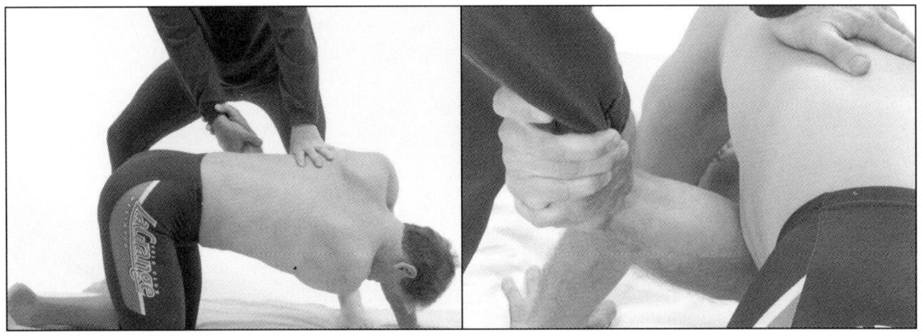

Mid trap and rhomboid CRAC stretch. Use 3 different angles of stretch.

Trapezius

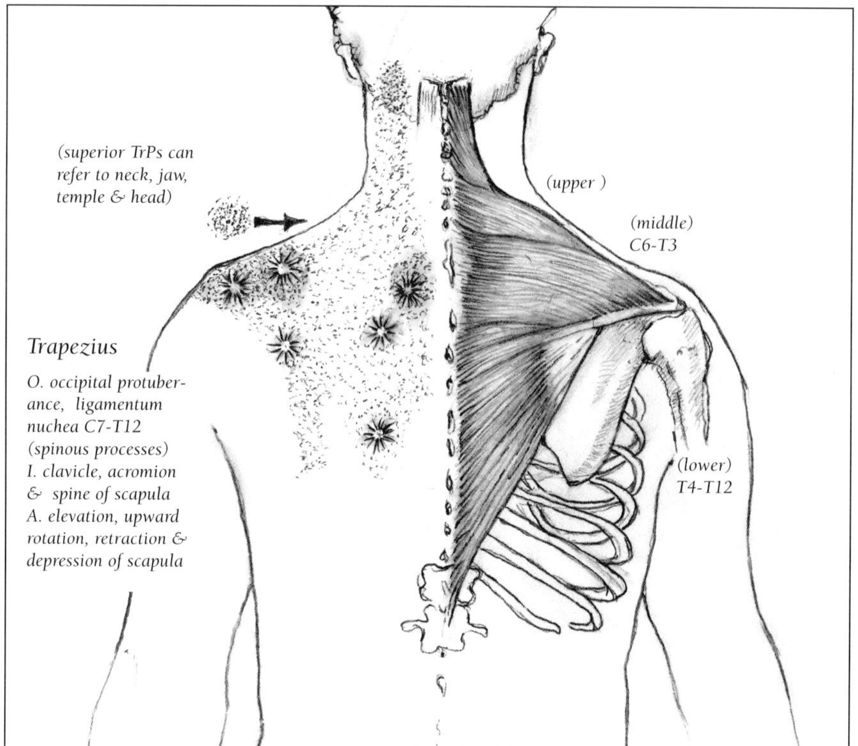

Trapezius & TrPs

Dr. Travell declares that the upper trapezius trigger point is almost omnipresent. Unlike most other trigger points, it will not shorten or weaken its muscle. The upper trapezius does, however, harbor trigger points that remain latent until stress-filled times when they can fire (become active) and cause temporal headaches. Numerous office workers experience this problem at deadlines. Unfortunately, sufferers often choose to treat the headache with over-the-counter (OTC) analgesics rather than with direct pressure or pincer palpation.

Trigger point headaches are often misdiagnosed as migraine headaches. This, in part, is due to their intensity. Trigger point pain may be as severe, but can be differentiated from classic migraines. They won't have the accompanying prodromal (indicating onset) symptoms.

We've rarely worked with a misdiagnosed migraine sufferer without finding trigger points in the upper trapezius. Trapezius trigger point referral patterns include the neck, ear, temple, and parietal areas. When treated, this pattern intensifies. As we squeeze our client's upper trapezius and their headache worsens, we know that we've found the primary trigger point. We expect that after a 20 second treatment, their headache will diminish or cease. Often there are several trigger points in close proximity that require treatment by pincer palpation or heel.

Neck pain is the second most common problem created by trigger points in the upper trapezius. However, more common sources of neck pain originate from trigger points in the levator scapula and posterior neck musculature.

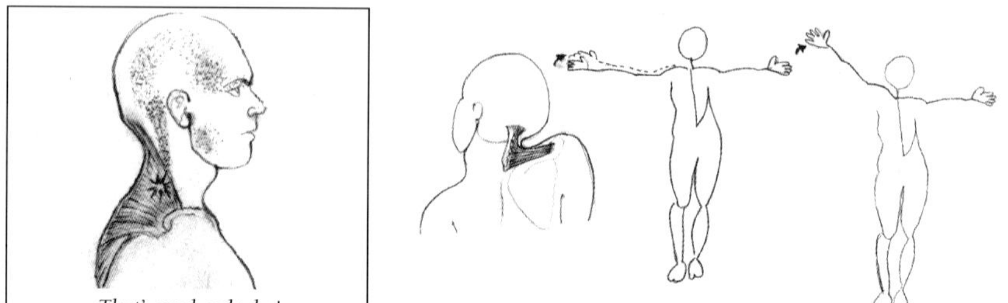

That's my headache!

> Vigorous Swedish massage can activate latent upper-trapezius trigger points resulting in client headaches. Pincer palpation to the trigger point (source of headache pain) for 15 or 20 seconds will often abort this problem.

When upper traps are hypertonic, they can create a shearing stress to the greater occipital nerve. This leads to tingling in the occiput – a numbskull? This occipital nerve entrapment can also occur in the semi-spinalis capitus muscle. Use caution – these symptoms can also result from an inflamed or ruptured disc.

The "squared coat-hanger" look of elevated shoulders quickly identifies hypertonic traps. Pincer palpation for trigger points and prolonged compressions for hypertonicity are the usual treatments. The upper trapezius is quite bulky in larger folks, and adequate pressure is sometimes hard to muster by hand – not so using your feet.

A family propensity towards squared shoulders is sometimes seen. Is it genetic or learned? Probably both, but this posture will not necessarily change with bodywork and, if not causing distress, should be left alone.

"Squared shoulders" should be differentiated from forward neck and shoulder posture. The neck forward problem can be addressed with pectoralis minor and major stretches, and mid-trapezius and rhomboid strengthening. Scapular winging (the vertebral border of the scapula riding off the ribs and visually readily apparent) will also require strengthening the serratus anterior. The above stretch and strengthen protocol generally improves shoulder mechanics and forward head posture, and reduces pain and permanent postural distortions.

Treatment

We combine several approaches for the treatment of the upper-trapezius. First, warm up the trapezius of your side-lying client with foot pressure. Therapist sits above the client's head. Put your back to the wall for support.

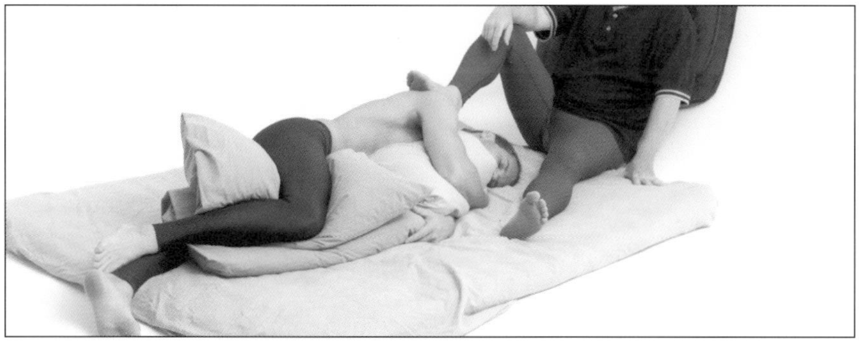

Support your back for prolonged upper trap direct pressure. Client should be comfortable for prolonged compressions.

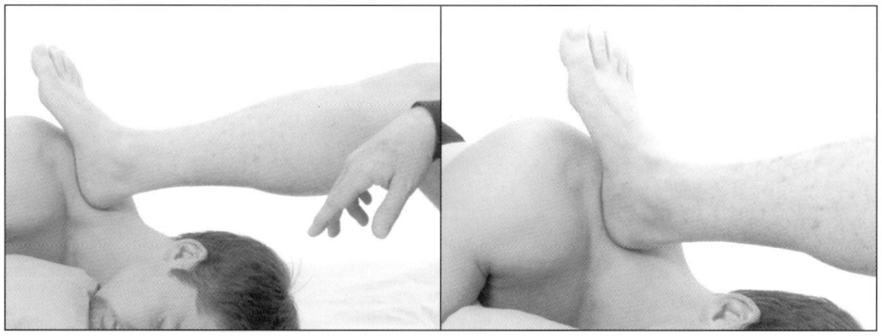

The heel can also be used for a warm-up.

Next use pincer palpation (prone or side-lying, on or off the table) to grasp the muscle between the thumb and index finger. If required, use both hands, one on top of the other, and hold for 10 seconds. We often find several trigger points on each shoulder. Remember, while the pain reference here is usually instantaneous, it can take several seconds of pressure on some trigger points before a referred pain is generated.

Compressing each trigger point for 15 to 30 seconds allows us to treat on alternative days without undue client soreness. If you treat each trigger point with longer duration and several times (three is our absolute maximum in a single session), treatments are best scheduled but twice weekly. Moist heat following trigger point treatments often diminishes post-treatment discomfort. Cold drafts following treatments should be avoided.

Post-treatment stretches should be done moderately. Extreme shoulder depression to stretch the upper trapezius can lead to post-treatment scalene soreness.

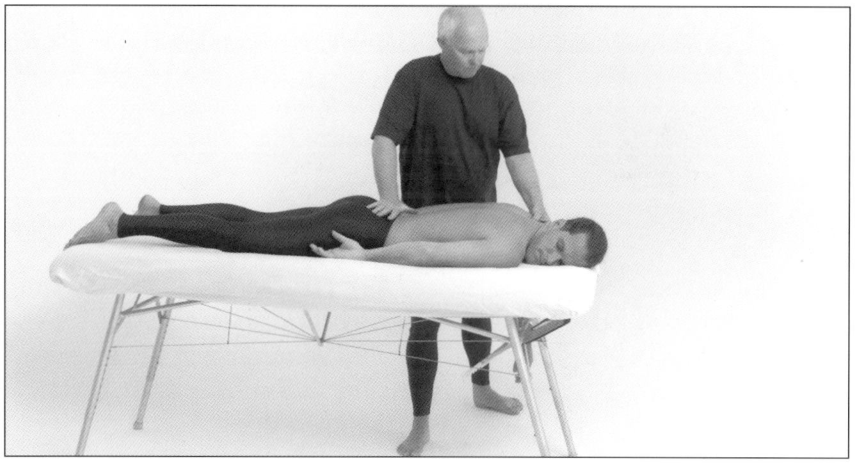

Good therapist biomechanics.

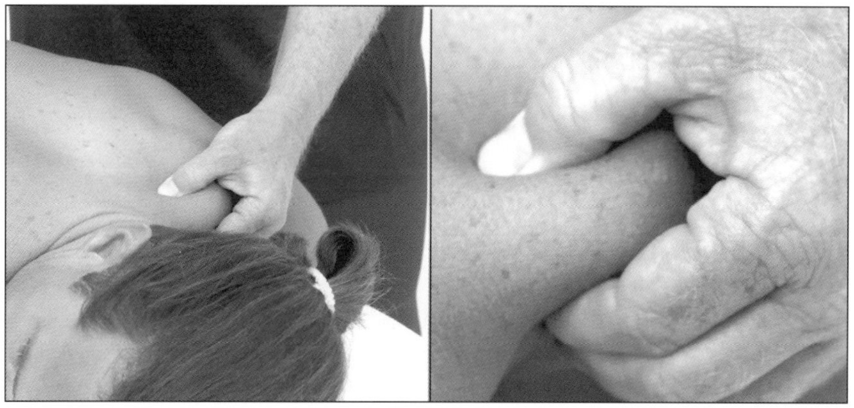

Grasp the upper trap with pincer palpation, Client faces away from the treatment. Pincer palpation must be in the thickness of the belly of the muscle. Treatment behind or in front of the belly has no positive effect.

The middle trapezius (overlying the rhomboids and serratus posterior) can have trigger points that refer to the thoracic spine and/or to the top of the scapula.

The lower traps refer to the top of the scapula and its medial edge. Treat by foot from the standing position or from a stool while seated. Press the trigger points against the underlying bone.

Causes or Factors Involved in Trigger Point Formation

1. Upper traps – Cradling the phone between your ear and shoulder fatigues the upper trapezius, particularly in stressful situations. Large-breasted clients who wear bras with narrow straps often have large, semi-permanent indentations in their upper traps. Equally troublesome are heavy purses. Both provide enough insult to create trigger points. Chair armrests that are too low to offer support place strain on the trapezius – the upper-trap is forced to support the weight of the arm for prolonged periods. Shoulders must be correctly supported with the arm rest neither too high nor too low.

2. Middle traps – Commonly associated with long periods of driving with hands resting on top of the steering wheel. The deltoids can also be adversely affected. Massage therapists who continuously bend forward and reach across their clients also stress the mid-traps.

3. Lower traps – Kids are quite susceptible to straining lower traps when carrying too many books in their tote bags and backpacks, or when they spend extended time slumping over their desks in boredom.

TEACHER'S STORY

A schoolteacher on medication for chronic earaches came to us. She was obviously tense, disliked her job, and had extremely elevated shoulders.

Using pincer palpation on her upper-traps immediately worsened her earache. This suggested that the cause of the pain in her ear could be related to her upper-trap trigger point. By the end of the session, the treatment had temporarily eliminated her symptoms. In our view, to permanently solve this problem, she would have had to either quit her job or change her attitude.

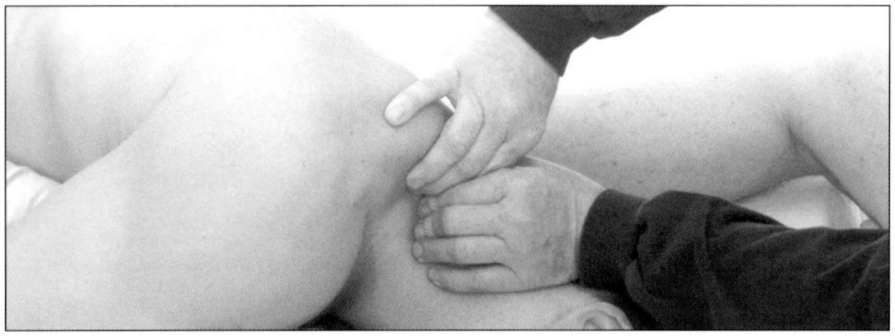

Two-handed pincer palpation to the side-lying client.

Treatment

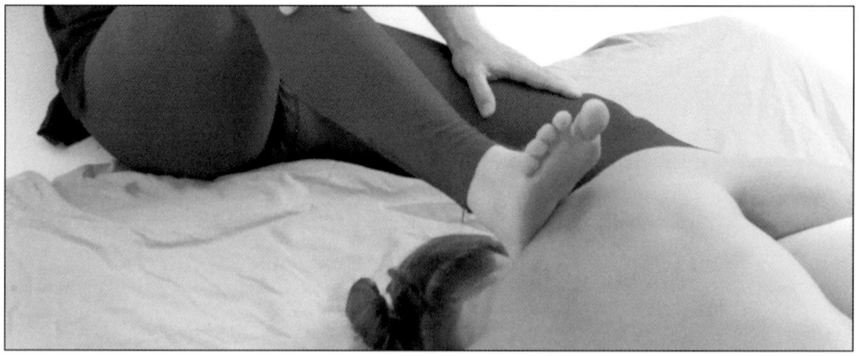

Direct heel pressure to the upper trapezius. Therapist maintains proper treatment leg alignment by resting his hand below his knee.

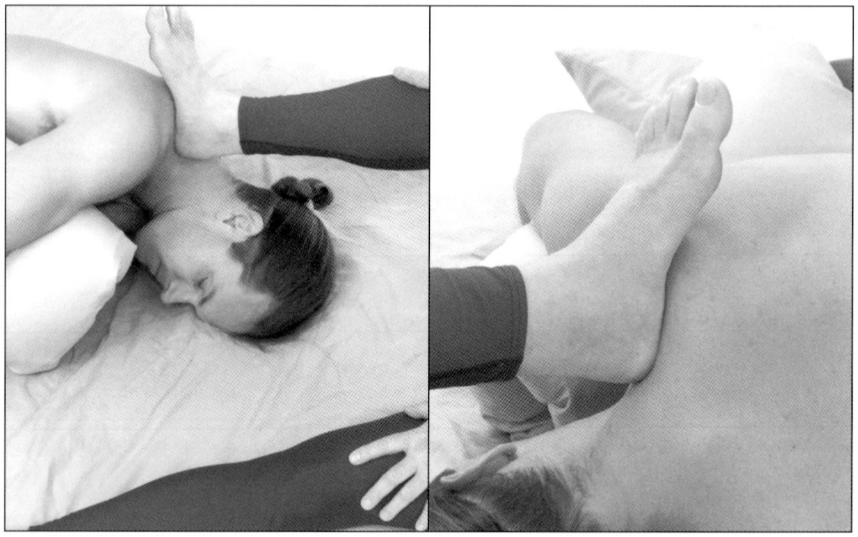

Direct pressure can be maintained for 2 or 3 minutes with great therapeutic results on hypertonic muscles and TrPs.

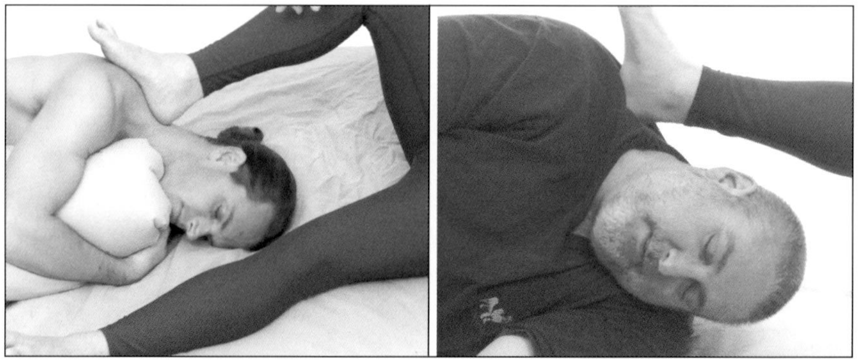

Direct pressure to a trapezius on a stretch is effective. See special caution – levator scap.

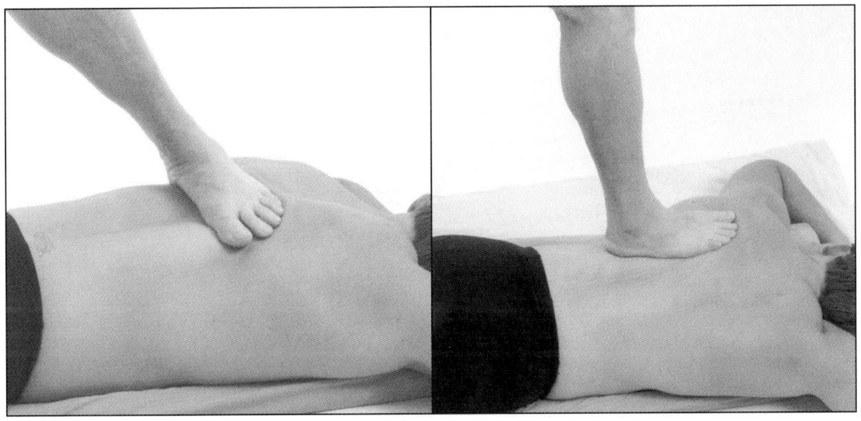

Mid trap stretch and warm-up.

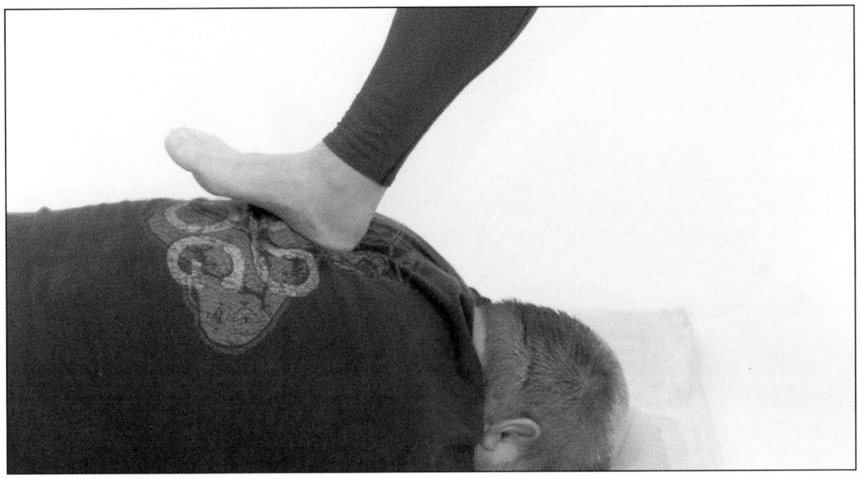

Direct pressure to the middle trapezius.

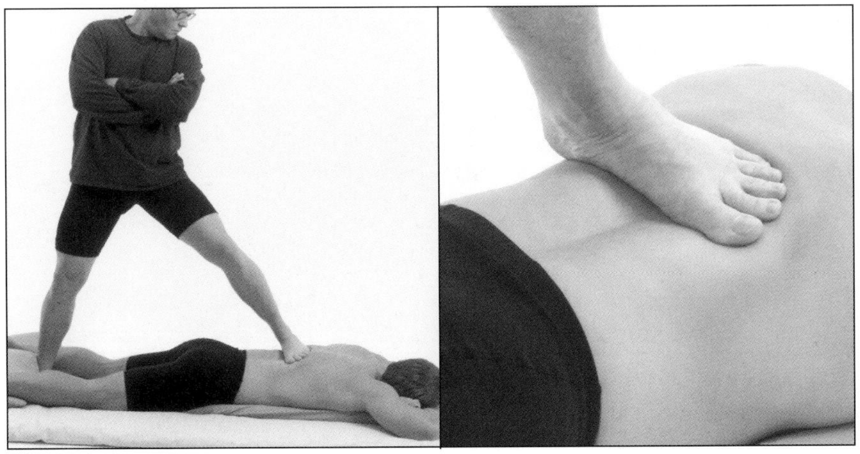

Stretch and warm-up to the lower trapezius.

CHAPTER 14

Shoulder Pain

THIS REGION ADDRESSES common tendon and trigger point problems of the supraspinatus, infraspinatus, teres minor and subscapularis – the rotator cuff.

The biceps and deltoid muscles are included here as they frequently contribute to shoulder pain.

While the upper trapezius, latissimus dorsi and levator scapula occasionally contribute to shoulder pain, we present them in chapter 13.

Quick-fix Guidelines are included to provide a quick overview and review.

Before You Begin

Safe, effective shoulder/rotator cuff treatments are enhanced by first reading the *Indications, Client Intake, Contraindications, Deep Compressive Massage, Endangerment Sites, Trigger Points, Cross-fiber, Fascial Release, Stretching* and *Hydrotherapy* sections.

Note the specific procedural notes and cautions. They will help you effectively treat your client without harm. Protocols and guidelines are included to help you know when to treat and when to refer.

Overview

Clients come to us with shoulder pain. After a medical history and a demonstration of what hurts (usually pain on humeral elevation), we palpate (absent any contraindications) their rotator cuff tendons and the muscle bellies of the supraspinatus, infraspinatus, teres and subscapularis. We primarily search for trigger points. We include the long head of the biceps and deltoid in this examination since they are often secondarily involved.

If a client exhibits possible pathologies, extreme weakness, probable neck involvement, or the injury is acute, refer for medical diagnosis. Be particularly careful not to treat clients with a whiplash, a blow to the head, or other neck problems without a medical assessment. Neck flexion or rotation involved in positioning the head for direct pressure could, in rare instance, move bone shards and possibly damage the spinal cord or other soft tissues. Hence, medical evaluation prior to treatment.

Use cross-fiber friction as the primary assessment and treatment tool. If no calcification is felt in the tendons, no indications of subdeltoid bursitis exist, and the injury isn't acute, use friction and direct pressure to address chronic tendonitis, scarred muscle bellies, and trigger points. Occasionally, use fascial stretching to free the joint capsule and surrounding fascial planes. Treatments are slightly painful, but reasonably non-invasive. The possibility of creating further injury is slight if the protocols and contraindications in this manual are followed. When in doubt, refer.

Expect good results. If client pain is reduced, and their movement is freer after the first visit, set an appointment for another treatment in 2 or 3 days. If your approach is well on the way to alleviating their shoulder pain within 3 visits, major progress will have been made, and a few more treatments should suffice. If not, refer for more exhaustive medical evaluation.

Rotator Cuff

The rotator cuff is four small muscles commonly referred to as the SITS group (the supraspinatus, infraspinatus, teres minor, and subscapularis muscles). Affixed to the scapula and the head of the humerus, they give movement and stability to the shoulder joint. This versatile and flexible joint is used every time we reach up, out, behind, and down – feed, wipe, scratch, and grab.

Tendonitis here is common, painful and, if left untreated, often results in the more intractable problem of frozen shoulder. Fortunately, rotator cuff tendonitis responds well to cross-fiber friction and direct pressure. A stretch and strengthen program to maintain balance in the shoulder girdle may be necessary for continued pain-free function.

Your understanding of palpatory and applied anatomy will make this an easy area to treat. Brief sessions become highly effective. Results are immediate – it either works or it doesn't. Clients, by attempting to do what they couldn't do when they walked in the door, will immediately know if there is an improvement.

Our original protocol for treating these tendons came from Dr. James Cyriax's *Illustrated Manual of Orthopedic Medicine, 1989*. Over the years, we have amended this protocol based on our own clinical experience.

Dr. Cyriax postulated that functional assessment was necessary to differentiate between pain in inert or contractile tissues. This differentiation was critical to proper diagnosis and treatment of bursitis, arthritis, or ligament strain (problems for which we routinely refer), and muscle or tendon pain, which we commonly treat. Functional assessment is used to diagnose clinical level problems, those problems severe enough to hurt during muscle and tendon functional assessment. Functional assessment does not, however, work as well for identifying the sub-clinical or intermittent problems which we also address.

Many of our clients have had sub-clinical or intermittent problems. While Dr. Cyriax admonished therapists to use functional assessment and not palpation as an initial diagnostic tool, we have chosen to disregard his admonition. We rely heavily on palpatory assessment. If it hurts, it's injured. The level of pain often indicates the severity and/or healing stage of the injury.

Cross-fiber friction works extremely well as a palpatory assessment tool in locating microtrauma. Finding and treating problems in their early stages, often provides quick results. This is better than treating the full-blown macrotrauma that eventually develops. Fewer sessions are needed to abort incipient problems.

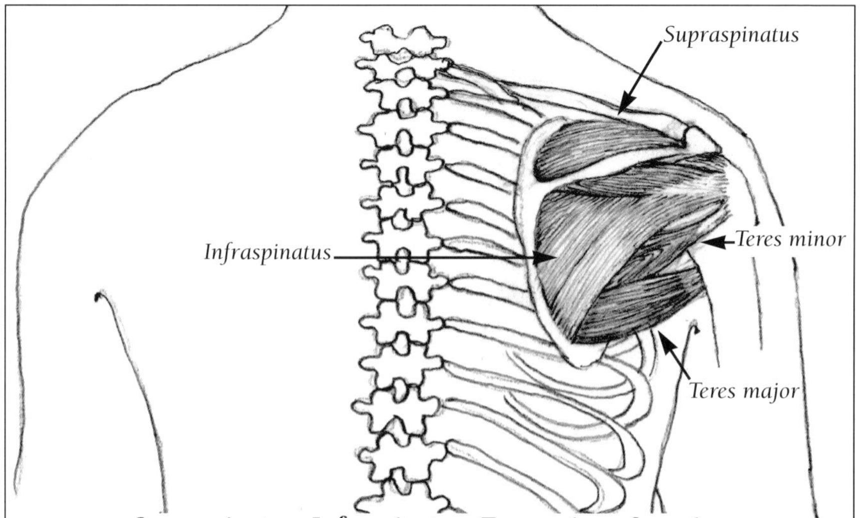

Supraspinatus, Infraspinatus, Teres minor & major

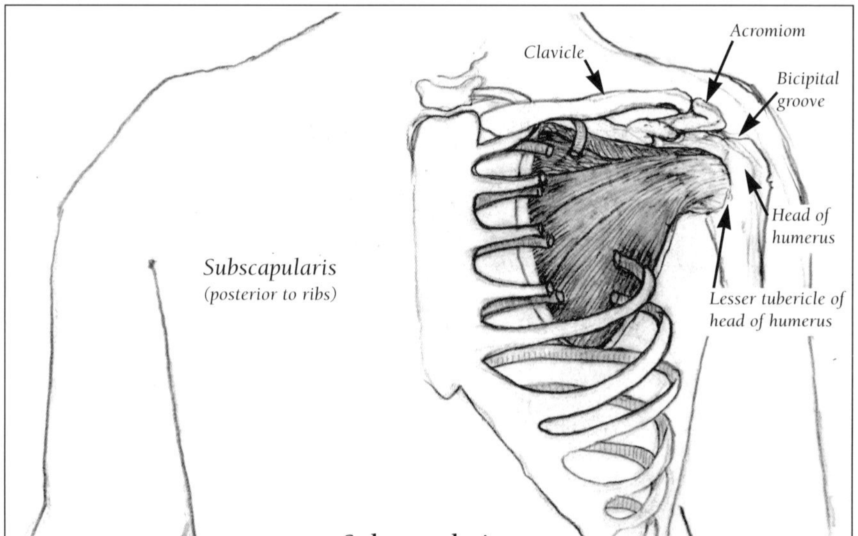

Subscapularis

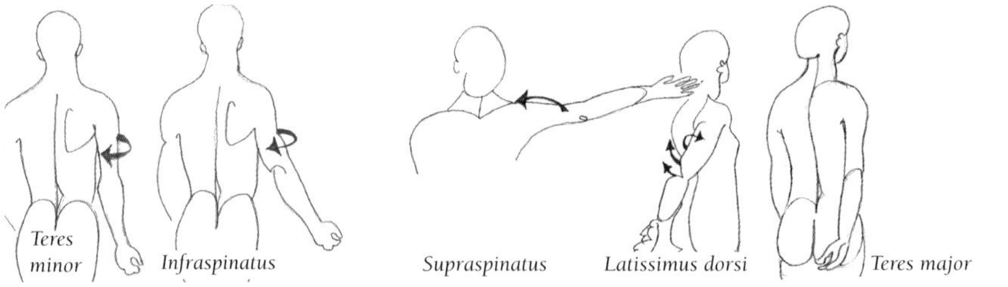

Most of the pain problems with the shoulder come from one type of impingement syndrome. As a client lifts their arm, inflamed rotator cuff tendons are squeezed between the bony acromion and the humerus as the arm is elevated. This impingement syndrome pain will temporarily disappear as friction massage creates a counter-inflammatory response, inhibits "Lewitt's P factor" (a neurotransmitter of pain) and releases endogenous morphines that reduce pain sensation.

The temporary respite in pain allows for non-weight-bearing and non-resistive (therapeutic) movement to speed healing. Clients are encouraged to be careful as over-taxing/overuse could worsen their condition. This healing process includes clients testing and exploring for positions they still might hurt in. They will find highly original and creative positions, but they won't find "their" pain. However, later that day, they may rediscover vestiges of earlier pain. This renewed pain can result from the treatment rather than the original impingement syndrome. At this point, to alleviate pain, client self-care with ice is important.

Several more treatments on alternate days generally give clients enough pain-free movement to sensibly begin using their arm again, and insure that the shoulder capsule won't shrink and progress to the much more serious "frozen" shoulder. Medical referral is necessary for clients with calcium growth in the rotator cuff tendons, bone spurs on the acromion, rotator cuff tears, subdeltoid bursitis, arthritis and frozen shoulder.

Quick-Fix Guidelines

Preferably, clients arrive with an accurate medical diagnosis of their soft-tissue problems. Realistically, however, many clients arrive without a diagnosis because they mistrust medical practitioners. However, in California, massage therapists can't diagnose.

Fortunately, you can, keeping all contraindications in mind, assess the rotator cuff with friction to each tendon as our massage assessment tool. Pain in a tendon is an indication, barring calcification or other contraindication, for friction massage. A reduction in pain following a conservative first treatment is an indication to follow-up with one or more treatments. Here are the guidelines to use for determining what to treat, what to sometimes treat, and what not to treat.

Treat:
Problem #1 – Rotator cuff tendonitis

Clients primarily present with pain when they raise their arm, as in eating, combing their hair, swimming a stroke, pitching a ball, scratching their head or waving good-bye.

Your Action – cross-fiber friction to all painful rotator cuff tendons (determined by cross-fiber friction).

Problem #2 – Trigger points (TrPs) and muscle strains

Clients present with pain on elevation, soreness, aching, and diminished strength and range of motion (ROM).

Your Action – pinpoint the trigger point source of pain by palpation and apply direct pressure by thumb or by heel.

Both these common problems respond positively to our protocols. Always assess each client for problems #1 and #2.

Sometimes Treat:
Problem #3 – Pre-surgical pain

Clients with major tears in their rotator cuff will need surgery. Even with medication, comfortable sleep may prove impossible for them. Altered shoulder mechanics will initiate trigger points and ischemia. Both can cause devastating pain.

Your Action – physician-approved pre-surgical therapy. Use direct pressure by thumb or heel for trigger points (client size determines mode) and foot compressions or massage to reduce or relieve general muscular pain and tension to promote sleep. Do not exacerbate tears by using friction massage or by putting your client's arm in positions of mechanical stress or pain.

Problem #4 - Post-surgical pain

Clients in the initial recovery period are often in pain.

Your Action – physician-approved post-surgical massage therapy. Massage to the neck and back will reduce suffering during immobilization of the shoulder. Fascial release may prove useful during the lengthy later stages of rehabilitation.

Do NOT Treat prior to diagnosis and then treat only if bodywork is indicated:
Problem #5 – Neurologic problems

Nerves can be compressed, entrapped, inflamed or otherwise damaged. Clients can experience decreased sensation, numbness, tingling, and mild to severe weakness – all with or without pain.

Your Action – refer for medical diagnosis. Following diagnosis, you may be of service to clients with muscular nerve entrapments. Gentle compressions and/or trigger point treatments to the hypertonic muscle can release muscularly entrapped nerves.

Problem #6 – Torn rotator cuff

Clients generally experience pain and/or weakness with a torn rotator cuff. With slight downward pressure on their elevated arm, these clients will be unable to keep their arm from dropping to their side.

Your Action – refer for medical diagnosis. Massage and trigger point treatment may help by keeping muscles supple, particularly if the client opts for surgery after a prolonged period.

Problem #7 – Acute or chronic subdeltoid bursitis

Clients will present with intense pain in acute subdeltoid bursitis. Over 3 days the pain will spread from the shoulder to the wrist. No sensible client will let you anywhere near their arm. If chronic, a small portion of the bursae is inflamed and can be mistaken for tendonitis. Functional assessment is often helpful to differentiate a bursitis from a tendonitis. The bursal pain won't increase with muscle testing, but will increase with passive movement, especially at the extremes of range-of-motion.

Your Action – refer for medical diagnosis. Medical treatment often is injection of corticosteroids into the bursae in conjunction with non-steroidal anti-inflammatory drugs (NSAIDS). Sometimes massage to surrounding muscles can enhance general blood flow and speed healing.

Assessment/Treatment Protocol Outline

1. Take a medical history with focus on shoulder history. Do not work on any acute (recent) injuries typified by pain, heat, redness and swelling.

2. Complete an optional Muscle and Tendon Functional Assessment.

3. Ask client to demonstrate what hurts; when, and where (in what position).

4. Assess by palpating the rotator cuff tendons and long head of the biceps using progressive cross-fiber friction. The head of the humerus itself will usually be tender with a rotator cuff tendonitis. Don't rub it.

5. Initially treat each painful lesion using cross-fiber friction for 30-60 seconds.

6. Have client repeat the previously painful movement. If there is a substantial diminution in pain, you are on the right track.

7. Search the bellies of the rotator cuff muscles (SITS) for trigger points.

8. Use hand massage or prolonged barefoot compressions to warm the surrounding shoulder girdle muscles – *levator scapula, upper trapezius,* lateral edge of *latissimus dorsi, mid/upper trapezius,* and *rhomboids.*

9. Treat all trigger points with direct pressure applied by thumb or by foot.

10. Have your client actively stretch his arm with a pain-free range of motion (ROM) in all planes - abduction, extension, elevation, adduction, lateral flexion and extension, and internal and external rotation.

11. If needed, fascial release, by hand or foot, may be used to encourage greater range-of-motion and pain-free movement.

12. Ask client to avoid activities that hurt.

13. Use moist heat to prevent post-treatment trigger point soreness. Use ice for any inflammation caused by cross-fiber friction.

14. Note postural distortions and refer for corrective exercises if needed.

15. Set next appointment in 2 or 3 days.

16. Refer or reevaluate treatment protocol if major improvements do not occur within 3 sessions.

IN GENERAL

Trigger points can often be a secondary source of pain around arthritic joints. Trigger point treatment is indicated in the case of rheumatoid arthritis during times of remission. Other forms of arthritis may need medical treatment combined with trigger point therapy. There is some conjecture that trigger points can contribute to rotator cuff tears. Continuous muscular overload (from trigger points shortening and weakening the muscle) stresses the tendon and contributes to tearing. M.D.s frequently prescribe NSAIDS, but these drugs can have dangerous side effects including bleeding, hypertension, and drug/drug interactions.

Do not stretch any shoulder muscles if there is a rotator cuff tear.

Acromial spurs, calcification in the tendon or bony anomalies in the acromion itself can predispose the shoulder joint to pain that doesn't respond to soft tissue therapies. Refer for medical evaluation.

Weakness noted with or without pain during functional assessment often denotes nerve impingement, torn ligaments, or more serious problems. Refer for medical diagnosis.

A stretch and strengthen protocol for balancing the shoulder joint is often essential for reestablishing efficient mechanics and continued pain-free use. Refer to physical therapist (P.T.) or certified athletic trainer (C.A.T). See "When Clients Won't Stay Better" appendix.

A continued restricted range of motion following treatment by progressive cross-fiber friction, compressions, and/or fascial stretching, may indicate a shrunken shoulder joint capsule. Serapin injections have helped some clients. Serapin, an extract from the pitcher plant, may help alleviate the need for painful and slow physical therapy stretch protocols.

Remember that shoulder pain can also originate from the thoracic region, cervical spine, and neck muscles.

Muscle and Tendon Functional Assessment (MTFA)

TO ISOLATE INJURED TISSUES, we occasionally use MTFA. Strong muscular contractions are used to stress muscle bellies and tendons. The involved joints are held in midrange and immobilized, keeping joint capsule or ligament pain from invalidating the test. Increased pain denotes either a muscle belly tear or a tendonitis.

Note: One way to determine if there is a tear is the "drop arm" test. Have client abduct to 90 degrees. Then ask them to slowly lower it to their side. If there ARE tears, the arm will drop to his side. The client will NOT be able to lower their arm slowly and smoothly. Secondarily, with the arm held in 90 degrees abduction, tap the client's forearm. With a rotator cuff tear, the arm will fall to his side.

TO TEST INERT TISSUES (bursa, joint capsules, and ligaments) we use passive stretches at the end of range-of-motion. Reduced ROM, an unusual joint end-feel (the typical hard or soft feel at the extremes of range of motion of a healthy joint as you feel it by taking your clients through passive range of motion, e.g., the hard feel of the elbow joint in extension and the soft feel of the elbow joint at the end of flexion) at ROM extremes, or an increase in pain in the stretched, inert tissues alerts us to bursitis, ligament sprains or arthritis. Refer.

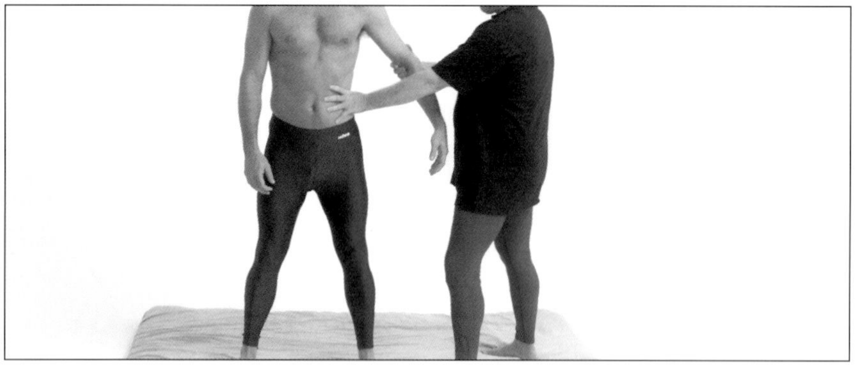

1. Pectoralis major, Latissimus dorsi, and Teres major and Teres minor Muscle and Tendon Functional Assessment (MTFA)

Client adduction of their arm against therapist's resistance tests for tendonitis and muscle belly tears in the pectoralis major, latissimus dorsi, and teres major and minor. Offer resistance above, not below, the elbow joint to preclude stressing non-contractile tissues (ligaments, bursae, and joint capsule) in the elbow joint.

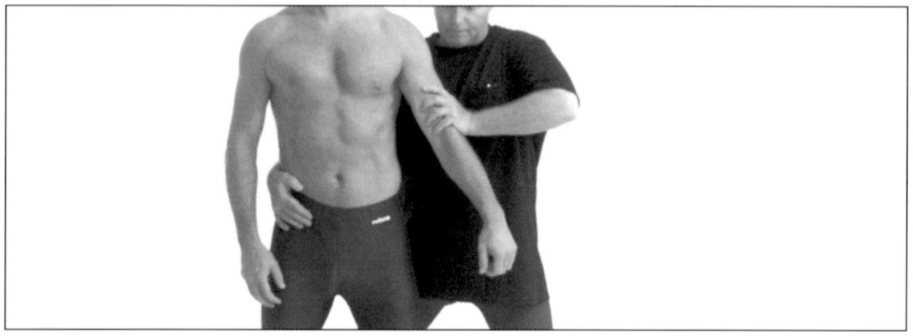

2. Supraspinatus MTFA

Resisted abduction tests the deltoid and supraspinatus muscles. Increased pain usually signifies supraspinatus tendonitis at the tenoperiosteal juncture. Offer resistance to client abduction above the elbow joint thus avoiding contamination of test from stress on the inert tissues of the elbow.

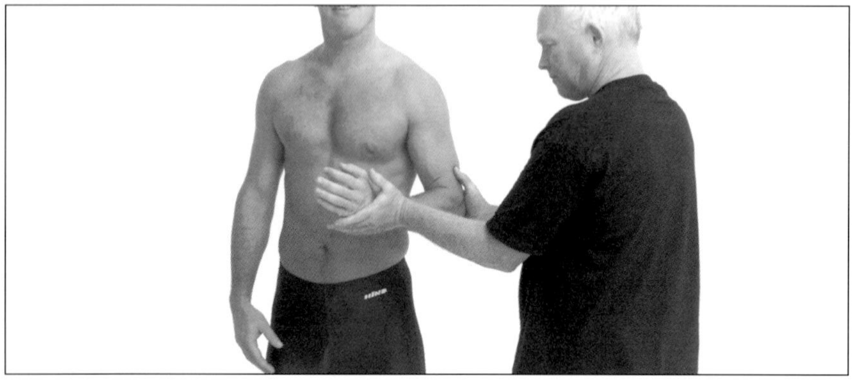

3. Infraspinatus MTFA

Resisted external rotation stresses the infraspinatus and teres minor. Increased pain will generally indicate infraspinatus tendonitis. Ensure that the client gives an external rotation of their humerus rather than humeral abduction.

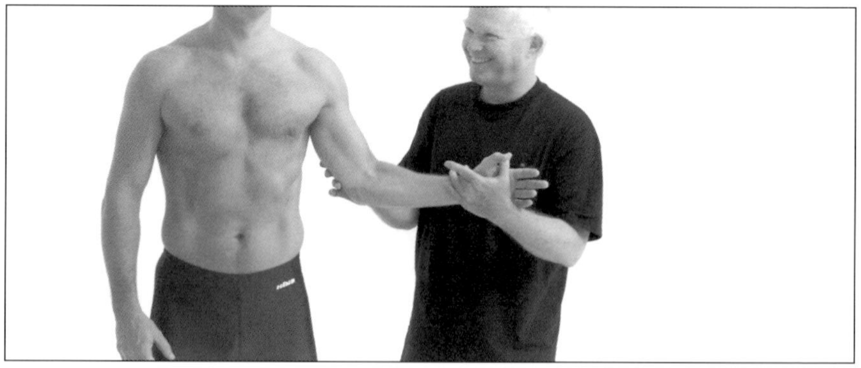

4. Subscapularis MTFA

Internal rotation primarily tests the subscapularis. Increased pain usually indicates tendonitis at the subscapularis tendon. If indicated, include a second arm position (starting with the client's hand closer to the belly) to stress the muscle/tendon complex more thoroughly.

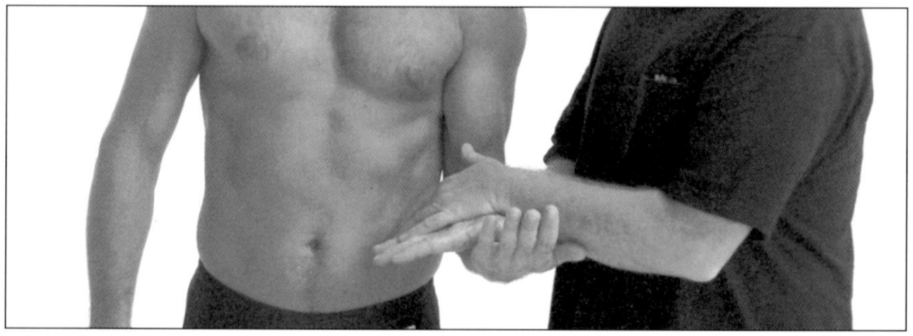

5. Long Head of the Biceps MTFA

Resisted elbow flexion tests for biceps tears or bicipital tendonitis. Offer resistance above the wrist on the forearm. Client gives a full contraction. Therapist allows no movement.

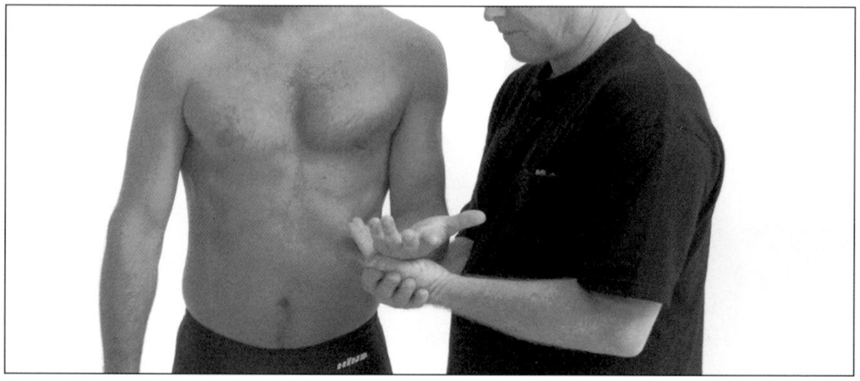

6. Triceps MTFA

Client attempts to straighten their arm against therapist's immovable resistance. Increased pain signifies tendon or muscle problems in the triceps. Severe weakness in any muscle suggests neurologic problems or severe tears. Refer for diagnosis.

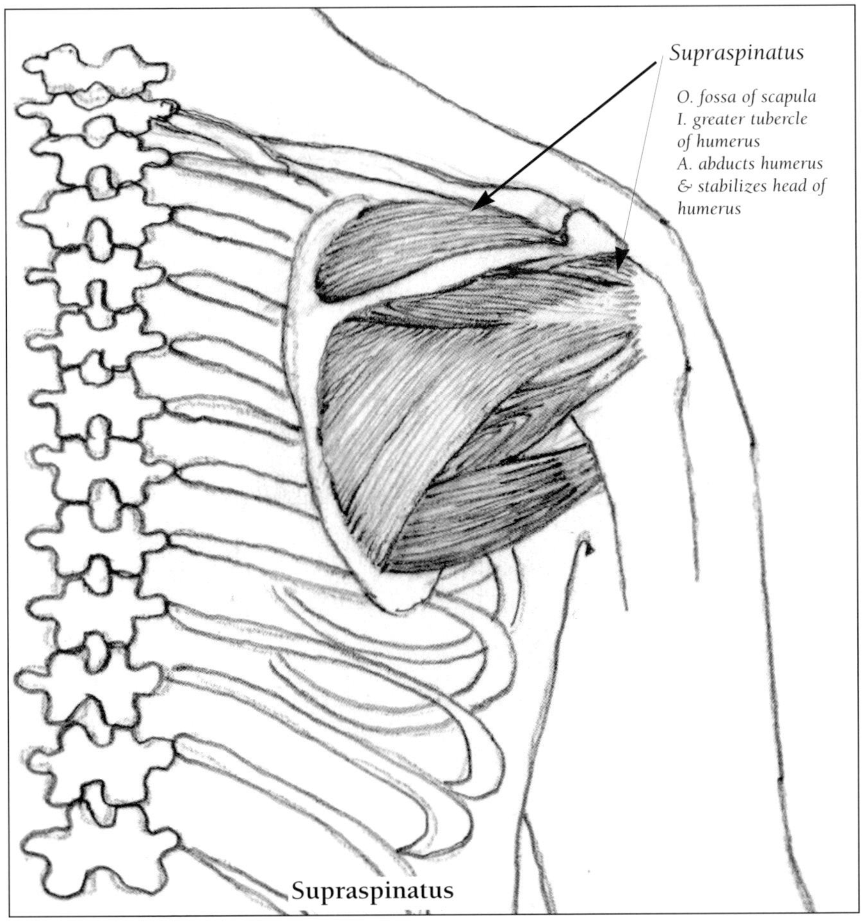

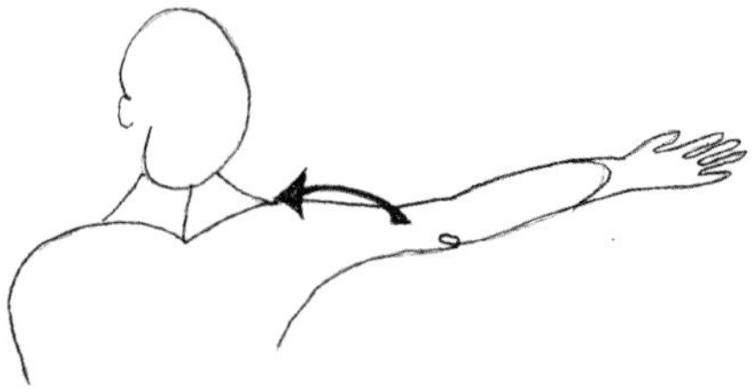

PALPATE THE SUPRASPINATUS TENDON FIRST – it's often the primary source of pain in rotator cuff tendonitis. The supraspinatus belly is also susceptible to trigger points. The supraspinatus tendon lies directly beneath the acromion process. To access this tendon with cross-fiber friction you must extend and internally rotate the humerus (the hammerlock position). Soreness indicates microtrauma; pain, macrotrauma. Friction the lesion for 30 seconds to a minute on the first visit.

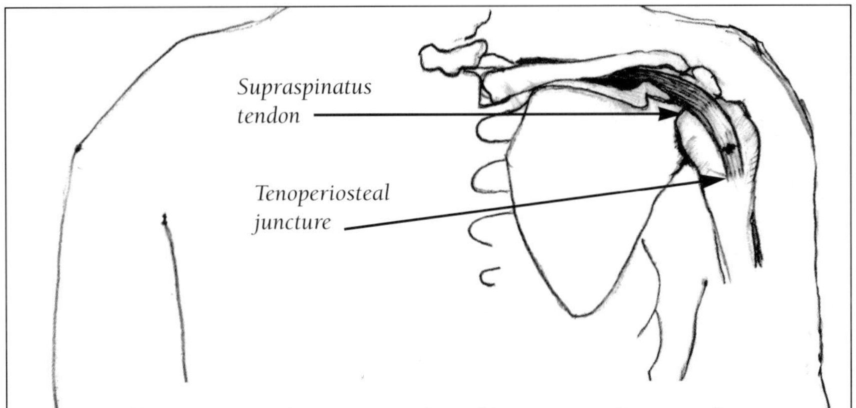

Treating supraspinatus tenoperiosteal juncture requires extension & internal rotation of humerus to expose tendon (a hammerlock).

On occasion there can be a tendonitis of the musculotendinous juncture of the supraspinatus. With no impingement pain present, resisted abduction will still create pain if there is a tendonitis here. Treatment must be with the client's humerus elevated passively to 90 degrees to move the musculotendinous juncture out from beneath the acromion process.

While swimmers and others who overuse the shoulder joint often have supraspinatus tendonitis, this problem is also present in folks who carry heavy briefcases. Since the supraspinatus initiates and sustains the abduction of the humerus required to keep from clipping oneself with one's own briefcase, it, rather than the larger, stronger deltoid, carries the major load. This slight, prolonged isometric humeral elevation will eventually cause microtrauma at the tenoperiosteal juncture. Reducing the briefcase weight or using luggage carriers with wheels is well advised.

A trigger point in the tendon responds to the direct pressure component of cross-fiber friction more quickly than tendonitis does. Keep in mind that trigger points can occur in ligaments, tendons, fascia and the periosteum of bone – not just muscle. Each has its own pain pattern. Trigger points in the supraspinatus belly can refer into the deltoid. Treat with direct pressure. Treating the trigger points in the belly of the muscle will also reduce hypertonicity and thereby, the pull on the tendon. This reduction of tension on the tendon speeds healing.

When treating the more lateral portion of the supraspinatus or the musculotendinous juncture, clients will occasionally complain of a temporal headache. These headaches result from direct pressure on a trigger point located in the overlying upper trapezius muscle. Use direct pressure or pincer palpation to deactivate the trapezius trigger point before continuing to treat the underlying supraspinatus.

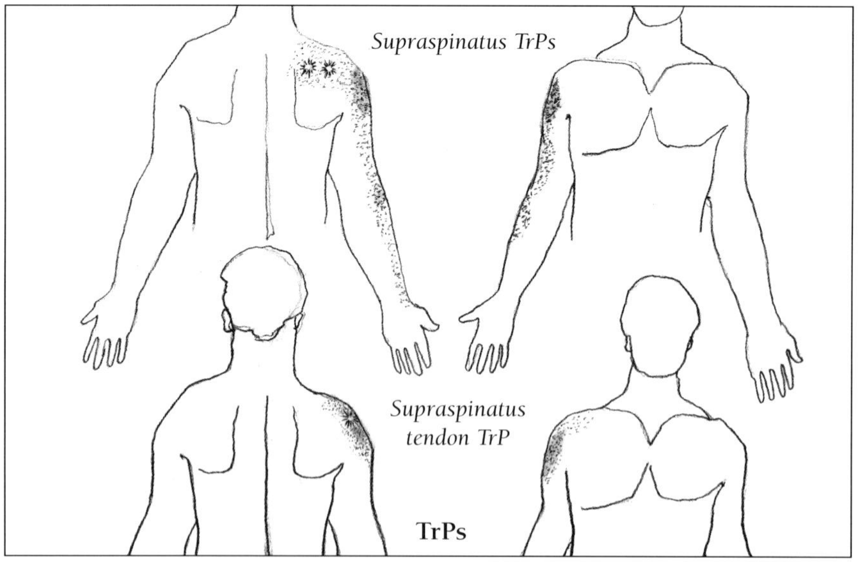

CONTRAINDICATIONS TO FRICTION TREATMENTS

Do not stretch any shoulder muscles if there is a rotator cuff tear.

Calcium deposits (bumpy or gritty-feeling tendons) can irritate the overlying subdeltoid bursa. Cross-fiber can exacerbate the irritation. X-rays are required to verify.

Subdeltoid bursitis (acute or chronic) is another contraindication to frictioning the supraspinatus tendon. Intense pain makes acute bursitis easy to identify. Your client won't move their arm, much less let you touch their shoulder. By the third day of an acute attack, their pain will run from shoulder to hand and be excruciating. Refer.

Chronic bursitis will be more difficult to ascertain. Functional assessment can help delineate between tendonitis and bursitis. Resisted abduction without shoulder joint movement will not increase pain with bursitis, but pain will increase with clinical level tendonitis.

X-rays or MRIs are required to determine the existence of calcium spurs on the underside of the acromion. Clients with these spurs may need medical intervention for removal. If left untreated, these spurs may shred the tendon, leading to major shoulder surgery. Cross-fiber is contraindicated.

Treatment

Supraspinatus – Muscle and Tendon Functional Analysis (MTFA)

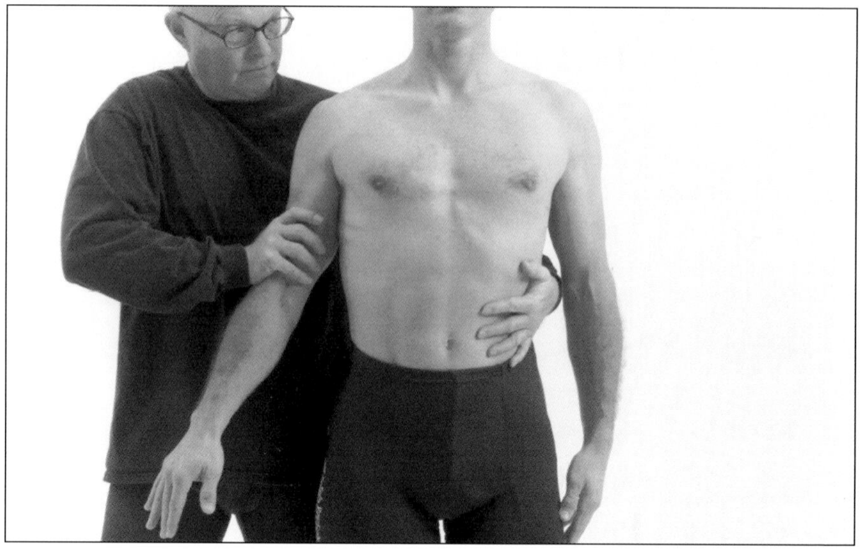

Resisted abduction tests the deltoid and supraspinatus muscles. Increased pain usually signifies supraspinatus tendonitis at the tenoperiosteal juncture. Offer resistance to client abduction above the elbow joint thus avoiding contamination of test from stress on the inert tissues of the elbow.

Friction Massage for the Supraspinatus Tendon

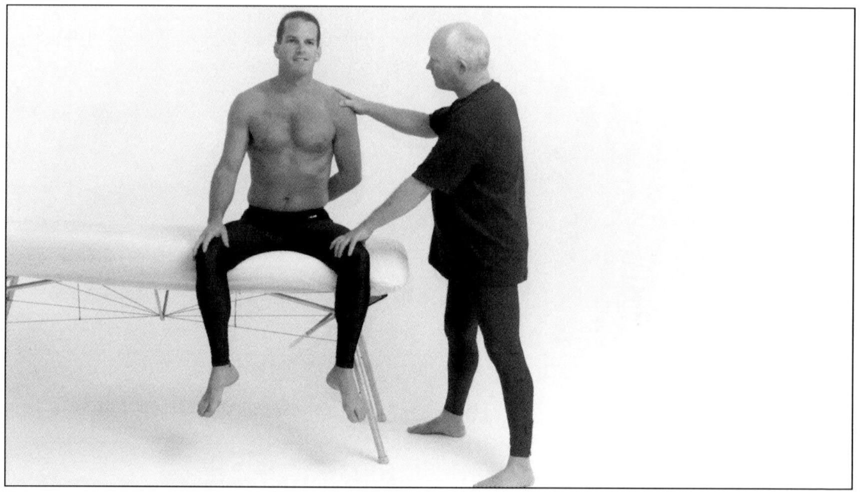

For treatment, client's arm is extended and internally rotated (hammerlock). Therapist's thumb now rests on the tenoperiosteal juncture of the supraspinatus tendon.

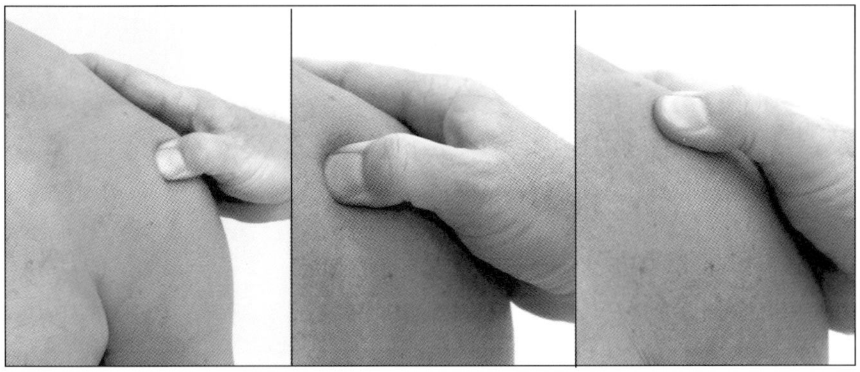

1. The thumb is slightly flexed and locked to give a "solid hand" with friction movement coming jointly from the wrist and arm. There is absolutely no movement in the joints of the thumb.
2.The therapist's wrist is alternately flexed and extended to create a friction movement across the supraspinatus tendon. Note that the thumb frictions below the acromion process and above the head of the humerus.
3. Remember that the client's arm must be in the hammerlock position to expose the tendon, bringing it out from under the acromion process.

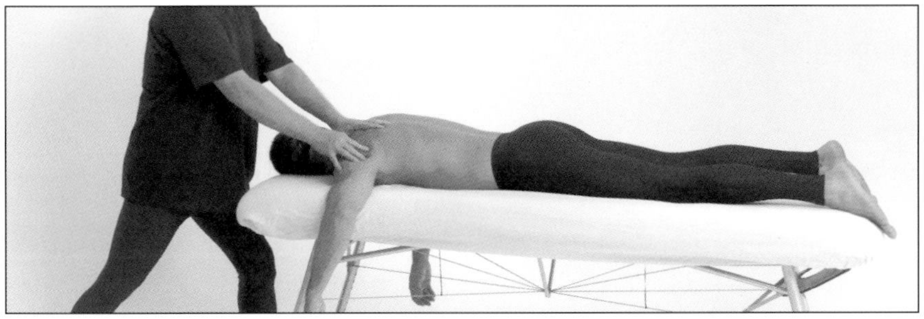

To friction the musculotendinous juncture of the supraspinatus, the client's humerus must be elevated to 90 degrees.

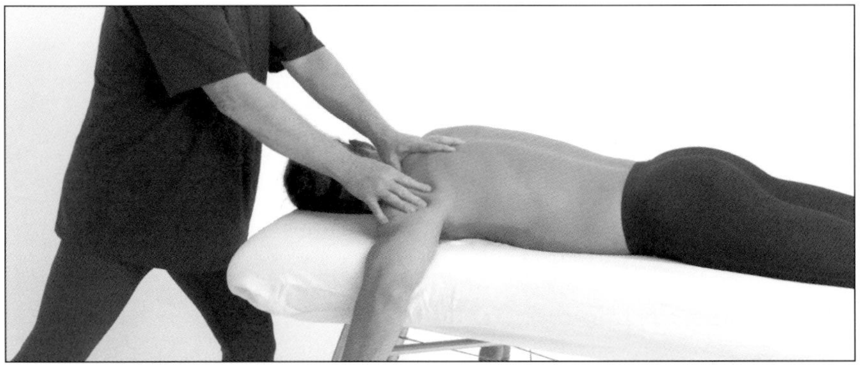

The left thumb administers the friction with the right thumb reinforcing it. The thumb pushes against the upper trap and into the supraspinatus in the "u" shaped space where the acromion, the clavicle and the spine of the scapula all meet.

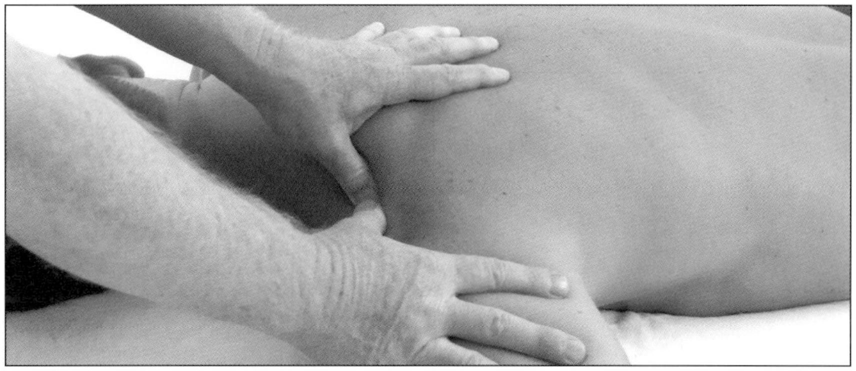

Thumbs are held straight and rigid – all movement comes from the wrist and arm. This is a rotational movement as if there were a rod through the center of the treatment thumb around which it rotates.

Trigger Point Treatment

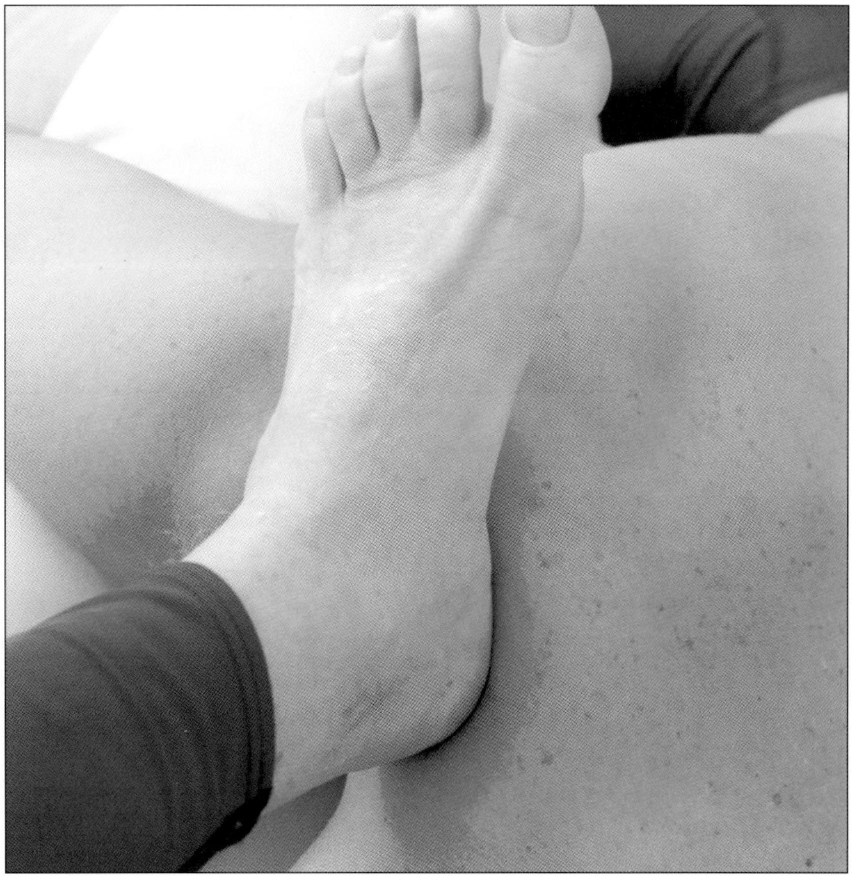

Direct heel pressure (from floor-seated position) into the most medial portion of the muscle through the trapezius to treat a supraspinatus TrP.

Infraspinatus

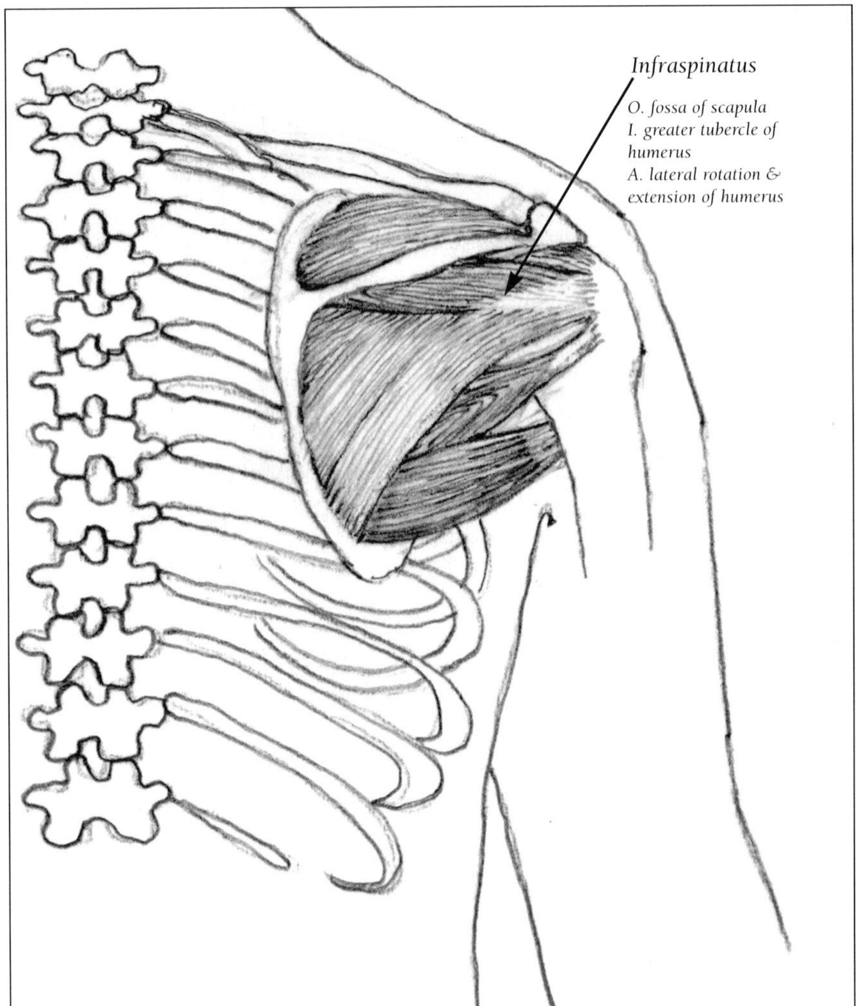

Infraspinatus

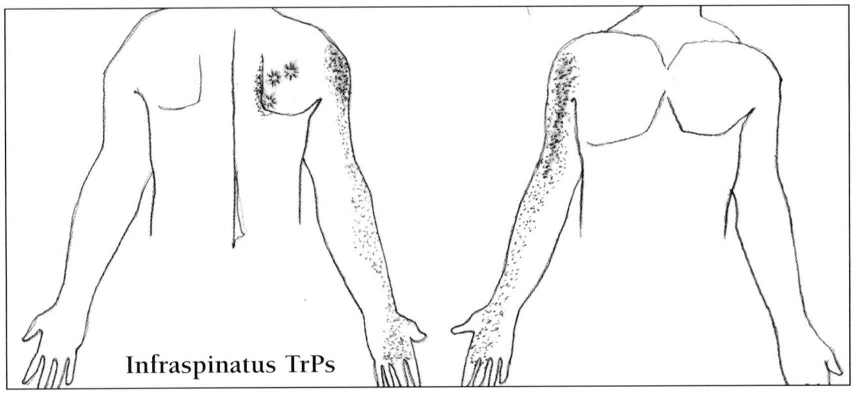
Infraspinatus TrPs

Infraspinatus pain often plagues people who paint ceilings and walls. The infraspinatus decelerates booming tennis overheads and is subject to overuse syndromes. This overuse leads to tendonitis. The "woe-is-me, alack & alas" position allows for easy tendon location and treatment.

The infraspinatus tendon and the supraspinatus tendon are often concurrently inflamed and painful. When inflamed, the infraspinatus tendon gets pinched and hurts with humeral elevation. On rare occasion, its sister muscle, the teres minor, will also have a tendonitis – quite rare, but don't overlook it.

Often, two or three short treatments of cross-fiber friction will end the pain of chronic tendonitis and return the shoulder to its normal, rhythmic, pain-free movement.

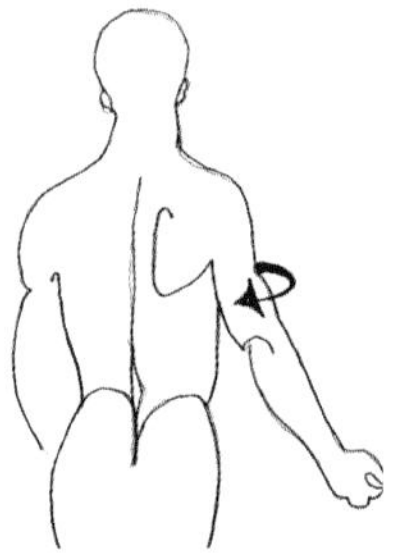

Infraspinatus trigger points are common and share a similar, but not identical, pain referral pattern to the anterior and middle scalene muscles. Assess both when your client has that long referral from the shoulder into the back of the hand. Trigger points in the infraspinatus can cause considerable grief with extreme local tenderness that often causes clients to feel nauseous or weak-limbed when treated. Use caution.

A few visits can move these trigger points from active to latent. Stretching and strengthening exercises help insure lasting cures although there are differences of opinion as to which should come first. Consider referring your client to a physical therapist or certified athletic trainer for the design of a stretch and strengthen program if you aren't qualified.

> When there is a rotator cuff tear, do not stretch any shoulder muscle.

Broad heel compressions on the well-bolstered shoulder are an easy way to treat – especially on the big folks. Enter slowly, even when using the broad surface of the heel. Too much pressure or too quick an entry can force the client to armor against the work.

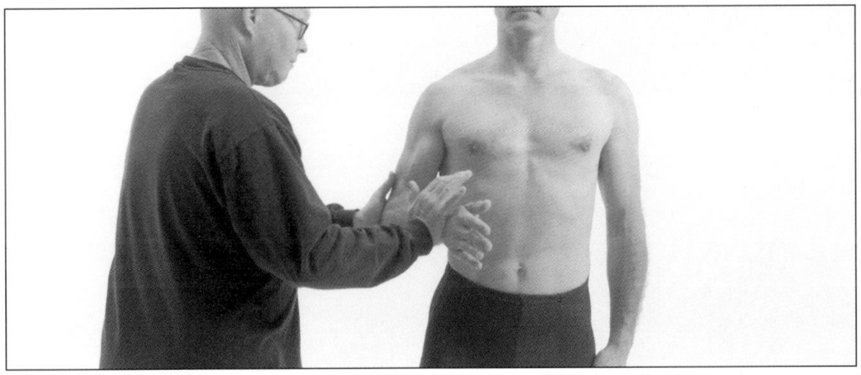

Infraspinatus MTFA: Resisted external rotation stresses the infraspinatus and teres minor. Increased pain will generally indicate infraspinatus tendonitis. Ensure that the client restricts the resisted movement to external rotation without humeral abduction.

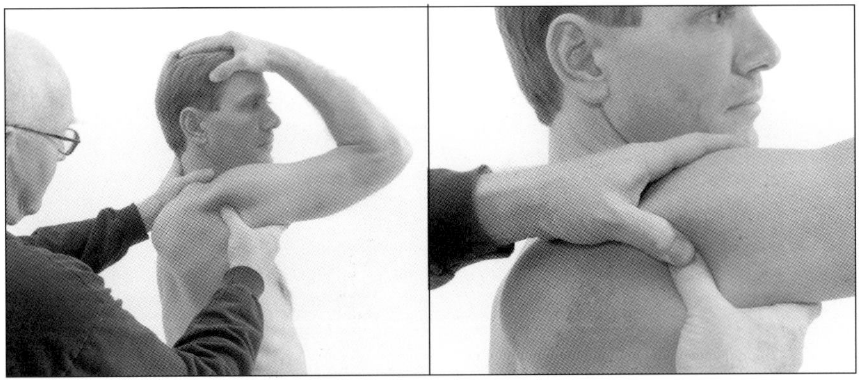

Woe-is-me, alack & alas position.

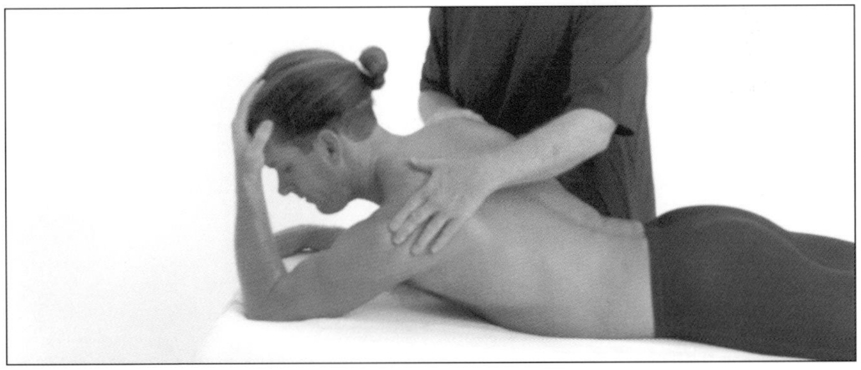

To find the painful portion of the infraspinatus tendon, stand on the opposite side of the client's body and place your index finger parallel to and just below the spine of the scapula. The tip of your index finger will be at the curve where the acromion process begins. Your middle finger will lie approximately on the infraspinatus tendon. This location protocol is a good way for beginning therapists to find the tendon. Slight corrections can be easily made for either large or small clients or large and small therapist hands.

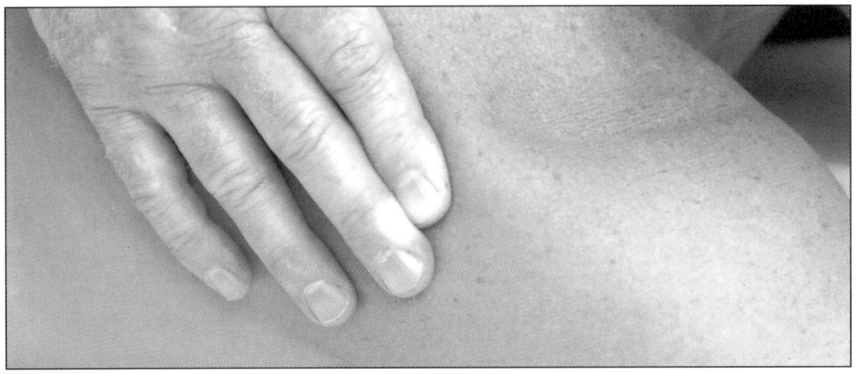

Finding the infraspinatus tendon.

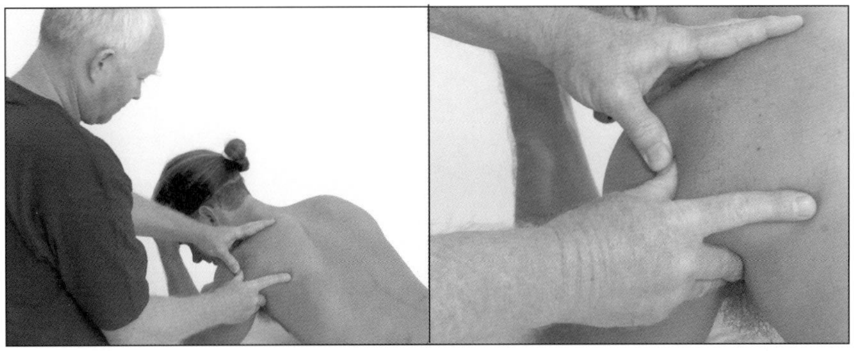

Use thumb-on-thumb cross-fiber to search through the tendon for the most painful spot. Then administer deep transverse friction to that exact spot.

Friction the most painful spot on the infraspinatus tendon 30 to 60 seconds on the first visit. There should be no thumb joint movement when frictioning. The thumbs are held immobile and function as a tool. Thumb movement comes from the arm and wrist.

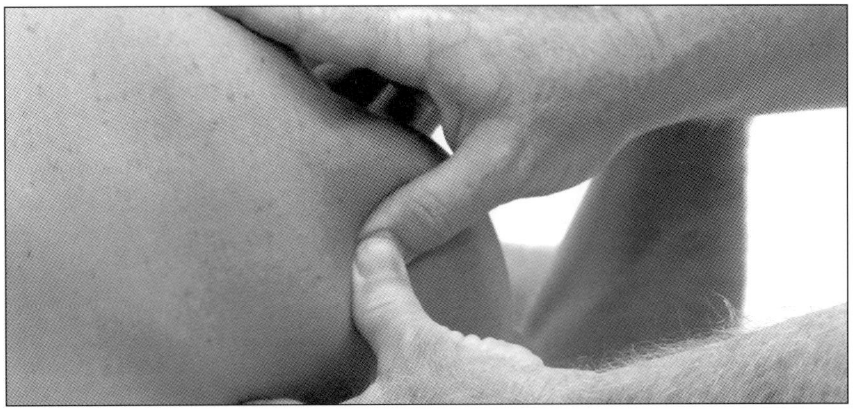

Good hand positioning for frictioning the infraspinatus tendon. The tendon will hurt if there is a problem. Begin gently. Deltoid TrPs often occur along with the infraspinatus tendonitis. Treat the deltoid and the infraspinatus belly with direct pressure from the thumb, heel, or ball of the foot.

Teres Minor and Teres Major

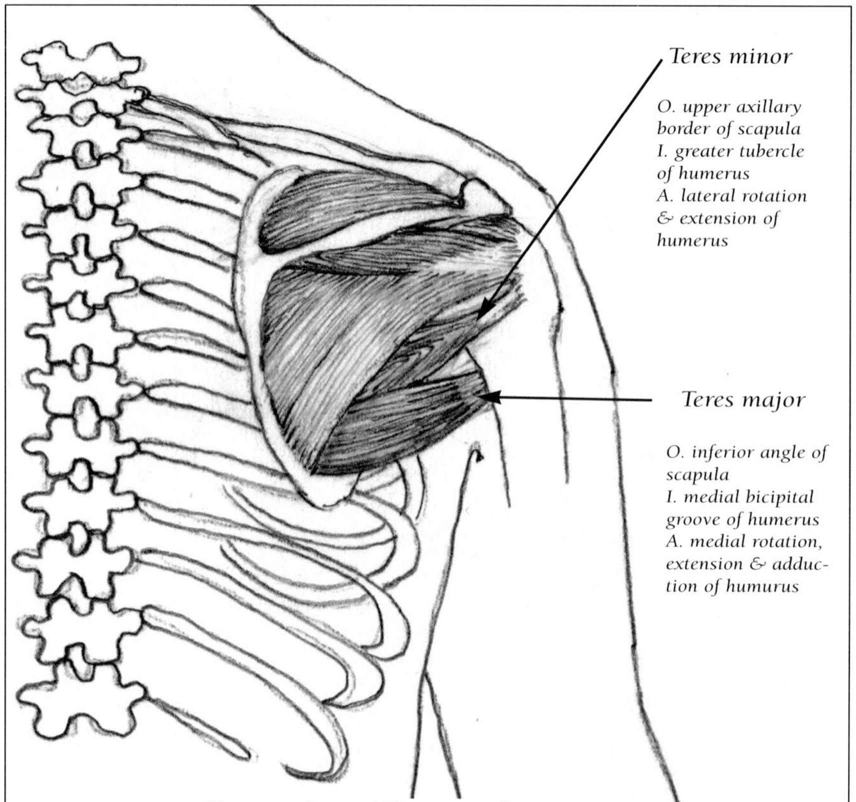

Teres minor / Teres major

The teres minor and/or the teres major occasionally cause shoulder pain. Even though the teres major is not a rotator cuff muscle, our shoulder protocol includes a palpatory assessment of the teres minor and the major. Use direct thumb pressure and pincer palpation to assess.

Rotator cuff problems proper often include trigger points in the teres. It may well be that the rotator cuff pain substantially interferes with rhythmic, fluid scapular and humeral motion. The altered shoulder mechanics seems to make the teres susceptible to trigger point formation. A well-placed heel to the teres of a side-lying client works wonders with trigger points and hypertonicity.

Some postural problems can set the stage for glenohumeral pain. Shoulder girdle mechanics are imbalanced by a kypotic thoracic spine, excessively protracted scapulae, or forward head position. Long-term recovery may necessitate a change in shoulder mechanics and habit patterns.

Do not stretch any shoulder muscles if there is a rotator cuff tear.

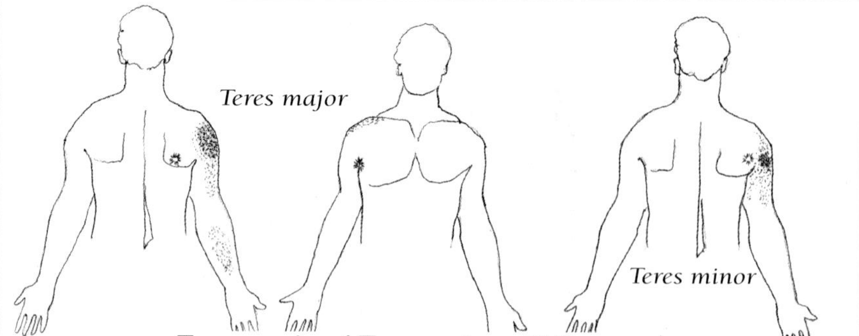

Teres major / Teres minor TrPs

Treatment

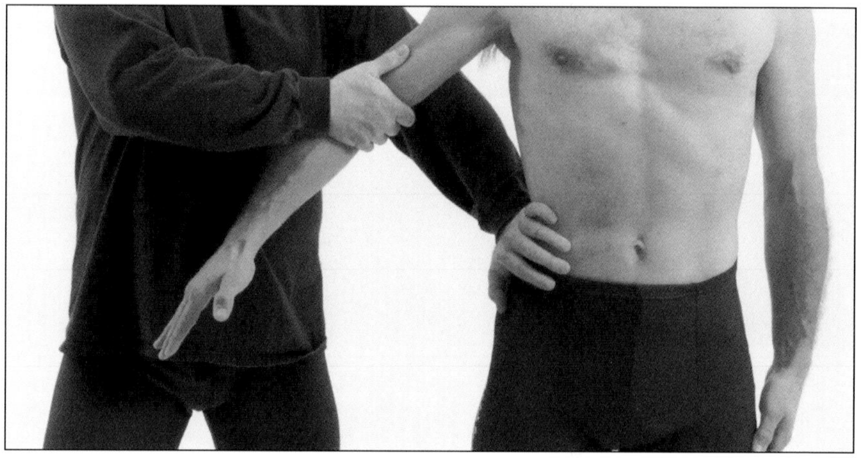

Client adduction of their arm against therapist's resistance tests for tendonitis and muscle belly tears in the pectoralis major, latissimus dorsi, and teres major and minor. Note that the therapist offers resistance above, not below, the elbow joint. This precludes stressing non-contractile tissues (ligaments, bursae, and joint capsule) in the elbow joint.

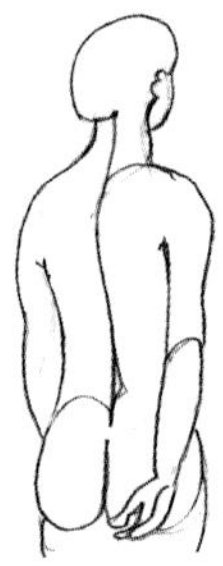

Teres major

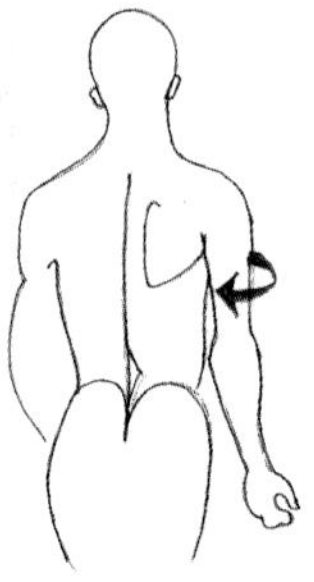

Teres minor

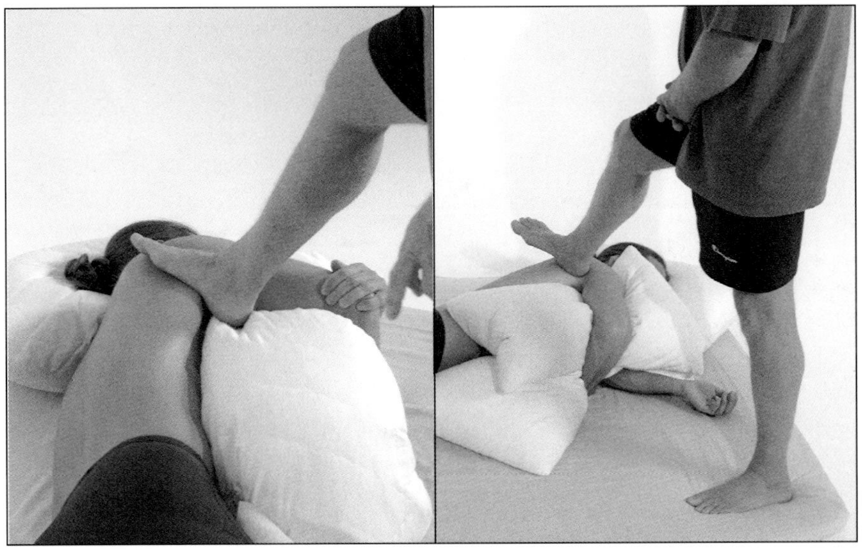

1. Lateral edge of therapist's foot directs pressure into the teres group.
2. Direct heel pressure to the teres minor. Note bolstering. Client "hugs" pillow to stabilize his scapula and provide good access for heel pressure.

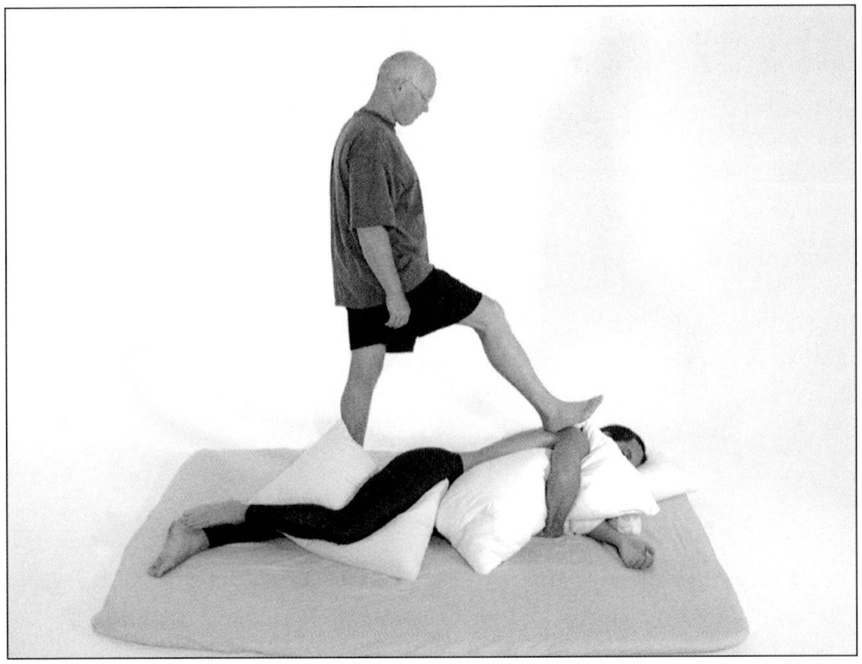

Posterior approach to infraspinatus and teres TrPs.

Subscapularis

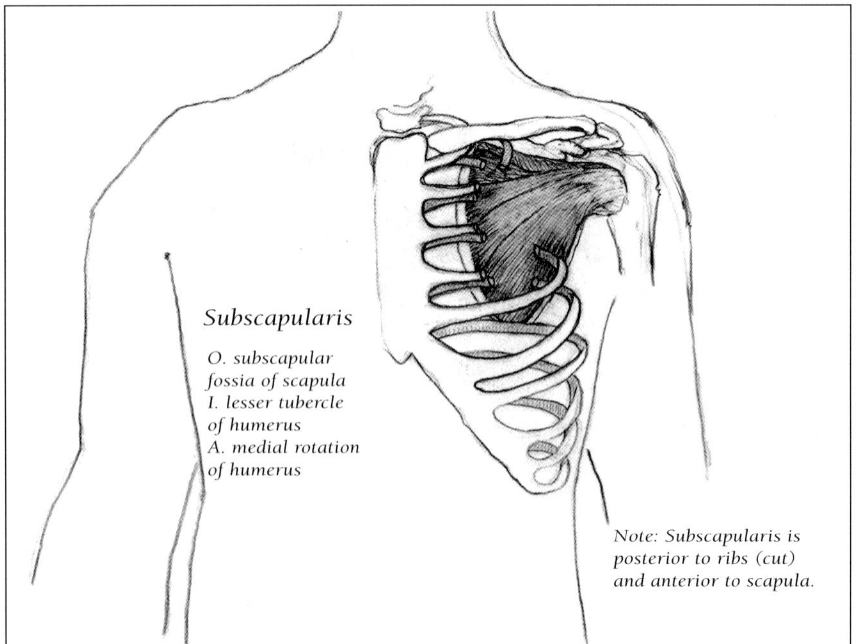

Subscapularis

The subscapularis internally rotates the humerus and is operative in throwing, swimming, house painting, and waving good-bye. We commonly see subscapularis tendonitis in house painters, plasterers and other men and women of the trades who continually internally rotate against resistance, e.g., the weight of the paintbrush. Overuse can result in both tendonitis and trigger points. Also, in many athletes, this muscle is underdeveloped for the demands placed on it.

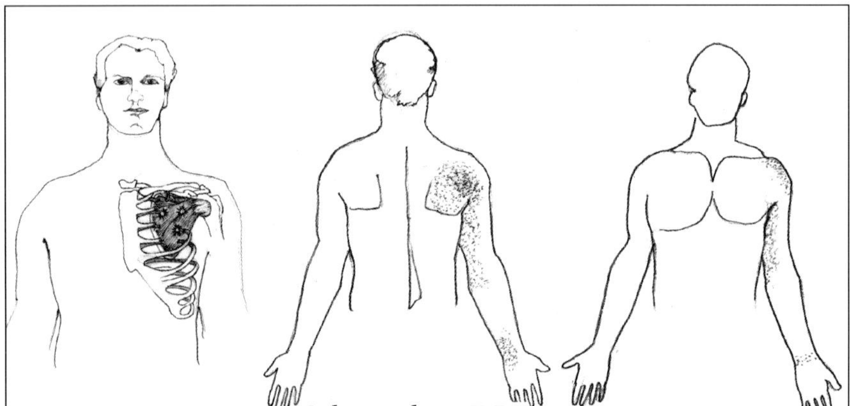

Subscapularis TrPs

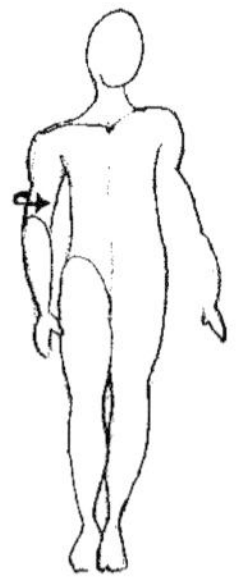

According to Dr. Cyriax, the inflamed subscapularis tendon is extremely painful. Begin treatment slowly and gently. The tendon is difficult to palpate even though it has a broad attachment on the anterior portion of the lesser tubercle of the head of the humerus. Knowing the bony landmarks of the shoulder will facilitate locating the lesion. Pain with friction massage to this tendon will be highly indicative of a tendonitis.

The current trend toward hypertonicity in the deltoids (as a replacement for the biceps as a sign of virility) often means more work for us. You have to move these highly developed anterior deltoids to gain access to the underlying subscapularis tendon. Don't be fooled by the striated nature and feel of the multi-pennate middle deltoid tendon fibers as you explore the shoulder. They may be sore, but they aren't the subscapularis tendon.

Confusion can also arise with trigger points referring from the subscapularis into the location of the infraspinatus or the supraspinatus tendon. So, be aware, trigger points in the subscapularis can mimic rotator cuff tendonitis. Frictioning the infraspinatus and supraspinatus tendons will prove futile. The pain will not diminish. When shoulder pain doesn't diminish with friction to a painful tendon, it is time to examine the belly of the subscapularis for trigger points.

If, in examining the belly of the subscapularis you find a trigger point that generates a predictable pain pattern into the anterior shoulder, suspect that the client's pain is from the trigger point and not from an inflamed tendon. As a standard part of treating any tendonitis, palpate for trigger points throughout the muscle belly.

With cross-fiber friction there should be a marked, if sometimes temporary, reduction in the pain caused by the tendonitis – a counter-inflammatory response. If the marked reduction of pain isn't present following the treatment, look elsewhere.

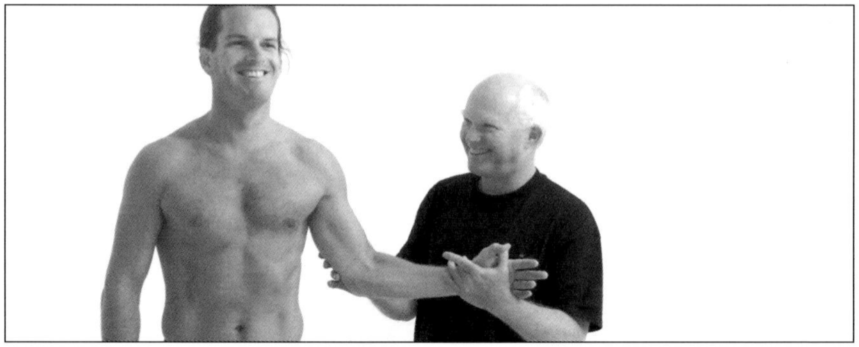

Internal rotation primarily tests the subscapularis. Increased pain usually indicates tendonitis at the subscapularis tendon. If indicated, include a second arm position (starting with the hand closer to the belly) to stress the muscle/tendon complex more thoroughly.

STUDENT'S STORY

One student who learned our rotator cuff protocol decided that he had a supraspinatus tendonitis. He spent the next 6 months rubbing his supraspinatus tendon with only a very sore tendon to show for his work. In another class a year later, he complained about the effectiveness of the treatment. We gave him two 15 second treatments to his subscapularis trigger points and completely cleared his "rotator cuff tendonitis."

The true culprit was a trigger point in the belly of the subscapularis that referred pain into the region of the supraspinatus tendon. Our student had completely forgotten the Three-Treatment Rule: If there is not substantial improvement in 3 visits, look for another source of the pain or refer.

The belly of the subscapularis can be particularly hard to access in people with tight shoulder girdle musculature. We often use contract-relax-antagonist-contract (CRAC) stretches to the mid-traps, rhomboids, long head of the triceps, latissimus dorsi, and teres minor and major to gain access to this muscle.

A trigger point can be as far back (medial) as 3/4 of the way to the vertebral border. This deep trigger point requires a careful yet firm entry. Remember, do not stretch any shoulder muscles if there is a rotator cuff tear.

When learning our approach to palpating and treating this muscle, be careful that entry is made anterior to the latissimus dorsi. Some therapists inadvertently try to push the edge of the latissimus beneath the scapulae and it just won't go. Trigger point injection by an M.D. with a long needle may be necessary for the deepest (most medial) trigger points.

In the sporting world, swimmers, pitchers and quarterbacks can all experience severe referred pain from trigger points in the belly of this muscle. Direct heel pressure across the posterior surface of the scapula will often compress any trigger points against the underlying ribs and give relief. Standing compressions can be used with big, heavily muscled clients. Seated compressions should be used to modulate the pressure against the underlying ribs on thinner or smaller clients.

In conjunction with examination of the subscapularis belly, use pincer palpation on the latissimus dorsi and both teres. Prolonged muscle and fascial stretching completes the treatment to eradicate pain from the scapular region.

PLAYER'S STORY

A young rugby player came in with a very weak and painful shoulder. Two weeks prior he had attempted to make a tackle by sticking his arm out in front of an opposing player's advance. He had not improved much after two subscapularis treatments. On the third visit, (our theoretical third and last visit) we reached deeper, medial and superior toward the vertebral border next to the axilla, and found the primary trigger point. Our earlier treatments had given minor results because we were only treating the nearby associated trigger points. Full recovery followed treating the primary trigger points.

Severe pain from the subscapularis – particularly with older clients – can stop them from using their shoulder. After a week or two this disuse can become habitual and the shoulder capsule begins to shrink. This can lead to a true "frozen shoulder" with all the medical consequences. Surgical procedures for adhesive capsulitis are not always successful. Conservative stretching by physical therapists can take a year or more.

Chronic hypertonicity contributes to pain. This hypertonicity can be mitigated by post-isometric relaxation (PIR) – prolonged contractions followed by relaxation of the affected muscles. PIR will enhance signaling, reset tonicity and often diminish pain. This method should be tried when simple stretching proves ineffective.

Treatment

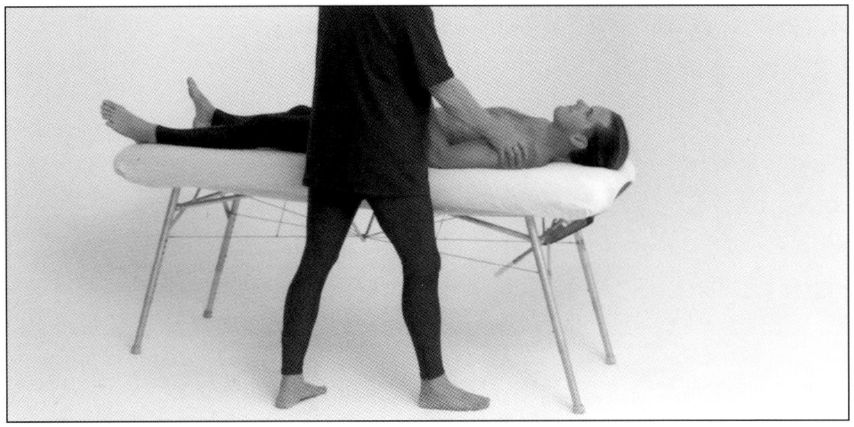

Good position for treating the subscapularis tendon at its insertion into the lesser tubercle of head of the humerus.

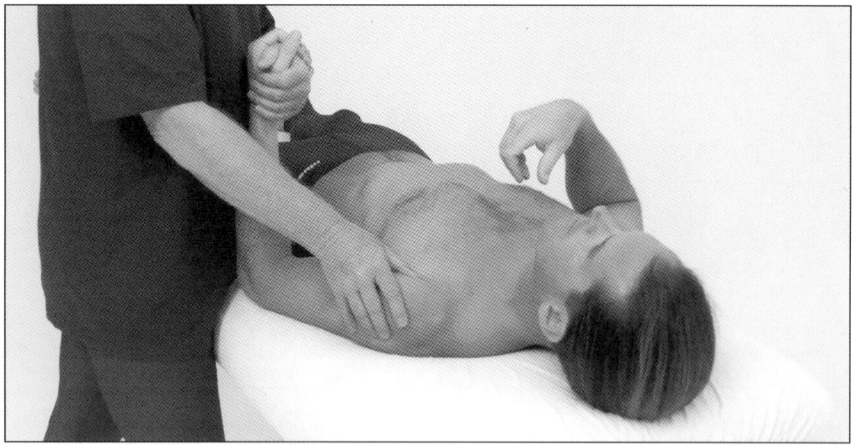

Dr. Cyriax claimed that the subscapularis tendon, when inflamed, was the most painful in the human body. Begin slowly and keep a good hold on your client's hand. Friction across the tendon is parallel to the humerus…up and down, up and down.

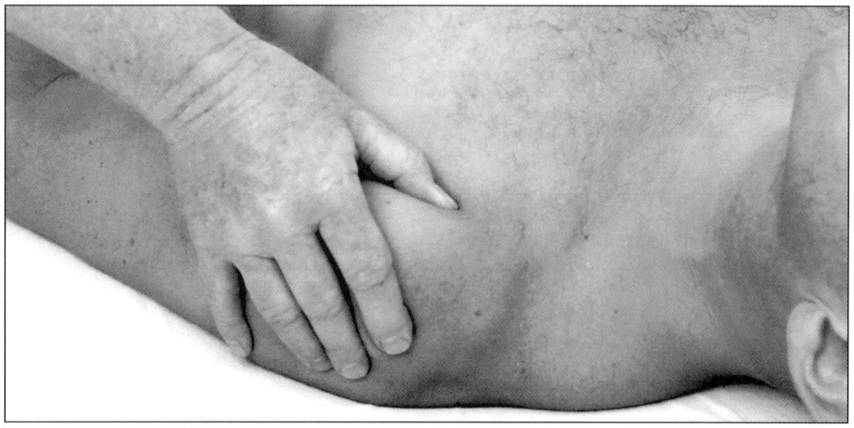

The subscapularis insertion is just medial and superior to the bicipital groove on the lesser tubercle of the head of the humerus. Finding the bony landmarks is critical. The tendon (adjacent to the bicipital groove) is thin and difficult to feel.

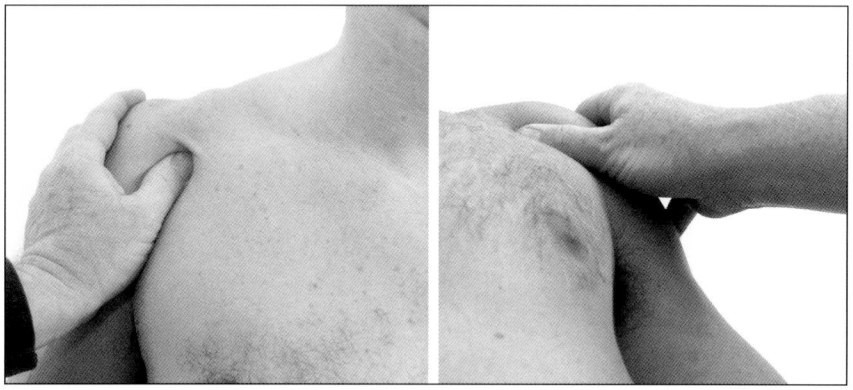

Push the deltoid aside to gain easier mechanical access to the tendon.

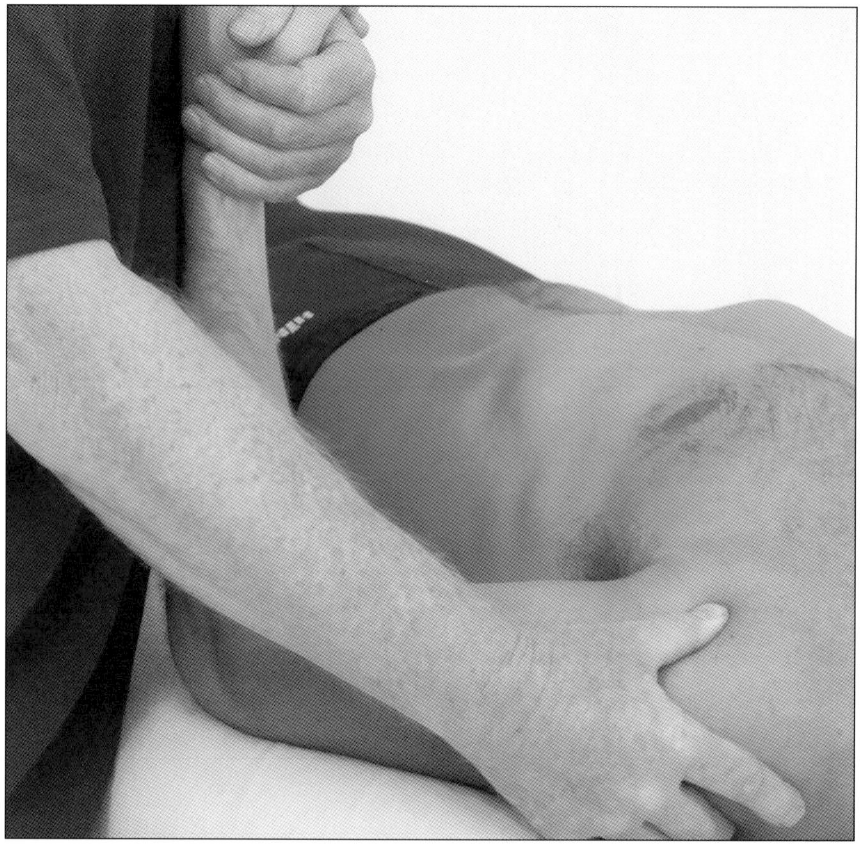

To find the long head of the biceps tendon, place your entire thumb across the head of the humerus and then internally and externally rotate the arm. You will feel a hard-soft-hard sensation or a bump-space-bump. The lateral bump identifies the greater tubercle of the head of the humerus. The softer space in between is the bicipital groove, and the medial bump is the lesser tubercle of the head of the. You will find the subscapularis tendon attachment on the lesser tubercle.

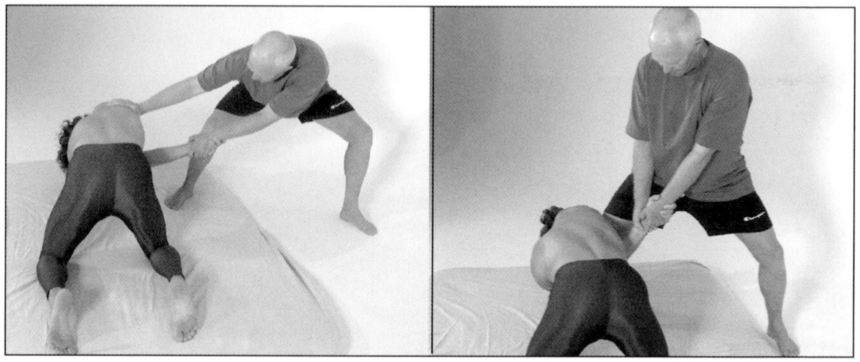

1. Stretch for teres, infraspinatus, posterior deltoid, mid-traps and rhomboids. Client's head hangs freely.
2. To get a slightly different stretch, change the angle of pull. This gives a deeper stretch to the infraspinatus, mid-traps and rhomboids. Clients with extremely flexible spines will benefit little from this stretch.

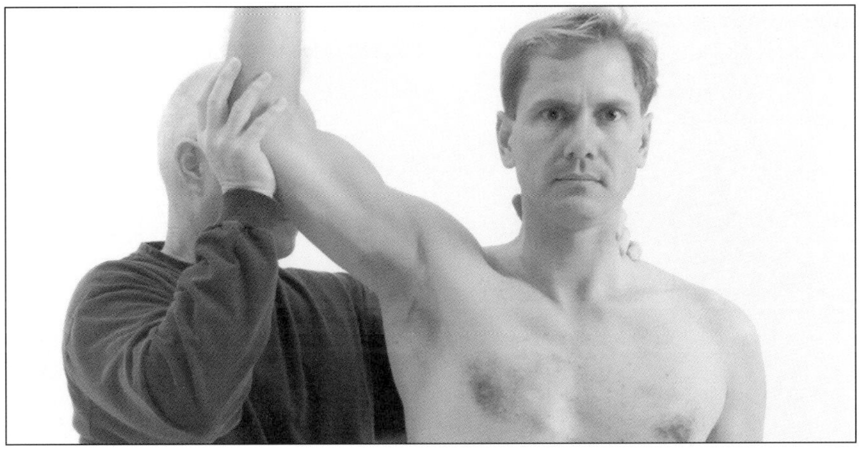

CRAC stretch to the latissimus and teres in preparation for easier entry into the subscapularis belly.

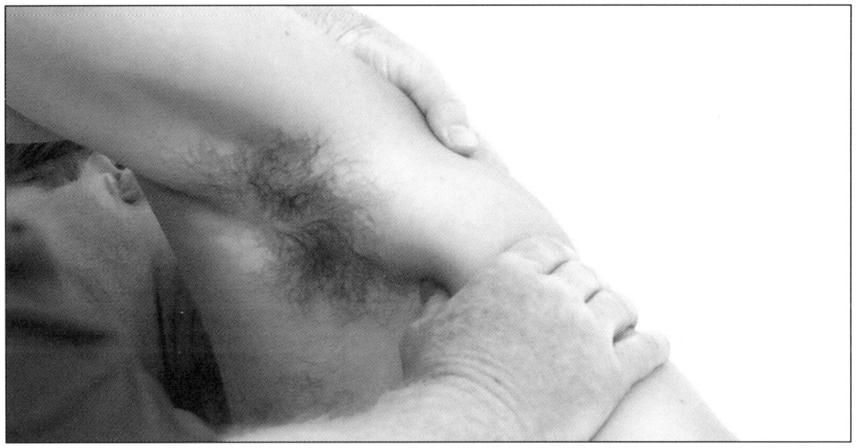

The thumb lies flat over the ribs and serratus anterior - there is absolutely no pushing or digging into the ribs. The therapist must push beneath (medial to) the edge of the latissimus dorsi. The latissimus cannot be pushed under the scapula. Remember you must push beneath the edge of the latissimus dorsi.

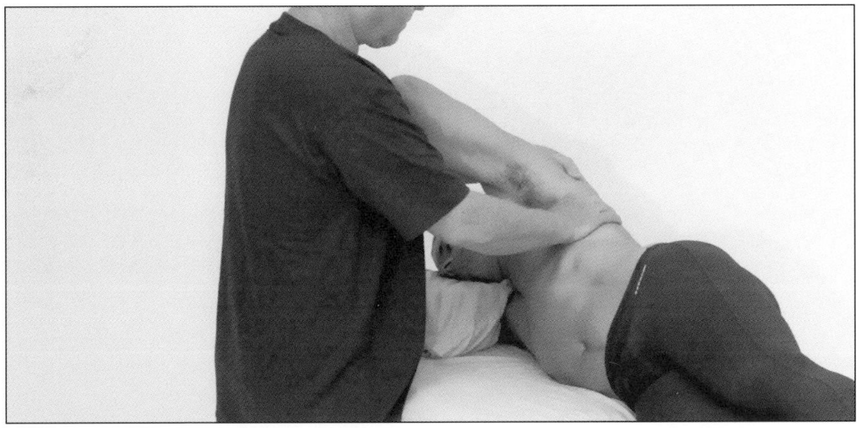

Access position for the belly of the subscapularis. The therapist's left arm is under and supports the client's freely hanging left arm.

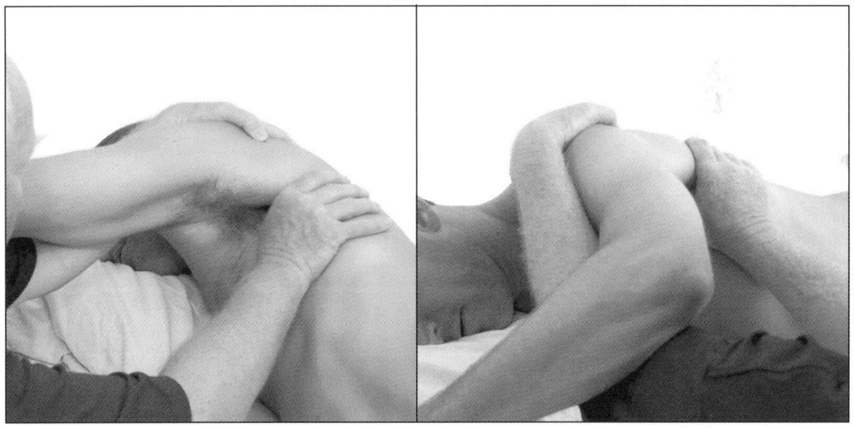

1. With the client's scapula protracted, push your thumb upward into the subscapularis muscle.
2. Enter slowly and search throughout the belly for jump signs. If access is difficult, we use CRAC stretches to relax shoulder girdle musculature. Use the arm drape demonstrated earlier.

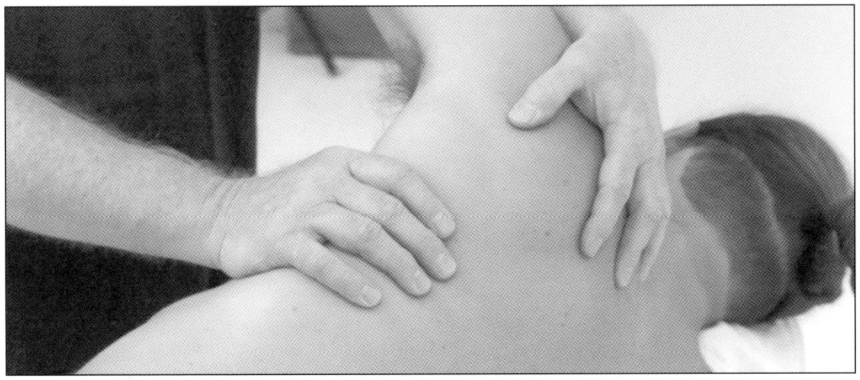

Hand position to control protraction and retraction of the scapula to facilitate access to the anterior surface of the scapula.

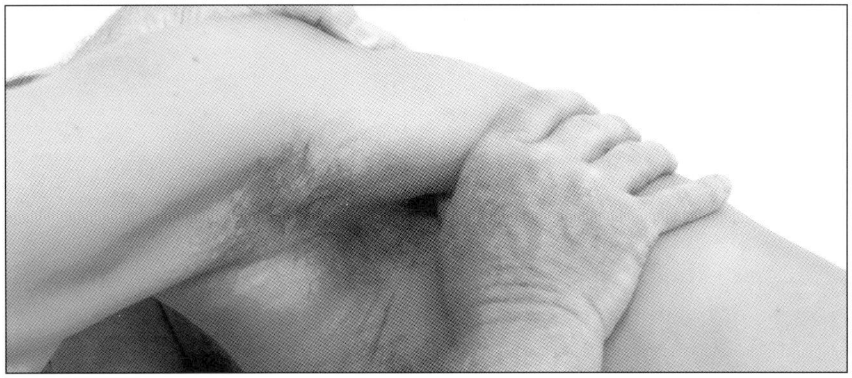

Avoid the axilla. Note the thumb is anterior and medial to the latissimus.

Long Head of the Biceps

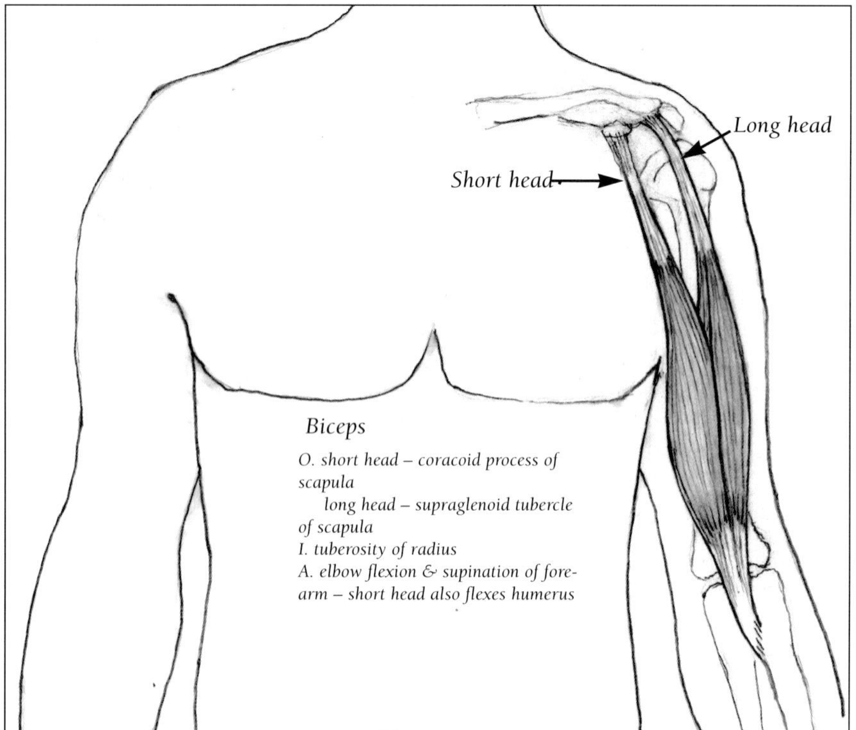

Biceps

An inflamed long head of the biceps tendon, while not part of the rotator cuff, hurts in the anterior shoulder. Palpate the entire length of this tendon to find the most painful spot. Treat the lesion with cross-fiber friction. Begin moderately. This tendon, like that of the subscapularis, can really hurt. Follow friction with the client performing whatever activity previously caused pain. A reduction or cessation of pain suggest an effective treatment..

Use pincer palpation to examine the belly of the muscle. Trigger points can refer up into the region of the tendon and cause confusion as to whether the problem is a bicipital tendonitis or a muscle belly trigger point. These trigger points can also refer into the radial attachment of both heads of the biceps.

Trigger points are generally found in the distal belly and are generally a secondary cause of pain. Tendonitis of the long head of the biceps is much more common.

You rarely need to use your feet on the belly of this muscle except in the cases of extremely large, well-developed clients. However, occasionally you can use prolonged direct pressure from the ball of the foot onto the anterior deltoid and the biceps tendon to provide a salutary effect. Avoid the nearby deltopectoral groove. Do not stretch any shoulder muscles if there is a rotator cuff tear.

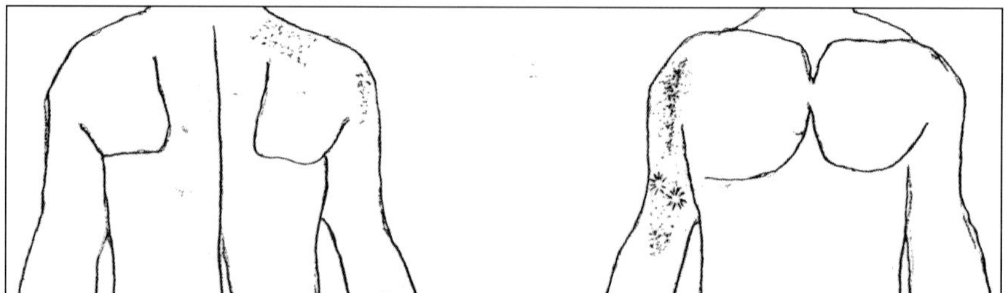

Biceps TrPs

Treatment

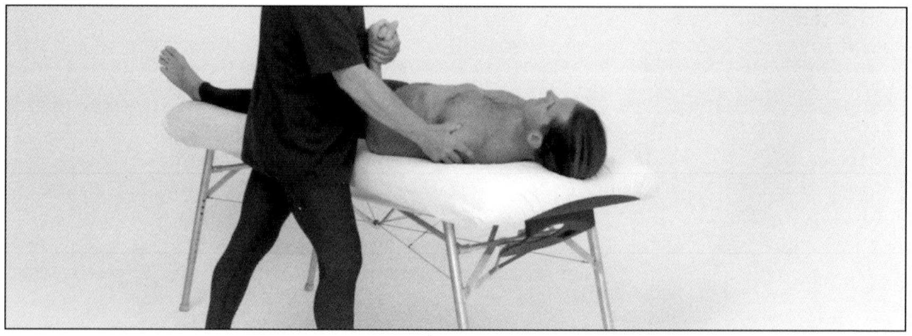

Treatment position for the long head of the biceps tendon – a common cause of pain in the rotator cuff area.

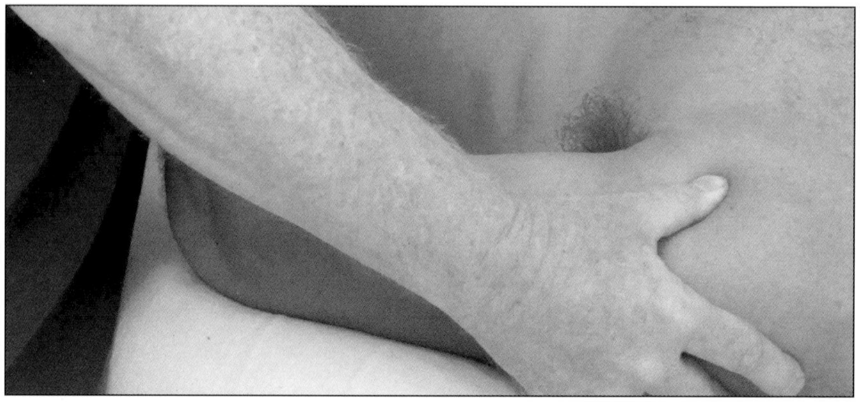

To find the long head of the biceps tendon, place your entire thumb across the head of the humerus and then internally and externally rotate the arm. You will feel a hard-soft-hard sensation or a bump-space-bump. The lateral bump identifies the greater tubercle of the head of the humerus. The softer space in between is the bicipital groove, and the medial bump is the lesser tubercle of the head of the humerus.

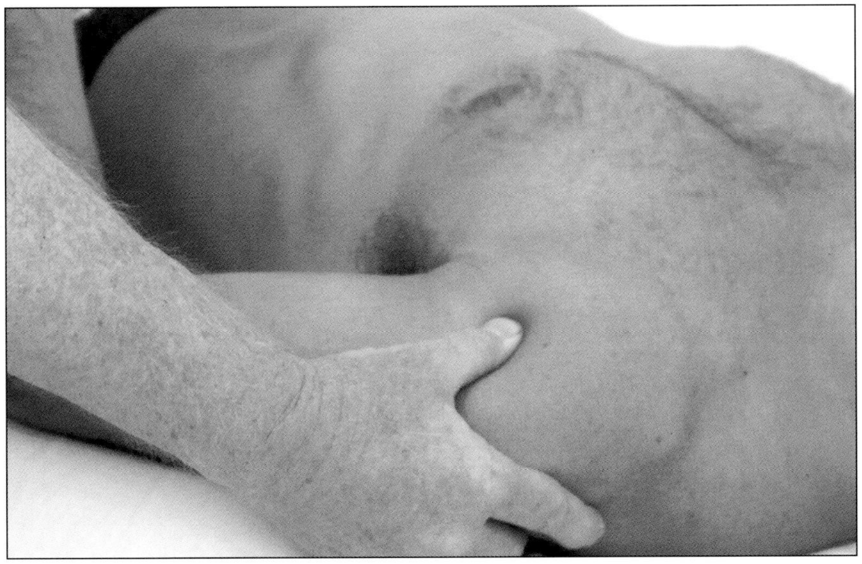

The thumb and fingers lock into "C-clamp" and the friction movement comes from a rolling of the thumb across the tendon with the fingers offering counter-pressure. There is no movement in the joints of the thumb or fingers. Movement comes from the wrist and arm.

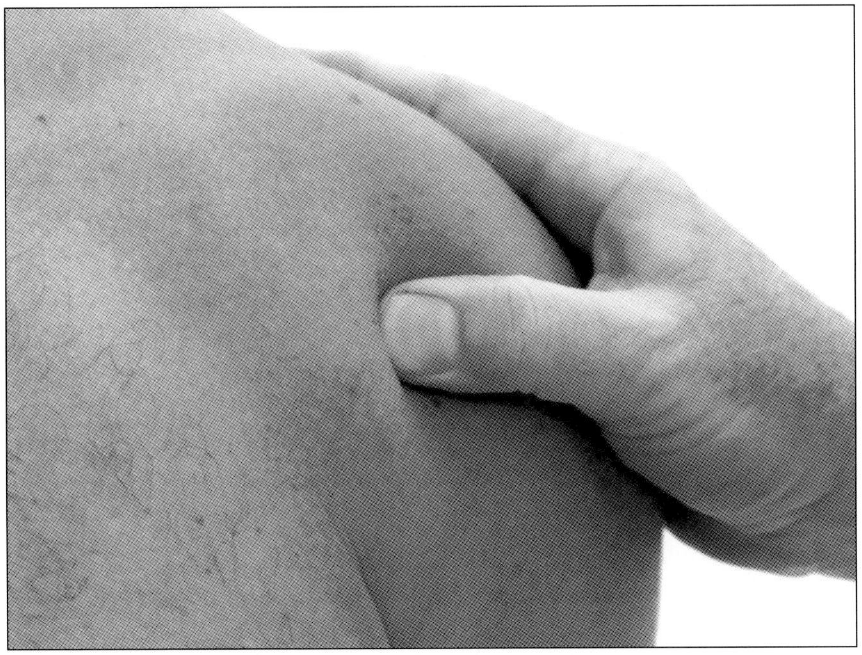

Close-up of friction to the biceps tendon. Note the thumb is slightly flexed and locked at the distal interphalangeal joint. The tendon is 2 to 3 inches long and may be painful along its length. Work the most painful area.

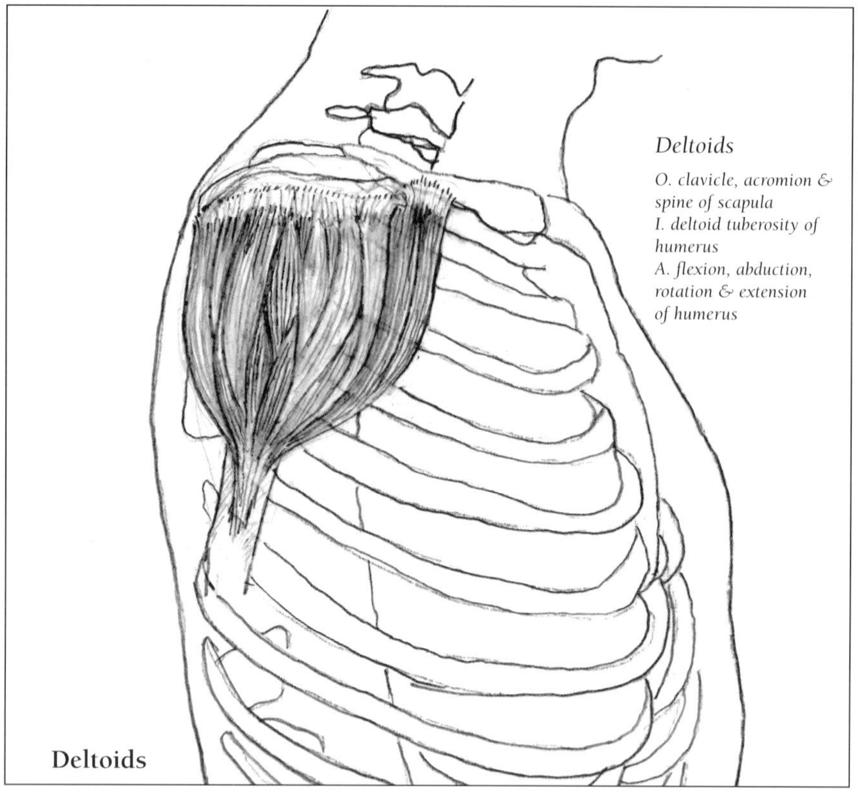

Deltoids

When we first started working with chronic pain years ago, it seemed that the deltoid was seldom a problem. A tendonitis of the long head of the biceps, the tenoperiosteal juncture of the supraspinatus or the infraspinatus tendon were often the quick and easy fixes for shoulder pain.

Now we see increasing numbers of deltoid problems. We think these problems result from overuse, primarily from poorly positioned computer keyboards, direct trauma and from over-training in the gym or pool. The senescence of our aging population plays a role, too.

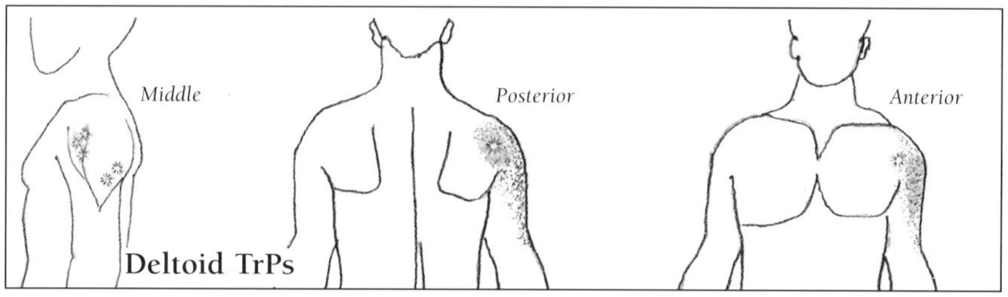

Deltoid TrPs

AUTHOR'S STORY

One of our very own senior authors developed an extremely debilitated deltoid while working with too much focus on his computer. Fortunately another senior made an astute observation and was able to diagnose the "ergonomics" problem. We used deep compressive massage to help him back to his machine where he is presently typing under ergonomically friendly conditions.

Trigger points caused by direct trauma and overuse usually occur in the anterior and posterior deltoids. Deltoid trigger points usually refer to the front or back of the shoulder. The pain can be so great as to completely inhibit deltoid contractions needed for humeral elevation. These trigger points respond nicely to direct pressure. Deltoid trigger points can also occur concurrently with an impingement syndrome. Cross-fiber friction massage to the tendons of the supraspinatus, subscapularis and long head of the biceps plus direct pressure to the deltoids may be necessary to end pain.

A suspected bursitis problem is often actually due to rotator cuff or bicipital tendonitis. Use palpation assessment (if it hurts, it's injured). Functional assessment may be necessary to differentiate a bursitis from a tendonitis.

Functional assessment is useful in determining clinical level problems (problems severe enough to hurt more under the stress of the resisted contractions of functional assessment). If possible, it's preferable to work with pain at an earlier stage, with a sub-clinical tendonitis. Sub-clinical problems are painful to the touch but don't necessarily respond with pain to functional assessment. Our work is most effective in aborting tendonitis in its earlier stages.

Small tears and adherent scarring are problems found in the more powerful middle deltoid. These areas are much more difficult to heal, and tend towards intermittent pain. This pain increases during strong contractions against resistance, and is not the result of an impingement syndrome. Cures are sometimes incomplete and require maintenance treatments for the client to stay pain-free, especially when the muscle is regularly overtaxed, as in weight training, long drives or hours at the keyboard.

Poor shoulder mechanics, primarily because of muscle imbalances, create problems that won't heal. An exercise and stretch protocol to balance the shoulder joint is desirable.

If the pain is caused by acute subdeltoid bursitis, your client won't want you to touch their shoulder – much too painful. By the third day of pain, your client will hurt all the way down to the hand. Cure comes with rest or corticosteroid injection(s). Massage is ineffective or exacerbates the problem. If well tolerated, ice helps with the pain. With bursitis, tendonitis or any rotator cuff tear, do not stretch any shoulder muscle. Pain on stretching is, again, a contraindication.

Medical treatments for bursitis usually include steroid injection and NSAIDS (non-steroidal anti-inflammatory drugs) such as Ibuprofin and some of the other over-the-counter (OTC) analgesics. However, current medical research suggests possible damage to cartilage can result from use of NS anti-inflammatories. In this case, steroid injections are not suspect of causing damage to cartilage, but can eventually cause damage to muscle tissue or tendons.

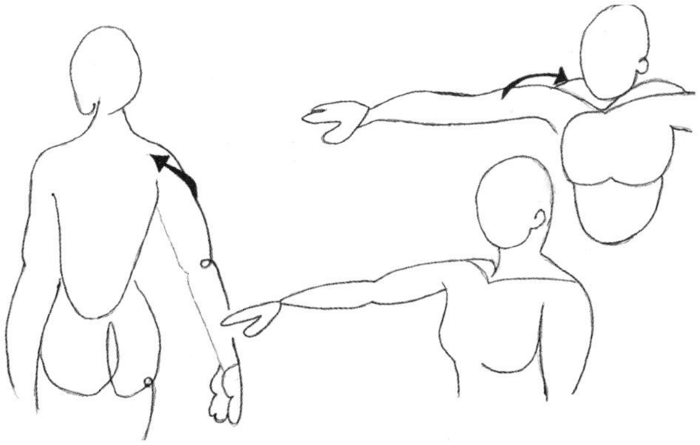

Query: Which contributes more to cartilage damage, the NSAIDS or the inflammation they reduce or eliminate? Medical questions and considerations quickly become very complicated – a practical reason that M.T.s do not diagnose or prescribe.

Treatment

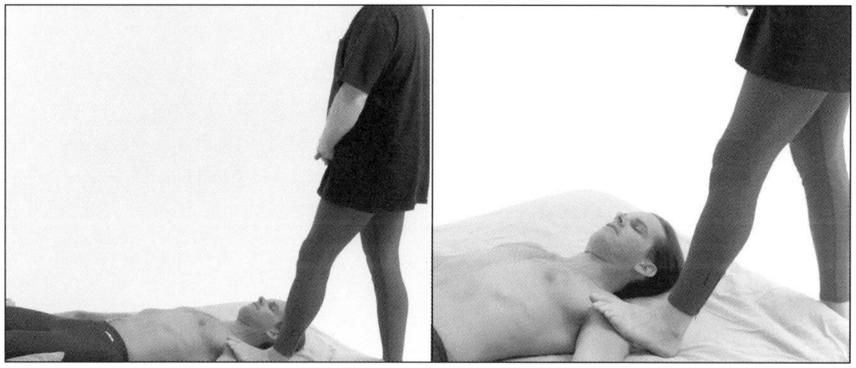

1. Direct pressure to the anterior deltoid. Note the therapist's planted heel to control pressure at the ball of the foot.
2. Anterior deltoid compression from the first ray of the therapist's foot.

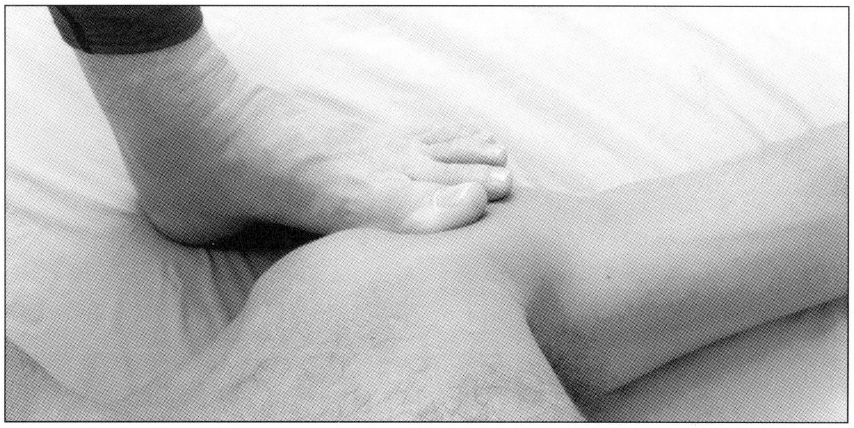

Dragging stretch and direct pressure to anterior deltoid.

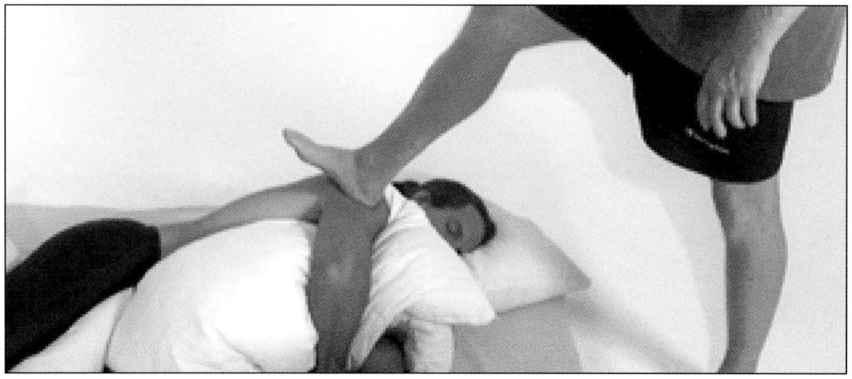

Direct heel pressure to middle/posterior deltoid.

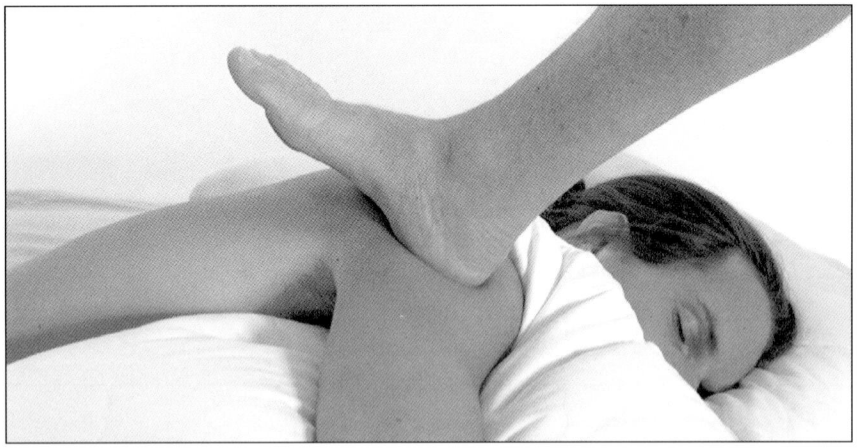

Close-up of direct pressure to the deltoid.

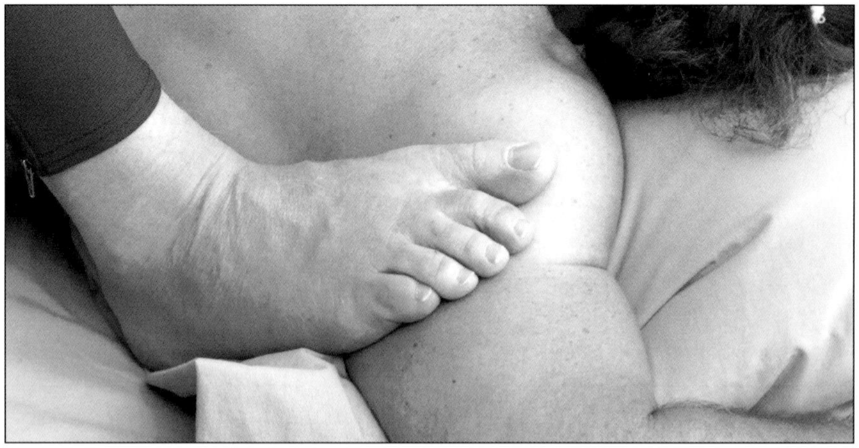

Direct pressure to posterior deltoid.

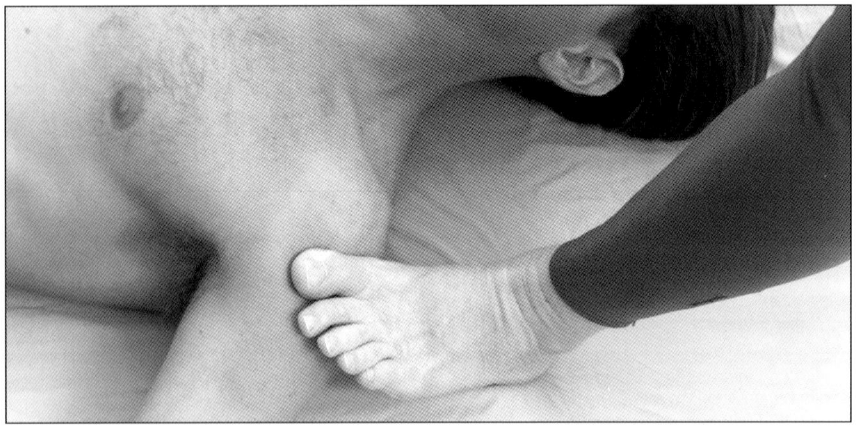

Direct pressure from first ray to middle deltoid.

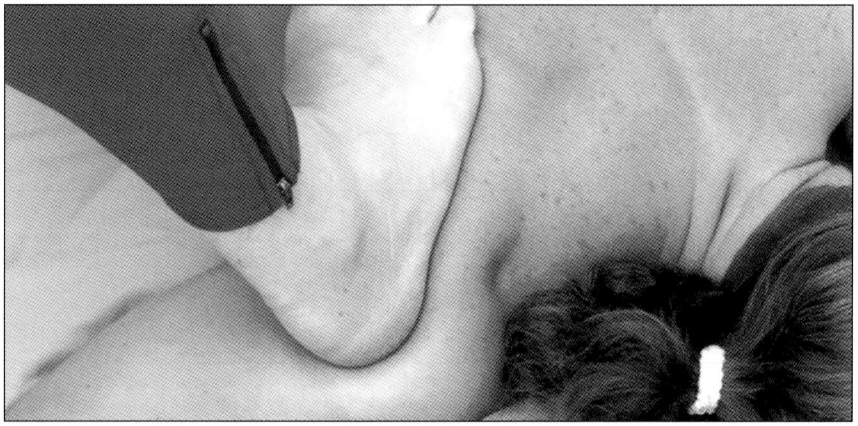

Heel compression into the posterior deltoid. Deep and strong.

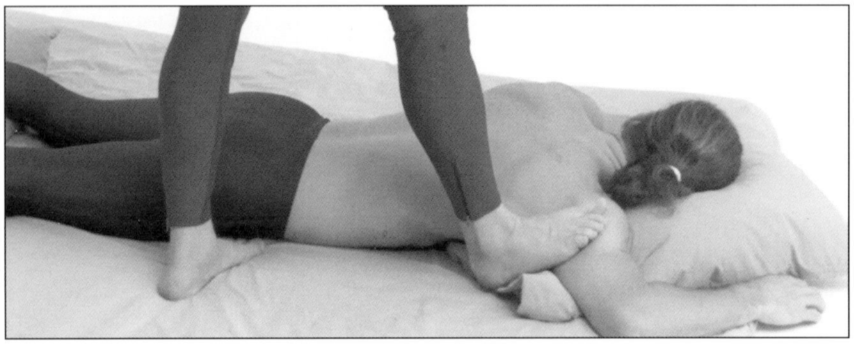

Clients with previous dislocations are vulnerable to another dislocation in this position. Shoulders dislocate anteriorly and need good bolstering to support against this posterior to anterior pressure.

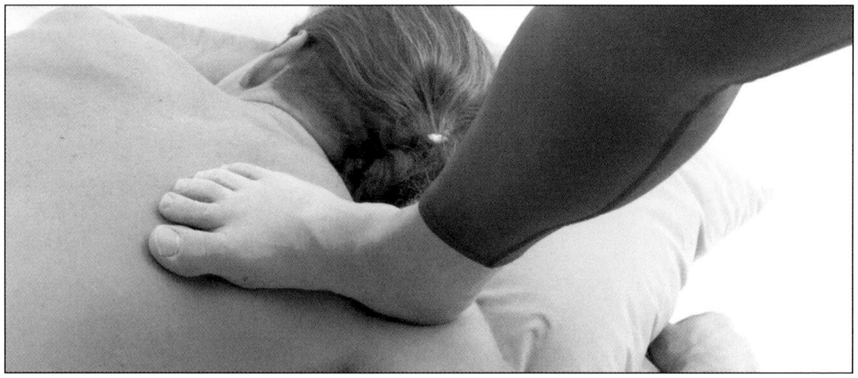

Shoulder joint is well-bolstered to prevent client's fear of shoulder dislocation.

PART 5

Appendices and Overviews

CHAPTER 15

Stretching for Bodyworkers and Clients

About Stretching

SWEDISH MASSAGE can be a highly effective tool for relaxation and restoration, but using it to relieve hypertonicity in muscles can be difficult and time-consuming. Many therapists rub and rub and rub in the hopes of relaxing tight muscles. Initially feeling good, this prolonged rubbing soon becomes an irritant. It is more effective and much quicker to stretch a muscle to submission that to rub a muscle into submission.

Prior to a Swedish massage, clever therapists stretch their client's problem areas. Stretched muscles are soft and can gain greater benefits from Swedish kneading and stroking. It's just more effective. Although there is some discussion about this, proper stretching most probably prevents injuries and reduces pain. Incorrect stretching, however, can shorten muscles and contribute to scar tissue formation, doing more harm than good.

Stretching can promote a healthy self-awareness. It provides for safe transitions from passivity to activity. Strength, balance and flexibility all increase from the improved range of motion resulting from stretching. We may also benefit from the meditative aspects of habitual stretching. A quiet stretch helps therapists center attention. It decreases our tension and increases our sensitivity.

Stretching has been shown by some research to prevent injuries when used before and after strenuous exertion. Regular stretching prevents the pulls, sprains and strains that inhibit maximum performance. Metabolites, the by-products of our muscles making energy, are more efficiently moved out of the body when muscle tissues are relaxed by stretching. Flushing of metabolites minimizes the nerve irritation that leads to delayed onset soreness. However, over-stretching after a maximal workout may worsen post-exercise soreness. Soreness resulting from torn muscle fibers following a strong workout won't be substantially helped by stretching and may be worsened by excessive or over-stretching.

When to Stretch

Stretch often. Stretching can be done almost anywhere and anytime. Stretch short, tight, tense muscles. They can cause postural problems. Muscles should be stretched prior to strengthening their weakened antagonists.

Some Examples:

- Stretch tight pectorals before strengthening rhomboids to properly position neck and shoulders generally found on clients with excessive mid-thoracic kyphosis.

- Stretch low back muscles and hip flexors to counteract excessive lordosis.

- Stretch hamstrings in flatback and swayback problems.

- Stretch the tensor fascia latae, illiotibial band and quadratus lumborum to correct lateral pelvic tilt.

- Deeper tissues and trigger points are easier to address after relaxing tense, hypertonic muscles. Stretching after direct pressure to trigger points helps prevent recurrence.

Over-stretching

Over-stretching (too deep or too quick a stretch) can trigger a stretch reflex, shortening rather than lengthening the target muscle. Muscle spindle cells, concentrated in muscle bellies, are the source of this protective reflex. When they sense muscles lengthening too much too quickly, they reflexively initiate tightening to prevent tearing.

Before You Stretch

"LET GO" is the attitude to assume for stretching. Effortless efforts are required – this means you don't compete with yourself. You may have to set some old attitudes aside about trying to assume more relaxed ones. Muscles with trigger points will not stretch properly. Known trigger points should be treated before stretching.

Relax soft tissues and warm them up before stretching as warm muscles release and stretch more easily. Fascial tissues also yield more comfortably and effectively when warm. Warming lessens the occasional occurrence of a stretch injury.

A 2 degree increase in body temperature is considered optimal for effective stretching. Some active exercise or work usually achieves this increase in body temperature. Noting when you first break a sweat identifies the 2 degree increase needed to draw blood from the viscera to the extremities, making them more amenable to stretching. Deep compressions, deep kneading massage, joint shaking and manipulation or direct applications of heat also effectively raise body temperature.

Refer to *Notes, Cautions,* and *Warnings* at end of the CRAC/PNF section before beginning your stretches.

How To ...Stretching Rules

1. Pay attention to the feeling of your stretch. Try to identify the feeling of muscle release, elongation. You are probably over-stretching if the feeling of the stretch doesn't begin to diminish after 10 to 12 seconds.

2. Be aware that there should be absolutely no pain. A successful stretch is not and should not be painful.

3. A simple stretch, usually from 20 seconds to 1 minute, can range from a few seconds to 5 minutes. Do it again, but this time with a slight pull into the stretch and you'll accomplish a developmental stretch.

4. Stretch as long as you like and as often as you like. Bigger and stronger muscles with more bundles of fibers need to be stretched for longer times. We increase ROM by lengthening these bundles.

5. Forget ideal posturing and distances stretched or degree of muscle elongation and try to feel. Most simply put, "Just let go" or "Feel the stretch."

6. Keep track of the rest of your body. All parts not being stretched must remain relaxed. This includes your breathing.

7. Do not over-stretch. Excessive stretching causes spasms or shortening. Too abrupt or forceful stretching violates proprioceptive mechanisms designed to protect tissues from injury.

8. Your body type, its structure, flexibility and attitudes should all be considered with regards to frequency, intensity and duration for optimal stretching.

9. After stretching has attained your desired result, consider how to best strengthen the antagonist muscle to achieve joint stability.

Proprioceptive Neuromuscular Facilitation (PNF)

CRAC (Contract Relax Antagonist Contract) is a form of proprioceptive neuromuscular facilitation that quickly lengthens muscles. Its effect on fascial restrictions is minimal. CRAC stretches can be done alone or with a partner.

How CRAC Works

In a normal static stretch, muscle spindle cells attached to the myofibrils are stretched along with the muscle. When stretched too quickly, the spindle cells send information to the central nervous system to stop the muscle from stretching. This mechanism, the myotatic stretch reflex, prevents tearing and over-stretching the involved joint. A static, simple stretch usually should be held for 30 to 60 seconds to disengage the spindle cells for a deeper stretch. CRAC can achieve greater gains more quickly. CRAC stretches utilize an isometric contraction followed by an antagonist contraction. These stretches, following basic physiological principals, give quick, deep stretches.

Principles

• Isometric contractions are used to warm the target muscle.

• The target muscle is mildly fatigued by the contraction and is better prepared to relax.

• The antagonistic muscle contraction inhibits the stretch reflex in the target muscle. Simply stated, when one muscle contracts, the opposing muscle is inhibited from contracting – the spindle cells disengage and the muscle is allowed to lengthen.

Assisted CRAC Stretching

1. Client stretches the target muscle to maximum pain-free length. To stretch the hamstrings, have your supine client contract their hip flexors to stretch the hamstrings. Keep the knee straight but not locked.

2. Position yourself against the upraised leg to provide resistance.

3. Your client contracts the hamstring into your resistance. No movement occurs in the client's hip. The contraction should begin gradually and build smoothly (from 10% to 50% exertion is used). Have your client breath normally throughout the contraction. Clients hold the contraction for about 6 seconds.

NOTE: Deconditioned muscles can spasm, create post-treatment soreness or even tear. Use a 10% to 20% contraction for deconditioned clients.

4. Following the hamstring contraction, the client relaxes and takes one deep breath. This "cleansing breath" following flexion and before extension of the hips prevents injury to the hamstrings – particularly with competitive athletes. A rapid change in direction following a maximal hamstring contraction sets the muscle up for a strain.

5. Client then contracts the antagonist muscles, in this case the rectus femoris and psoas, and pulls the hams into a deeper stretch.

6. You then move up to the leg in its new, lengthened position, to again offer resistance for another isometric contraction.

7. Repeat the process 3 times. Remember deconditioned people should usually start with less effort and with 1 or 2 repetitions to avoid post-treatment soreness.

8. CRAC stretches must be PAIN-FREE. If pain is experienced, try repositioning the limb, or use less force during the isometric contraction of the target muscle. If pain persists, do not use CRAC for that particular muscle until you have determined and treated the cause.

CRAC stretches make dramatic changes in muscle length. They are used to increase flexibility and decrease pain while softening tight, hypertonic muscles prior to massage or trigger point work. Occasionally a trigger point laden muscle will cause pain and spasm when stretched. Generally treat active referring trigger points first and then passively or actively stretch the muscle. Save the CRAC stretches for when the trigger point is inactivated.

Important Note

In bodywork, moderate gains are preferred to dramatic changes in muscle length. Large, rapid increases in flexibility permit antagonist muscles to contract into new foreshortened positions. This leads to the problems of spasm, cramps, and activation of trigger points in the antagonist muscle. When the hamstrings were lengthened through PNF, the rectus femoris was able to more fully contract. This new shortened position can induce new problems. We can prevent most of these problems by remembering to stretch both agonist and antagonists and treating any trigger points.

Recommended Stretching Manuals

Robert McAtee, NCTMB, CSCS, provides clear and careful instruction on specific PNF work in his manual, *Facilitated Stretching* (1999). McAtee uses ample illustrations and includes essential definition. Readers can order the book directly from him at Pro-Active Massage Therapy, Colorado Springs, CO., or from Human Kinetics Publishers. McAtee also has a web site: stretchman.com

Bob Anderson's manual, *Stretching* (1986), Shelter Publications, Random House, is a good text to consult for explanations of simple and developmental stretches. Detailed examples cover stretches required for many popular sports

Warnings and Contradictions

- Don't stretch hypermobile joints.

- Confer with your client's physician before using stretches which could effect recent surgical procedures.

- Never stretch acute or current joint injury sites or inflamed, bleeding or swollen tissues.

- If pain is encountered, understand the source before deciding whether to proceed.

- When stretching leads to any sharp pain, STOP!

CHAPTER 16

Hydrotherapy

HYDROTHERAPY (the use of hot and cold) decreases the pain of injuries, reduces post-treatment soreness and speeds healing. Clients can be safely trained to use hydrotherapy when needed. A comprehensive handout will ensure safe and effective client use.

Heat

Heat effectively relieves chronic muscle pain and spasm. Warmth increases both muscle flexibility and joint mobility. It loosens arthritic joints and effectively reduces chronic muscle tightness. Since moist heat penetrates, we prefer moist heat over dry sources.

Never use heat when dealing with acute (inflamed) injury. Heat is always reserved for the post-inflammatory period generally defined as 48 to 72 hours after the onset of acute pain – usually resulting from a trauma. No heat source should be so hot as to cause pain.

Clients respond distinctively to trigger point treatment. Use conservative first treatments and recommend clients follow-up with moist heat to reduce post-treatment soreness.

To relieve headaches by reducing intra-cranial arterial pressure, have your clients place their feet in tolerably hot water. The heat dilates blood vessels which, in turn, draws blood from their head to their feet. The resultant blood pressure reduction relieves certain types of headache.

.

Moist Heat Sources

• Moist heating pads, covered with flannel that leaches moisture from the air, are clearly superior to dry pads whose heat is mostly carried off by capillaries. Moist heating pads are available in a variety of shapes and sizes from medical supply outlets. Velcro can hold the one designed to attach around the neck snugly in place. Somewhat less effective, but also less expensive, moist heating pads utilize a sponge dampened prior to use.

• There are several brands and sizes of hydrocollator pacs (sand-filled canvas bags) and compresses filled with gels that can be heated in hot water or microwaves. They can be used by themselves or, preferably, placed on a moist towel.

• Sitting in the shower with a towel over the sore area provides an immediate, inexpensive source of moist heat. This form of heat application is especially effective on the neck. You can also soak a towel in hot water and place it directly on the painful site, or simply wrap a moist towel around a hot water bottle.

Cold

Cold is used for pain and soreness following deep transverse friction and during acute sprain or strain. It is also used to help eliminate tendonitis, acute backache, swelling, inflammation and even chronic muscular pain.

Notice how injured athletes are being iced practically before they're off the field or court? Putting ice on an area of acute injury speeds recovery, especially if quickly applied to injured, inflamed areas.

The primary action of cold is contraction of the skin's unstriated muscles. Contraction squeezes the tissues and removes capillary blood and lymph from the injured area. Pumping action lasts for 5 to 8 minutes after the cold is removed. Action of the capillary walls themselves is much the same.

The reaction (secondary response) to cold is dilation (expansion) of blood vessels. Dilation brings in additional arterial blood which, in the acute stage, is contraindicated. Note that heat produces a similar momentary reaction when applied to chronic problems. When using cold or heat, post-treatment diameter of blood vessels is greater than before their application. This action/reaction is also true for foot compression, but, as with heat, do not use DeeperWork compressions on recent (acute) injuries.

How Cold Works

Cold (icing) decreases secondary or hypoxic tissue death following injury by slowing metabolism and constricting capillaries which minimizes secondary cell death caused by pooling of excessive fluids from ruptured tissues. Excess fluids starve tissues of oxygen as they pour from damaged tissues into areas of acute injury, thus flooding them with unbalanced nutrients. This is known as hypoxic tissue damage. Essentially, cold promotes cell hibernation, so to speak, and limits the number of cells drowning in unregulated fluids.

The cold also has an analgesic effect. A decrease in pain relaxes tissues by diminishing the reflex arc while it also calms the injured person. The swiftest healing, however, occurs during sleep.

Splinting spasm is reduced when less pain is felt. Icing reduces the afferent signal (input side of the reflex arc) so the amplified efferent signals (those going out to fire motor neurons which leads to the spasms) are also reduced. Icing allows increased, pain-free movement and speeds injury recovery.

Clients can usually apply ice to painful, acutely injured areas for 10 to 15 minutes. People respond very differently to cold. For some fair-skinned or hypersensitive types, 5 minutes proves optimal. Some cannot tolerate more. When dealing with acute injury, our general guide indicates ice for 10 to 15 minutes once every 1 to 2 hours for the first 2 to 3 days. For chronic problems, apply ice less frequently (once every 5 to 6 hours) for the same period of time (5 to 15 or 20 minutes). Many clients won't follow this regime, but any application of ice can prove beneficial.

Sources of Cold

- Reusable cold compresses are available from drug stores or a hospital supply. Keep them in your freezer. To avoid complications, always put a thin, damp cloth between any ice source and the skin. A very cold source will freeze a damp cloth. Use care to avoid frostbite.
- Ice cubes in a plastic bag will do in a pinch, but it's best to never apply ice directly.
- Injured (inflamed) tissues, e.g., tendons beneath integral skin, benefit when placed in ice water. Be careful as numbing can occur in seconds, not minutes. To prevent possible damage, remove before the area is numb.

Alternating Hot and Cold

Alternating between heat and cold is tedious but highly effective in rapidly reducing swelling. Tissues react to changing temperatures by expanding and contracting – "pumping" blood and lymph. Constrictions and dilations take place quickly and strongly. A general timing guide is 4 minutes of heat followed by 1 minute of cold. Make the change from heat to cold gradually. Slowly heat to a maximum, pain-free temperature and then cool to ice temperature. Remember to end the alternating hydrotherapy treatment with cold.

Except for the admonition not to apply heat to an inflamed area, either heat or cold may be used on chronic problems. Use whichever proves most effective.

ROGER'S STORY

Roger loves to play the piano – his playing reflects it. His musical feelings are expressed with intensity. After years of occasional playing for amusement, Roger renewed a more serious interest, hired an inspiring instructor and began to practice in earnest. Some phrasings demand considerable force. His older body reacted to a call for youthful vigor by developing trigger points and tendonitis in his forearms and at finger extensor attachments.

I treated my friend Roger by applying direct pressure to all obvious finger and wrist extensor trigger points. Wanting to fix him completely, I also employed some deep transverse friction to erase adhesions on some select forearm musculotendinous junctures.

Two plastic bags containing magic "microwave-it or freeze-it" stuff were used to ice the inflamed attachments. One compress was sitting directly over the freezer coils. This more solid bag was placed on the left forearm and the other on the right. Both were wrapped with a towel to keep them securely in place.

While the ice did its trick, we did some neck work, checking the scaleni for additional triggers that might be adding to his arm pain.

Seven minutes later we checked the iced tissues. Except for the area directly over the inflammation, the right arm was cold. The left arm, while less inflamed initially, was very cold. It actually appeared sort of gray where the ice compress had been placed. The skin's texture resembled a drippy popsicle… felt like one, too.

Roger wanted to move along – he had an important appointment. His arm was numb so it didn't hurt. His therapist, however, was in a panic. Fortunately, remembering a survival school admonition to minimize frostbitten areas, he convinced Roger to stay a bit longer. Beginning with the temperature near freezing (he put the ice bags in a pan of cold water) he repeated brief cold towel applications, slightly warmer each time. The thawing took 25 minutes.

Embarrassing frostbite was narrowly avoided. Roger would have suffered significant damage if we had put hot or even warm water on frozen tissues. Cell walls would have surely ruptured and skin or possibly even muscle damage could have been severe. Fred carefully reconsidered his short-lived career in cryogenics and hopes you will benefit from his embarrassment.

Lessons Learned

• Do not apply ice over too broad an area – localize cold over the inflammation. Areas of more severe inflammation can handle colder temperatures without damage.
• Remember that ice comes in different temperatures, even from the same freezer. A compress sitting directly over the cooling coils can be much colder than its neighbor.
• It pays to check your client's iced area every couple of minutes to avoid trouble.
• People are different – some of us have higher rates of metabolism. More/increased circulation delays frostbite and freezing.
• It is a good idea to warn your clients about the inherent dangers involved in applying ice.
• Don't count on total cures in a single session. If it takes years to develop problems, you can't expect to fix them all in a single session.

Hydrotherapy – More Cautions and Contraindications

• Avoid adding heat to heat. Heat is contraindicated in acute soft tissue injury, since it would increase swelling and subsequent cell morbidity. Use ice on acute injuries and inflamed areas.
• Do not apply ice directly to tissues – cover with thin cloth and examine frequently to avoid frostbite. Ice for a maximum of 5 to 20 minutes every 2 hours. Exact timing varies with metabolism and skin type.
• Cold must be felt (very cold) to be most effective. Use care to avoid tissue damage.
• To prevent tissue damage (frostbite), immediately remove the cold source/ice as soon as any area being treated becomes numb.
• Avoid icing superficial nerves often located in joint cavities; e.g., the superficial peroneal nerve.
• Avoid icing (or heat) on numb or infected tissues or areas with open wounds.
• No ice on diabetics without a doctor's approval since their circulation can be compromised.
• Do not ice anyone suffering from Raynauds Syndrome (defined by excessive pain in hands and feet upon contact with cold).
• Some people simply hate cold – ice is contraindicated for these people and for anyone whose pain worsens when it is used.

CHAPTER 17

Acute Injuries: RICE

ALL ACUTE INJURY to muscles, tendons and ligaments, regardless of severity, should be given prompt attention to forestall further damage from hypoxic tissue death. Generally, the earlier the application of ice, the quicker the recovery. Massage at the sight of the lesion is contraindicated for acute injuries. Clients should know how to use RICE – (R)est, (I)ce, (C)ompress and (E)levate.

Ice can be applied to the affected area immediately (for 10 to 15 minutes) and every 60 to 90 minutes thereafter (until bedtime) to help reduce the inflammatory response, limit the spread of secondary injury and control pain. Continue icing for 2 to 3 days – 10 to 15 minutes once every 1 to 2 hours.

There is some empirical evidence that fair-skinned, fair-haired people need only 4 to 6 minutes of ice treatment and that 10 to 15 minutes may lead to a paradoxical reaction causing the body to warm the iced area to avoid damage. The goal is vasoconstriction, not vasodilation.

Compression and elevation of the injured area will also reduce swelling and facilitate faster healing. In some quarters compression is viewed as more significant than ice in aiding recovery.

Rest of the injured area and appropriate massage therapy at the appropriate time will insure normal functioning to the damaged tissue by preventing the development of weak, inflexible, painful scars and their subsequent effect on performance.

Post-acute recovery utilizes non-resisted, non-weight-bearing, pain-free movement to speed healing and produce more resilient scars.

CHAPTER 18

When Clients Won't Stay Better

SOMETIMES OUR CLIENTS won't stay better. Some folks respond well initially but then remain only partially pain-free. Some don't respond at all. It is important to stop treating that modest number of clients who don't improve.

Failure to address perpetuating factors can keep clients from gaining permanent relief. These factors include mechanical stresses from repetitive work, work requiring stressful postures held for long periods, unrelenting emotional stress, poorly designed or ill-fitting furniture, postural distortions, and structural abnormalities primarily consisting of short leg length or small hemipelvis.

Part of our task is to help clients identify their perpetuating factors and assist them in eliciting changes. Once these factors are recognized and brought under control, stretching and strengthening regimes are followed to keep muscles pain-free and efficient.

Nothing works all of the time when trying to help people with chronic pain, and many things help only some of the time. In this section we have included some of the less familiar approaches to chronic pain. While chiropractic, osteopathy, physical therapy, acupuncture and acupressure or shiatsu and movement therapies such as Feldenkrais, Alexander, and Hanna's Somatics are valuable therapies, they are generally familiar to bodyworkers. The approaches we have chosen to include in this section are some you might be less familiar with.

Situations that often perpetuate pain but are generally out of our purview include:

- Nutritional Deficiencies
- Tension Myositis Syndrome
- Extreme Hypermobility, Recurrent Disc Herniations, Sacroiliac Pain and Traumatized Ligaments
- Lack of Nerve Mobility
- Rehabilitative Exercise and Chiropractic
- Hidden Hyperventilation syndrome / Paradoxical Breathing
- Posttraumatic Stress Disorder

Nutritional Deficiencies

Nutritional factors can prevent a client from improving or healing from myofascial pain syndromes. Drs. Travell and Simons state that, "Nearly half of the patients that we see require resolution from nutritional inadequacies for lasting relief." They indicate vitamins C, B1, B6 and folic acid are important to keep at optimal levels for soft tissue healing. Calcium, potassium, iron, and several other trace minerals are also required for a lasting healing accompanied by normal, pain-free function.

Santa Barbara nutritionist Robin Marzi goes even further in her approach to muscle health:

"Minerals are critical for optimal muscle function. Even more than vitamins, people tend to have mineral deficiencies. I recommend that people use chelated minerals, as those are best absorbed and tolerated.

Magnesium is probably the most important mineral for muscle function, even more than calcium. I find people do best when they get a 1:1 ratio of magnesium to calcium. Many people are not getting adequate magnesium for the amount of calcium they are ingesting. I have found this to be especially true for my patients with fibromyalgia.

Malic acid is also beneficial for muscles (especially when in combination with magnesium). The malic acid helps the magnesium to get into the Krebs cycle (the cycle in which many nutrients convert into energy). This combination, which usually is sold as Magnesium malate, really helps diminish pain and the tightness of the muscles.

Essential fatty acids (i.e. flaxseed oil, evening primrose oil, etc.) are also beneficial in aiding muscle release. The fatty acids regulate and balance our prostaglandins. When prostaglandins are out of balance, we have more cramping, pain, and inflammation.

Lastly, sometimes general dietary recommendations that help people incorporate more alkaline food (avocado, apricots, almonds, lima beans, millet, most vegetables, etc.) can help the muscles to become less acidic."

Robin can be reached via e-mail: r.l.marzi@att.net

Massage therapists and other bodyworkers are cautioned not to make nutritional suggestions unless they are trained nutritionists and are able to complete screening laboratory tests. As an example, excess magnesium can create problems for those with kidney or heart problems.

Tension Myositis Syndrome – (TMS)

In our experience, TMS is one of the most common causes of chronic musculoskeletal pain that doesn't self-resolve over six weeks or abate with DeeperWork protocols.

J. Sarno, M.D., coined the term "tension myositis syndrome." He proposes that, in the absence of cancer, kidney problems or other disease processes, repressed fear and anger are the primary causes of chronic back and neck pain.

Dr. Sarno has found that certain perfectionistic personality types are most prone to this syndrome. Their pattern can often be exacerbated by fears generated inadvertently by the medical profession. Conventional wisdom stresses the idea that the back is weak and vulnerable. This leads to the poor prognosis of back problems from medical treatment and simply creates more suffering. Dr. Sarno claims most back pain is caused by local ischemia that is, in itself, physically harmless. It is, however, highly painful, and can create devastating physical and psychological problems when left untended.

We've know of dozens of persons who have been cured by the understanding they garnered by attending Dr. Sarno's lectures, some of them personally. There are only a few West Coast practitioners. Los Angeles physician, David Schechter, M.D. is one (email SchechterD@aol.com). His website, MindBodyMedicine.com, offers a relevant workbook and audio program. While Dr. Schechter attended medical school on the East Coast, Dr. Sarno treated him successfully. Dr. Schechter has been successful in working with chronic neck, back, and shoulder pain using Sarno's method.

As a corollary to this healing of low back, neck and shoulder pain, clients also experience spontaneous resolution of tennis elbow, collateral ligament knee pain and other common forms of tendonitis concurrent with the healing of their back pain.

Dr. Sarno suggests that this pain serves as a defense mechanism to avoid awareness of largely unconscious hostility and fear – keeping a person's awareness focused on a physical pain rather than on unacceptable and frightening feelings. We view the mechanism somewhat differently – that we use back or neck pain to alert ourselves that all is not well; that our attention to unresolved issues in our lives is needed.

But whether or not any of us are correct about the purpose of the pain, the treatment remains the same:

- Develop an awareness of the unconscious mechanism, i.e., that unconscious feelings or the belief that mechanical problems are the cause is the cause.
- Discontinue treatments for mechanical causes. This includes massage, unless it is received for relaxation alone.
- Resume normal activities as soon as a reduction in pain becomes evident.

This relationship between unexpressed, unresolved feelings and chronic pain is familiar to all of us who work with clients in pain.

JIM'S STORY

Jim, with a Ph.D. in psychology and debilitating sciatic pain, spent over $5000 (at a time when that sum was meaningful) on massage, acupuncture, physical therapy, NSAIDS, homeopathy, psychics, faith healers and a dash of psychotherapy. We were intrigued by Jim's instantaneous healing concurrent with the safe birth, healthy first child and still-living wife. That's all it took. Jim's fear had all gone to his leg.

JULIE'S STORY

Julie, single mom and sole support for her young child, had to work hard to make ends meet. Her job required plenty of physical exertion. She awoke one morning with extremely painful sciatica. Julie could not walk in our door without tears running down her face. Acupuncture and cortisone didn't help. The strain/counterstrain position that we showed her helped her to sleep better at night, but relief was only temporary and completely unsatisfactory. Piriformis trigger point work also provided only short-term relief.

On her subsequent visit, we presented her with a copy of Sarno's book. Our experience suggested she might benefit from this approach.

On the next visit, Julie said, "The book kinda makes sense." We then asked what good, new things were happening in her life. She said, with a smile, "I have a new boyfriend." While momentarily thinking of him, she noted that the pain in her leg was gone – elapsed time was about one minute. When asked about what was not so good, she replied, "I haven't told my old boyfriend yet." Her pain came back with a vengeance – additional lapsed time, about 30 seconds.

Julie was able to increase and decrease her sciatic pain depending on what she was thinking about. In our minds, another graphic example of how quickly the anatomic nervous system can relax or constrict peripheral circulation resulting in local tissue ischemia and pain. The research from many cases of ideas transducing into physiology is well explored by E. L. Rossi in *The Psychobiology of Mind-Body Healing*. Unfortunately his work, written in the mid-'80s, has not been updated.

Extreme Hyper-mobility, Recurrent Disc Herniations, Sacroiliac Pain and Traumatized Ligaments

Up to 5% of the population is estimated to be hypermobile. This laxity can result in periodic episodes of intense pain – particularly from the spine. This type of pain does not respond to or resolve with massage or bodywork.

We generally don't use Deep Tissue or Compressive Massage on hypermobile clients – particularly in the area of the lumbar spine and pelvic region. Ligament laxity makes it too easy to over stretch the cervical or lumbar spine or move the pelvis and cause problems in the sacroiliac (SI) joint. Although these folks seldom have trigger points, they're easy to treat by hand.

There is also a real need to be careful not to overextend joints in hyper-mobile clients. We do not do follow-up stretches following the trigger point release, but we do have the client go through a gentle range of motion. Finally, we recommend client strengthening. Hyper-mobile people need to be in the gym and not in the yoga studio.

What can prove useful to hyper-mobile people is proliferant or slerosant therapy. The injection of a dextrose solution into the affected ligaments causes them to tighten. Until recently there have been few doctors in the U.S. experienced in what is now called "prolotherapy." In Santa Barbara we have two of the American pioneers of this primarily European approach to these problems – orthopedic practitioners Robert Klein, M.D. and Bjorn Eek, M.D.

Dr. Klein adds insight to our overview. He offers other areas where prolotherapy is proving effective.

"Patient's with recurrent disc herniations can often be treated successfully with prolotherapy and any patient who has sacroiliac pain can be treated successfully. Patients who have repeat manipulations and in whom the manipulation fails to 'hold' can also be successfully treated with prolotherapy. One of the most powerful uses for this form of treatment is in the patient with a whiplash injury. If the patient fails to quickly respond to routine therapy then we have been very successful in stabilizing the traumatized ligaments with the injections. We generally sedate patients for our back and neck injections and this minimizes the discomfort of the shots.

We do not have a web site, but I do have an email address if anyone has a question that they wish to address to me. It is rklein42@aol.com."

In our experience, the injections in prolotherapy can be quite painful without local anesthesia, but they have dramatically helped patients who were destined for a life on the couch and TV accompanied by a steady diet of ever more potent pain meds. Some of these people have been in pain for years and have highly acidic paraspinal muscles. Massage can be helpful in rehabilitating the back muscles after prolotherapy. Massage must be gentle for at least for the first 3 or 4 weeks, as strong massage will leave these tissues extremely sore.

PATRICK'S STORY

The conditioning coach of an Australian professional Rugby League football team sent Patrick to me. At times during the game, for no outwardly apparent reason, he would drop to his knees with agonizing back pain.

When Patrick came in, I conducted a thorough palpatory evaluation using the protocols described in this book for low back pain. This well-muscled young man had not a single trigger point in his quadratus lumborum, gluteals, or hamstrings. I found nothing to treat. However, when he got off the table and stretched, I noted a sharp angle in his lumbar-thoracic junction. This extreme bend indicated hyper-mobility. What was happening on the field suddenly became clear.

Spinal ligament laxity impinged the cord or nerve roots causing extreme pain and splinting spasm. This hyper-mobility cannot be treated by massage, chiropractic or pain medications. Strengthening and prolotherapy can help.

Lack of Nerve Mobility

Occasionally we've worked with clients whose symptoms strongly suggest one problem, but with treatment, no progress is evidenced. A possible answer we find few people yet know about is pain caused by a lack of nerve mobility.

Physical therapist Jean DeBettignies of Precision Biomechanics (email: JeanDeBe@aol.com) and her staff have done some seminal work in restoring nerve mobility. According to Jean:

"Lack of mobility in the nervous system is an often overlooked cause of pain. When central and peripheral nerves do not slide within their sheaths as we move, nerve irritation patterns can be created. They can mimic other types of pain that are not nerve related, causing confusion for the therapist.

The nervous system consists of the central nervous system (brain and spinal cord) and the peripheral nervous system (the nerves that serve arms, legs, and trunk). They are continuous – without structural breaks. The entire nervous system is 'sheathed' creating long tubes where the spinal cord and peripheral nerves live.

As we move, our nerves slide in their coverings. Nerves become taut and painful if they don't slide as we move. Consider a person wearing a long sleeve shirt. As the arm is raised, the sleeve slides down. Try it. If you hold your sleeve with the involved hand and raise your arm, the sleeve becomes taut and the arm's motion is limited.

Chronic inflammation, such as sciatica or carpal tunnel syndrome, can decrease nerve mobility. A stiff back or traumatic injuries such as whiplash also decrease mobility.

Any lack of motion in a portion of the body over a long period of time decreases nerve movement. However, nerve mobility can be regained. We identify the area of immobility and design exercises to gently work the nerve free.

Case Study

John L. is a 55-year-old gentleman who carries his own golf clubs and walks the course to get more exercise. His left heel began to hurt after playing a particularly hilly course. Soon his heel hurt every day, especially in the morning when standing after a period of sitting.

John searched the Internet for information. He found his symptoms to be those of plantar fasciitis. Logically, he felt that his heel pain was due to an irritated plantar fascia.

On evaluation, I found palpable tenderness over the plantar fascia insertion. His heel hurt in the morning upon arising or after sitting, and it hurt with extended walking, especially uphill – all symptoms of plantar fasciitis. But, he did not have excessive pronation or any of the other biomechanical symptoms of plantar fasciitis. He did have palpable tenderness over the tibial nerve under the calf muscle.

While sitting in a straight leg position, dorsiflexion of his left foot caused a feeling of pulling all the way through his calf up into his posterior thigh. This finding indicates limited nerve mobility. If dorsiflexion of the ankle were eliciting calf tightness, the pulling would only go to the knee.

Lack of nerve mobility in the calf will often elicit symptoms while walking or going up hill because the tibial nerve is not sliding in its tube as the foot goes into dorsiflexion. Lack of nerve mobility can imitate plantar fasciitis because inflammation of the medial branch of the calcaneal nerve lies in the vicinity of the plantar fascia insertion. Treating the nerve mobility problem directly resolves heel pain much more quickly than following a plantar fasciitis protocol.

As therapists, we routinely evaluate strength, flexibility, movement and structure. We feel mobility of the nervous system is a possible contributing factor. When therapists at Precision Biomechanics search for the cause(s) or treat clients with pain or movement dysfunction, we add mobility of the nervous system to our list of evaluating procedures."

Rehabilitative Exercise and Chiropractic

Kevin Fisher is a D.C. and champion power-lifter who teaches sports chiropractic. We include his work here because he uses a wide range of soft tissue modalities to gain homeostasis – not manipulation alone to address client pain.

"Corrective or rehabilitative exercise can be a powerful tool to combat pain, particularly if muscle tears and painful tendonitis have been rectified prior to initiating corrective exercises.

First, rule out articular dysfunction before prescribing exercises. The 'end feel' of most synovial joints is our easiest tool for determining joint health. We look for springy end feel, which is normal, as opposed to a hard end feel that suggests pathology. Initially massage and stretching may relax the joint enough for it to resume normal function. However, if the aberrant end feel doesn't change in a few visits, then adjustment by a chiropractor or osteopath trained in manipulative techniques should be utilized.

If, after three or four visits, the client remains in pain and pathology and articular disease has been ruled out, it's time to include an exercise regime.

Compliance can be a real problem when prescribing exercise. While athletes are generally well motivated and will follow recommendations, the general population is often too busy, too weak and too stressed out. The key to successfully getting out of pain is to focus on what is weak and suggest exercise in small manageable increments. Occasionally, only one or two corrective exercises can make a significant difference.

Common Problems

Within the musculoskeletal/fascial system imbalances can occur between agonist/antagonist, anterior/posterior, speed of contraction/flexibility, use/overuse, strength/weakness and scar tissue/healthy tissue. All of these parameters play an integral role in the pain control and bodily function. If there were one primary word that can be used to set a health goals, it would be balance. Homeostasis, the medical term for balance, is what I work towards with clients in pain.

Fix Pain *has most all the necessary tools for the manual treatment of various myofascial problems. These approaches will be successful in the majority of clients. However, when altered function or diminished athletic performance persists after deep compressions, transverse friction and stretching have failed, therapeutic exercises is often the answer.*

For example, weak abs, gluts and tight (strong) hams, hip flexors and thoracolumbar junctions characterize the typical lower-body imbalance. While short-term relief from low back pain is a real possibility, long term relief and the prevention of recurrence will entail finding the balance, the homeostasis that will allow proper musculoskeletal function. My protocol is to reduce inflammation, treat muscle and joint dysfunction, then stretch what's tight, and strengthen what's weak.

Manipulation is often an absolute wonder for correcting joint dysfunction and, at times, useless. If the hamstrings are hypertonic and the low back facets and sacroiliac joints are mobile, the treatment should concentrate on facial release and strengthening.

The number of manipulation treatments necessary for articular dysfunction varies from a couple per year to two times a month, depending on acute or chronic presentation. The U.S.A. Visa Decathlon team gets adjusted after every event during a competition, a form of treatment for prevention and peak performance.

As in the upper body, there are some general movements that can help the majority of low back patients.

Stretches
1. *Knee to chest*
2. *Hamstring stretch*
3. *Psoas stretch*
4. *Back extension or reverse extension*

Exercises
1. *Abdominal crunch*
2. *Squat*
3. *Lat pull down*

There are a few more specific movements that are also very helpful
1. *Bridge*
2. *Q-Ped*
3. *Lateral ball stretch*

One of the keys with low back strengthening is to control the torso and add controlled extremity movement. The list can go on and on.

Upper Body

If your client sits at a desk or computer an ergonomic assessment is crucial. All the good bodywork will be for naught if the client returns to the same dysfunctional setting. While you will remove trigger points and fascial problems in the sternocleidomastoid, subscapularis, sub-occipital triangle, para-vertebral muscles, levator scapula and C-t junction, my experience indicates that manual manipulation will be necessary for articular dysfunction.

Notes

Manipulation following exercise is easier, less painful and holds longer. While the gym is the most effective setting in which to gain strength, in some cases elastic tubing can be a satisfactory substitute.

The cornerstone to this upper body syndrome is weak scapular retractors. Patients are rarely able to isolate the muscles that roll the scapula posterior and inferior. With the patient prone or standing, place your hand on the inferior medial border of the scapula. They will be unable to push your hand down and across toward their opposite pant pocket. In addition, they will probably have contracted shoulder rotators that will prevent the scapula from rotating posteriorly.

This is the typical bench press posture you find at the gym. This lifter will work the chest and shoulders to death with virtually no posterior deltoid, external rotators or inter-scapular strength to balance all the forward anterior pressing movements. The result, an unbalanced posture with a shearing at the shoulder that predisposes future rotator cuff problems.

Outside of the gym, we typically see:
1. *Forward anterior head weight bearing*
2. *Bilateral internally rotated shoulders*
3. *Weak interscapular muscles*
4. *Hypertonic trapezius/levator scapula*

Stretches to counteract this problem include:
1. *Corner stretch*
2. *Hanging dumbbell stretch*
3. *Pullover stretch*

Initial exercise prescribed should be:
1. *Lat pull front - close grip*
2. *End-range scapular retraction*

This all too common problem caused by modern work and play habits leads to dowager's hump, chronic neck and shoulder problems and a view that most of the world takes place somewhere down by your feet. Finding the elusive trigger point, weakness or altered joint function can be a trying process. Experimentation with various creative techniques and movements enables you to help people find their own path to health."
(email: KFisher54@aol.com)

Paradoxical Breathing or Hidden-Hyperventilation

One of the easiest to treat and least recognized syndromes that affects both muscular pain and a sense of well being is hidden-hyperventilation. Hidden hyperventilation often is noted in clients who breathe paradoxically.

As bodyworkers we are easily able to identify paradoxical breathing. With a relaxed client, we can readily note their neck muscles tightening and their belly being sucked in on inhalation. Both of these actions are called paradoxical breath and they are indicative of hidden-hyperventilation. Clients will often seem to struggle for a deep breath and complain of feeling as if they can't get that last little bit of breath they need. In fact, the cure is to decrease both breathing rate and volume.

Hyperventilation blows off excessive amounts of carbon dioxide and destabilizes the body's homeostatic mechanisms. This leads to compensatory mechanisms – endocrine, chemical, and neurologic. As we observe the client, we note hypertrophied and tense neck muscles – sternocleidomastoid and scaleni.

The physiology of this problem has been well explained by the Russian doctor, Constantine Buteyko. His research over 40 years has profound implications for hidden-hyperventilation and asthma, high and low blood pressure, diabetes and other chronic diseases. The Russians use this modality to successfully treat over 150 different syndromes.

People can be trained over time to stop paradoxical breathing or hyperventilation. This can be an extremely valuable self-help tool for clients with panic disorders, pain syndromes that are exacerbated by lack of sleep, and sympathetic dominance characterized by flight or fight responses. Learning hypoventilation can enhance the health of many clients. The Australian osteopath, Dr. Rosalba Courtney (email: crthouse@geko.net.au), has produced a video to teach the Eucapnic-Buteyko technique – a refined form of treating hidden hyperventilation.

JENNY'S STORY

Jenny was an outdoor-loving young woman with a dog and three cats. She also unfortunately needed 10 to 12 hits a day on her puffer medication for asthma prevention. Within three days of practicing Eucapnic-Buteyko, she was able hike and be with her cats without medication. Sound extreme? Many doctors think so, but both medical tests and our personal experience with asthmatics, sleep apnea sufferers and athletes bear out the healthy effects of breathing retraining and hypoventilation.

Compression Massage combined with hypoventilation can do wonders for tense necks and shoulders and other respiratory muscles. It is, however, illegal, immoral, and unethical to treat asthmatics – particularly those using medications – without professional level training in the Eucapnic-Buteyko method. Tapes are now available from Dr. Courtney and others on this technique. Dr. Buteyko doesn't recommend learning from a tape, but the need is so great for help for asthma and other hyperventilation problems that the number of practitioners can't meet the pent-up demand. There are currently few practitioners in the U.S.

Current Findings

Recent research indicates that chronic pain that responds poorly to pain-killing drugs, standard mechanical approaches, and Compression Massage, could result from a "modulation disorder" in the sensory nervous system. Modulation disorders take place in the brain rather than the soft-tissues. Some information related to this view is found under the heading of Myofascial Pain Modulation Disorder in Volume 1 of *The Trigger Point Manual* by Travel and Simons. While there, read the section entitled "Posttraumatic Hyperirritability Syndrome" on the following page.

The implication for us as bodyworkers is to think in terms of how, if at all, our work can modulate (regulate, temper, change or vary) neural hyper-excitability. The newly postulated "neural modules" theory (a neural network linking components from every region of the brain, including memory, emotion, sensory input, and others) could have a great influence on our therapies. See the September 21, 1998 issue of

The New Yorker magazine medical dispatch (pg. 98) for a remarkably clear description of chronic pain and the brain.

If this new hypothesis proves workable at some point, the dance of bodywork may acquire a new step. We'll be re-focused on finding new ways to play the brain through the soft tissues in order to change the brain to control pain.

CONFUSING STORY

I was called in to consult by an Australian M.D. who was interested in trigger point and fascia release techniques. The patient was a woman presenting with pain and tenderness everywhere on her body. After considerable palpation, we were able to find one spot the size of a quarter on her left arm that wasn't hypersensitive.

Beginning there, we worked out (slowly and gently) with what, in our minds, was an attempt to use touch to desensitize hypersensitive areas. Our original thinking was that this approach would work as a counter-irritant and thereby decrease the pain. Over time, we had success in significantly decreasing her general level of pain. Later, however, she suffered a serious setback following the trauma of a dog attack.

A question remained. Was this decrease in pain due to the emotional support she felt or was it from desensitization caused by increasing the pressure to just below the threshold of creating greater pain? Could it have been from endogenous morphines released from the touch itself? Was her "idea" of pain changed? We know that the perception of pain is in part cultural and familial. Did we influence a modulation disorder?

Posttraumatic Stress Disorder (PTSD): Acute and Chronic Psychological Distress Following Traumatic Events

New findings suggest that trauma in its many guises can create anatomic and physiologic changes along with accompanying changes in function in our brains. Addressing trauma, usually within a day or two, through cathartic processes, recounting the trauma, and other healing interventions seems to prevent these changes. For those clients who have not had the benefit of early intervention and support, symptoms of pain, suffering, dissociation and other troubling symptoms may occur.

In our experience, clients with untreated posttraumatic stress disorder may prove unable to resolve trigger point pain. Not always, but in some instances, a combination of psychotherapy and bodywork may find the key to resolving ongoing trigger point pain.

In light of these new findings, bodyworkers have had to re-evaluate their approaches for recognizing and treating clients suffering from the long-term results of physical or emotional trauma.

Working with the admonition, "first do no harm," we have had to rely on more than a compassionate heart and competent hands. For many trauma victims, relaxation is tantamount to danger, and pleasure is a sin or sensation that must be punished – punishment administered almost invariably by clients to themselves. With this mind set, what we as bodyworkers normally attempt to accomplish – relaxation and pleasur – can be a source of pain and distress to our clients.

> Some clients won't heal from myofascial pain until they have both awareness and healing around childhood trauma – often sexual.

Nightmares, hyper-alertness, flashbacks, irritability, feelings of hopelessness, extreme emotionality with prolonged sobbing or shaking, heavy sweats, unrelenting anxiety, inability to concentrate, and, most particularly, dissociative states/detachment (what we sense in clients on our table as a "nobody's home" feeling) are common residual symptoms that result from severe trauma. This affliction, now commonly called posttraumatic stress disorder, can easily be exacerbated by even well-meaning, competent bodyworkers.

Posttraumatic clients often enter dissociative states during bodywork. This "leaving the body" seems to function as a protective state during frightening or stressful situations. It is a learned response that carried over from the original trauma. Unfortunately, while in this protective state, clients can be further traumatized without either initial recognition of this new trauma or their ability to interrupt the process.

Even giving a Swedish massage to a client in a dissociative state is risky. Appropriate feedback is sometimes difficult for the client to give. For example, clients who have been molested as children may not feel themselves able to ask you to stop kneading their gluteals, even though it is causing them distress. The therapist may have properly draped the client and be touching them in an entirely neutral manner with moderate pressure and still be breaching client boundaries. All of this good will and skill is meaningless if the client is being re-stimulated to past trauma.

The clients themselves may be unaware of how touch is stirring the pot. The effects of this touch may become painfully evident on their trip home or later that night when strong flashbacks surface. These flashbacks can be extremely frightening to the client and may certainly result in late night phone calls to you, the unsuspecting therapist.

We are obligated to recognize these clients and the stress they are experiencing even while they may not possess such recognition themselves. We need the capacity to identify behaviors or states without diagnosing or working outside our scope of practice. Initially, when we sense their distress, our usual response will be to get them back in their body and present awareness.

ALICE'S "SET AND SETTING" STORY

Our clients bring with them ideas of what should be accomplished in a session. The interplay between their ideas and the physical and emotional setting we present as therapists can strongly influence the course of our work.

Alice, a posttraumatic stress disorder client, tried using bodywork to help heal her anguish. In session, while clothed, even touching her hands or arms would result in Alice fainting. After fainting four times in one session, it became apparent to both client and therapist that at this healing stage, this work wasn't proving helpful.

However, the following week Alice received (from the same therapist) a sports massage for a marathon to be run in two days. The massage was given in her home and not the therapist's office. Our therapist was duly alert for any signs of disassociation. Alice comfortably and thankfully received this massage. Signs of distress never surfaced.

Note that in this instance the client felt safer in her own home. More often a client suffering with posttraumatic stress disorder feels safer when dealing with either touch or potentially frightening material if in a more neutral or professional setting. Altered states may result in clients falling back into their sense memories, which can be traumatizing. Hence the power of set and setting.

In most instances, referral to suitable professionals (usually a psychologist, psychiatrist, or family therapist trained in PTSD) is the best course of action. Various forms of bodywork can be helpful adjunctive therapies, but considering our experience in this field, we suggest that the primary therapist needs to be in the field of psychology. This is for ethical, legal and compassionate reasons.

Standard forms of bodywork, even of a gentle nature, may prove to be initially invasive. Very potent work can be accomplished with just simple touch – often with the client seated and clothed. The older idea that cathartic processes always lead to healing has not shown itself to be true as regards PTSD. It is often imperative for clients with this syndrome to learn to tolerate more physical and emotional contact without entering into either dissociate or emotionally charged states. Bodywork, done by patient and knowledgeable therapists, can be a valuable adjunct to psychotherapy. Bodywork without understanding the client's special needs can be a disaster for both.

If you find a client who dissociates on your table and is not simply in a very deep state of relaxation, you may choose to bring to their attention their seeming lack of awareness of your work. Remember that the dissociated client has the "nobody's home" feel. We sense this emotionally and feel it with our hands – an "empty feel" that comes from our client.

The tricky part is talking with clients who don't enter into flashbacks or extreme distress, but still show some of the signs and symptoms of posttraumatic stress disorder. The question of whether to suggest that something may be amiss is one that you will have to decide on a case by case, client by client, basis. If you do decide to refer or suggest medical evaluation, you should do so without entering into great detail or diagnosing any mental state. Unless you are licensed as a psychiatrist, psychologist, family therapist or other recognized mental health professional, this evaluation would qualify as a scope of practice violation.

Because of the unresolved controversy concerning recovered memory and posttraumatic stress disorder in relation to childhood sexual abuse, and the pain and disability associated with the healing process, there is a substantial responsibility placed on the shoulders of the massage therapist who chooses to address this subject. If you are uncertain as to what you see and feel, you may well chose not to mention your hunch. It may prove more salutary to "keep the clients in their bodies" by asking questions of them relating to the feel, pressure and tempo of your touch. Because this can be a delicate or difficult subject to broach for both the client and therapist, we recommend that you receive training to help you to recognize posttraumatic stress disorder and alert the client as necessary.

Final Notes

Bodyworkers are sometimes misled into treating problems that are medical in nature. Visceral disease can refer pain to surface areas of the body. Apparent muscular problems that are in fact visceral in origin (eminating from internal organs) can be serious and occasionally life threatening.

Muscular problems associated with sudden onset and with no apparent physical cause, with or without intense pain, and which don't resolve or shift in intensity or location with our soft-tissue intervention are all suspect.

If there are any concomitant signs of illness such as excessive fatigue, a low-grade fever or nausea accompanying the pain, refer for medical evaluation. Prolonged massage treatment can mask symptoms and prevent clients from receiving timely medical treatment.

In those cases that do not respond positively in 3 or 4 visits, it remains important to refer your client. Time is of the essence in cases of pain caused by possible disease processes either undiagnosed or unrecognized.

The nature of chronic pain is being re-thought. Clinical results are still not good enough; many people remain in pain, and there is much we do not understand. "Do No Harm" is a complex concept.

For updates and to express your own case observations and conjectures, please contact us at Press4Health.com or DeeperWork.com. We are particularly interested in the relationship between pain and social support, satisfying work, recreational outlets and healthy relationships.

Partial Bibliography and Recommended Reading

Biel, Andrew: *Trail Guide to the Body* (1997) Books of Discovery

Birnbaum, Jacob: *The Musculoskeletal Manual* (1986) W.B. Saunders Company

Cailliet, Rene: *Soft Tissue Pain and Disability* (1988) F.A. Davis Company

Calais-Germain, Blandine: *Anatomy of Movement* (1993) Eastland Press, Inc.

Chaitow, Leon: *Modern Neuromuscular Techniques* (1996) Churchill Livingstone

Chaitow, Leon: *Muscle Energy Techniques* (1996) Churchill Livingstone

Chaitow, Leon: *Palpatory Literacy* (1991) Thorsons

Chaitow, Leon: *Positional Release Techniques* (1996) Churchill Livingstone

Chaitow, Leon: *Soft-Tissue Manipulation* (1988) Healing Arts Press

Cyriax, James and Patricia: *Illustrated Manual of Orthopaedic Medicine* (1989) O M Publications

Fritz, Sandy: *Fundamentals of Therapeutic Massage* (1995) Mosby

Greenman, Philip: *Principles of Manual Medicine*, ed. 2 (1996) Williams & Watkin

Guyton, Arthur: *Textbook of Medical Physiology* ed. 7 (1986) W. B. Saunders Company

Hoppenfeld, Stanley: *Physical Examination of the Spine and Extremities* (1976) Appleton-Century-Crofts

Kapandji, I.A.: *The Physiology of the Joint, Vol. 1-3* (1982) Churchill Livingstone

Kendall, Florence & McCreary, Elizabeth: *Muscles, Testing and Function* ed. 3 (1983) Williams & Wilkins

Meagher, Jack & Boughton, Pat:: *Sportsmassage* (1980) Dolphin Books

McAtee, Robert: *Facilitated Stretching* (1999) Human Kinetics

Mannheim, Carol: *The Myofascial Release Manual* ed. 2 (1994) John Bond

Netter, Frank: *Atlas of Human Anatomy* (1989) CIBA-GEIGY

Nimmo, Raymond L.: *Receptor Tonus Technique*, workshop notes

Simons, David and Lois, Travell, Janet: *Travell and Simons' Myofascial Pain and Dysfunction, The Trigger Point Manual (Upper Half of Body), Vol. 1* ed. 2 (1999) Williams & Wilkins

Snider, Robert: *Essentials of Musculoskeletal Care* (1997) American Academy of Orthopaedic Surgeons

Travell, Janet & Simons, David: *Myofascial Pain and Dysfunction, the Trigger Point Manual (Lower Extremities), Vol. 2* (1992) Williams & Wilkins

Turchaninov, Ross & Cox, Connie: *Medical Massage* (1998) Aesculapius Books and Stress Less Publishing, Inc.

Turchaninov, Ross: *Therapeutic Massage, A Scientific Approach* (2000) Aesculapius Books

Solveborn, Sven-A.: *The Book About Stretching* (1985) Japan Publications

List of Illustrations

Index

Notes

Notes

Notes

Notes

Notes

Notes